Control of Head Movement

Control of Head Movement

Barry W. Peterson, Ph.D.
Northwestern University

Frances J. Richmond, Ph.D.
Queen's University

New York   Oxford
OXFORD UNIVERSITY PRESS
1988

Oxford University Press

Oxford   New York   Toronto
Delhi   Bombay   Calcutta   Madras   Karachi
Petaling Jaya   Singapore   Hong Kong   Tokyo
Nairoba   Dar es Salaam   Cape Town
Melbourne   Auckland

and associated companies in
Beirut   Berlin   Ibadan   Nicosia

Published by Oxford University Press, Inc.,
200 Madison Avenue, New York, New York 10016
Oxford is a registered trademark of Oxford University Press

Library of Congress Cataloging-in-Publication Data
Control of head movement.
    Bibliography: p.
    Includes Index.
    1. Head—movements.   2. Human mechanics.   3. Muscular
sense.   I. Peterson, Barry W.   II. Richmond, Frances J.
QP310.H43C66 1988   612'.76   87-7787
ISBN 0-19-504499-1

9 8 7 6 5 4 3 2 1
Printed in the United States of America
on acid-free paper

Preface

Head movement is a complex motor behavior that has never attracted a great deal of scientific attention. In the past, most considerations of head movement have been incidental to research on oculomotor control, vestibular function, or the control of posture and gait. Thus, information on head movement is scattered widely throughout the scientific literature. However, in recent years it has become apparent that head movement is a unique and complex motor system in its own right. In the summer of 1986, a satellite symposium of the XXX Congress of the International Union of Physiological Sciences was held to address "The Control of Head Movement." This symposium brought together scientists of many different backgrounds, each with a particular viewpoint to express. From the symposium grew the contents of this book.

The chapters presented here are not a collection of symposium proceedings but an attempt to bring together, in one volume, the many types of research that have contributed to our understanding of head movement. Each chapter provides a survey of research that has been undertaken on a single topic over the last several years. Material for each chapter was originally provided by the chapter authors. The editors then worked with the authors to harmonize the scope and style of each chapter, in order to create a book that would serve as a comprehensive review of the field: a book that could be read by anyone with a broad background in the life sciences.

Some chapters have a strong flavor of history. Others deal with fields so new that the information presented in them is only a few years old. The chapters are ordered so that the peripheral organization of the head-movement system is considered first; the nature of different neural pathways and control mechanisms is considered later. The book deals primarily with the physiological mechanisms responsible for head movement. However, the breadth of the field is also reflected in chapters that deal with modeling of the head-movement system, with psychophysical experiments, and with pathophysiology.

We must acknowledge the help of Drs. V. Abrahams, A. Berthoz, and D. Guitton, who helped us to define the scope and content of this book, both directly and through their organizational assistance of the IUPS Satellite Symposium on Head Movement. We are particularly indebted to Dr. V. Wilson for his advice and assistance with Chapters 6 through 10. We thank the Departments of Physiology at Queen's University and Northwestern University for financial and administrative support. However, the greatest credit for this volume must go to the contributors themselves. We are grateful for their patience and flexibility during the protracted editorial process.

Chicago, Illinois   B.W.P.
Kingston, Ontario   F.J.R.
November 1987

Contents

Contributors

V. C. Abrahams
Department of Physiology, Queen's University, Kingston, Ontario, Canada K7L 3N6

J. Baker
Department of Physiology, Northwestern University, Chicago, Illinois 60611 U.S.A.

D. A. Bakker
School of Nursing, Laurentian University, Sudbury, Ontario, Canada P3E 2C6

A. Berthoz
Laboratoire de Physiologie Neurosensorielle, Centre National de la Recherche Scientifique, 75270 Paris Cedex 06, France

E. E. Brink
The Rockefeller University, New York, New York 10021 U.S.A.

M. Crommelinck
Laboratoire de Neurophysiologie, University of Louvain, UCL 5449, B-1200, Brussels, Belgium

N. Dieringer
Institut fur Hirnforschung, Universität Zurich, Switzerland

J. H. Fuller
Department of Oral Anatomy, College of Dentistry, University of Illinois, Chicago, Illinois 60612 U.S.A.

A. Grantyn
Labortoire de Physiologie Neurosensorielle, Centre National de la Recherche Scientifique, 75270 Paris Cedex 06, France

D. Guitton
Montreal Neurological Institute, Montreal, Quebec, Canada H3A 2B4

B. Hannaford
Jet Propulsion Laboratory, California Institute of Technology, Pasedena, California 91109 U.S.A.

N. Hirai
Nihon University School of Medicine, Tokyo, Japan

R. E. Kearney
Biomedical Engineering Unit, McGill University, Montreal, Quebec, Canada H3A 2B4

S. A. Keirstead
Montreal General Hospital Research Institute, Montreal, Quebec, Canada
H3G 1A4

A. J. Pellionisz
Department of Physiology and Biophysics, New York Medical Center, New
York, New York 10016 U.S.A.

B. W. Peterson
Departments of Physiology and Rehabilitation Medicine, Northwestern University, Chicago, Illinois 60611 U.S.A.

O. Pompeiano
Dipartimento di Fisiologia e Biochimica, Universitá di Pisa, S6100 Pisa, Italy

F. J. R. Richmond
Department of Physiology, Queen's University, Kingston, Ontario, Canada K7L
3N6

P. Rondot
Service de Neurologie, Centre Hospitalier Sainte-Anne, Paris, France

P. K. Rose
Department of Physiology, Queen's University, Kingston, Ontario, Canada K7L
3N6

A. Roucoux
Laboratoire de Neurophysiologie, University of Louvain, UCL 5449, B-1200
Brussels, Belgium

R. H. Schor
Departments of Otolaryngology and Physiology, University of Pittsburgh, Pittsburgh, Pennsylvania 15213 U.S.A.

M. I. Stacey
Department of Zoology, University of Durham, Durham, DHI 3LE England

L. Stark
Department of Physiology, Optics and Engineering Sciences, University of
California, Berkeley, California 94720 U.S.A.

P. P. Vidal
Laboratoire de Physiologie Neurosensorielle, Centre National de la Recherche
Scientifique, 75270 Paris Cedex 06, France

C. Wickland
Department of Physiology, Northwestern University, Chicago, Illinois 60611
U.S.A.

V. J. Wilson
The Rockefeller University, New York, New York 10021 U.S.A.

J. Winters
Department of Chemical, Bio- and Materials Engineering, Arizona State University, Tempe, Arizona 85287 U.S.A.

W. H. Zangemeister
Department of Neurology, University of Hamburg, Hamburg, Federal Republic of Germany

Control of Head Movement

The Motor System: Joints and Muscles of the Neck

F. J. R. RICHMOND and P. P. VIDAL

Head movement is a complex motor task. It can seldom be achieved by changing the position of a single joint, but usually is the result of movements across several cervical and thoracic vertebrae. Head movements are controlled by the activities of more than 20 pairs of muscles that link the skull, spinal column, and shoulder girdle in a variety of configurations. The actions of these muscles are constrained by the physical properties of the vertebral column, whose articulations differ in their ranges and directions of mobility. The mechanical organization of both the muscular and skeletal structures must dictate the way that the nervous system will organize its neuronal output.

ORGANIZATION OF CERVICAL JOINTS

Structure

The cervical vertebral column has seven vertebrae in most mammals (including such diverse species as the giraffe and whale, but excluding the tree sloth, which has 9). It can be divided into two parts that have different structural and bio-mechanical features. The upper or superior cervical spine is composed of the first and second cervical vertebrae (the atlas and axis, respectively). These bones are highly modified morphologically. The ring-shaped atlas has relatively large lateral masses that bear articular facets on their superior and inferior surfaces and extend laterally into strong, wing-like transverse processes (Fig. 1.1). Unlike other vertebrae, the atlas has no spinous process and no vertebral body. Instead, the body of C1 appears to have become dissociated from the atlas and has fused with the ventral part of the axis, where it forms a long, pointed process called the odontoid process. The odontoid process lies within the vertebral foramen along the anterior aspect of the atlas and forms a specialized pivot joint around which the atlas can rotate. The atlas and axis also articulate with one another at broad, shallow joints on either side of the odontoid process (Fig. 1.1).

The lower or inferior cervical spine includes the remaining five cervical ver-

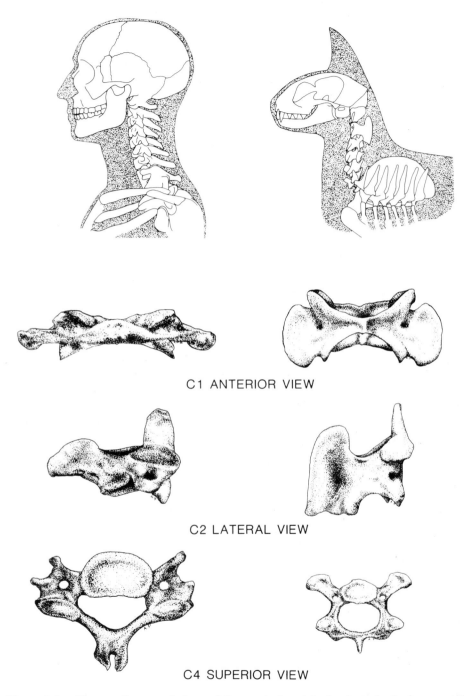

C1 ANTERIOR VIEW

C2 LATERAL VIEW

C4 SUPERIOR VIEW

Figure 1.1.   Comparative morphology of the cervical vertebral column in the human and cat. The normal relationships of the bones are shown in the top panel. The line drawings below show the structures of vertebrae C1, C2, and C4.

tebrae which have structural features more typical of vertebrae at other spinal levels. They are linked ventrally by intervertebral disks and have gliding synovial joints on either side of their dorsal arches. Each vertebra has a spinous process that projects dorsally, paired articular processes on their dorsolateral surfaces, and paired transverse processes that extend ventrolaterally from their vertebral bodies (Fig. 1.1).

The anatomical features of cervical vertebrae show a number of interspecies variations as shown in Figure 1.1, which compares the cervical column of cat and man. Differences in bone and joint structure undoubtedly introduce a degree of variability into the biomechanics of head movement from one species to another. Nevertheless, there remains an underlying similarity in the configuration of the cervical spine in many bipeds and quadrupeds. Furthermore, fluoroscopic studies (Vidal et al., 1986) have shown that the cat, rat, rabbit, and guinea pig all hold their cervical columns in a "humanlike" vertical orientation when they are sitting or standing quietly (Fig. 1.2). This posture has the obvious advantage of reducing the energy required to support the head against gravitational forces. It is also probable that the curved spine, embedded in long springlike muscles, will behave in some respects as a shock absorber for the head.

Description of Head–Neck Movements

The diverse range of mobilities at different cervical joints is important to ensure that the head can be moved in almost any direction. In man, head movements are usually categorized as flexion–extension (nodding), lateral bending, and rotation (turning), according to the principal plane of movement in one of three orthogonal axes (e.g., Jackson, 1977) (Fig. 1.3). In the cat, head movements are more commonly described using the vestibular terms of pitch (flexion–extension), yaw (lateral bending), and roll (rotation) (e.g., Baker et al., 1985; Suzuki et al., 1985). However, the vestibular terms have generally been applied in experimental situations in which the cat is held in a stereotaxic frame with its cervical column oriented parallel to earth and its skull angled 20° downward from this plane. When the cat is removed from this reference frame and placed in a different posture, the movements required to elicit pitch, yaw, or roll will change. For example, a rotatory movement around the C1–C2 joint will elicit "yaw" when the cat is sitting with its cervical column perpendicular to earth, while the same rotatory movement will be described as "roll" when the cat is standing with its head extended in front of its body and its cervical column parallel to earth. The descriptive terms of flexion–extension, lateral bending, and rotation may provide a more useful method of categorizing head movements in the quadruped as well as in humans because they do not depend on a particular relationship between posture and a gravity-related reference frame. However, even this descriptive terminology may be oversimplistic for purposes of head-movement analyses. A single head movement often represents the end point of a combination of joint movements at different levels of the serially linked vertebral column. In strict physiological terms such combined movements are best described by providing specific information about the motions taking place at each cervical joint. As one solution to this problem, Panjabi and colleagues (1974) have suggested that an orthogonal coordinate

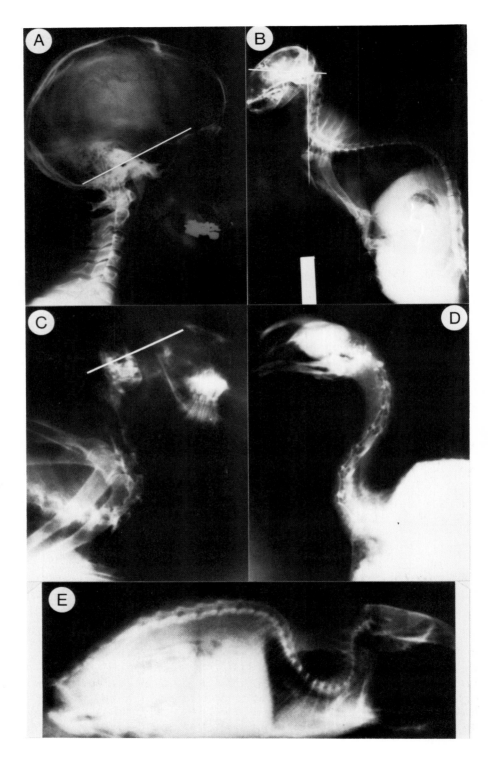

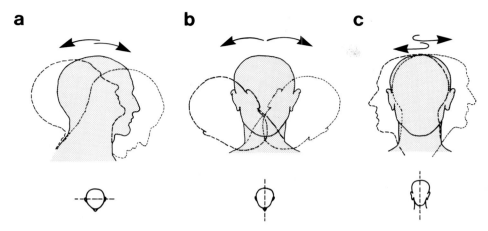

Figure 1.3. The three axes of motion normally recognized for the human head: (a) flexion—extension, (b) lateral bending, and (c) axial rotation. (Modified with permission from Jackson, 1971.)

system might be used to describe the movement of each vertebra with respect to its subjacent counterpart. However, the requirement for detailed information about vertebral movements can pose a challenge to the experimenter, because the articulations of the neck are deeply buried in soft tissue, and their motion can be difficult to monitor without highly specialized techniques.

Analyses of Joint Movements

Cervical articulations are organized similarly in humans and in most experimental mammals. For example, the atlantoaxial joint is specialized for axial rotation whereas the atlantooccipital joint has little freedom in this plane. However, quantitative data on the relative motions permitted at different cervical joints are so far available only for humans. In humans, the maximum range of motion permitted at different cervical levels has been studied in some detail because it provides an important base of information for clinical assessments of musculoskeletal dysfunction. Table 1.1 shows the maximum amplitudes of movements estimated for different joints of the cervical spine according to Kapandji (1974) and to Jofe and colleagues (1983). There is some variability in the reported values and these may

Figure 1.2. Orientations of the skull and cervical vertebral column in several species including (A) human, (B) cat, (C) rabbit, (D) chicken, and (E) rat. Radiophotographs in each case provide a lateral view of the head and neck when the animal is resting quietly. In all species, the cervical column is held vertically. The white lines in (A) and (C) indicate the orientation of the horizontal semicircular canals. Those in (B) show the orientation of the horizontal semicircular canal (horizontal line) with respect to a line perpendicular to earth (vertical line).

Table 1.1. Range of mobility at different cervical joints

	Flexion–extension		Lateral bending (from midline)		Axial rotation (from midline)	
	a	b	a	b	a	b
Skull/C1	13°	15°	8°	3–8°	0°	12°
C1/C2	10°	5°+	0°	0°	47°	12°
C2/C3	8°	100°+	10°	37°	9°	56°
C3/C7	58°		27°		42°	

Source: (a) Jofe et al. (1983) and (b) Kapandji (1974).

stem in part from the use of different techniques, such as examinations of cadavers, radiographic and cinefluoroscopic analyses, and indirect estimates derived from information about head and neck posture. The data suggest that the atlantooccipital joint has at least two degrees of freedom; it can undergo flexion–extension and will permit a small amount of lateral bending. However, there is disagreement about whether the atlantooccipital joint has a third degree of freedom in axial rotation. Although many investigators consider that significant axial rotation does not occur between the skull and C1 (cf. Jofe et al., 1983), others conclude that the joint will permit up to 10° of axial rotation (Kapandji, 1974; Worth, 1980).

The atlantoaxial junction also has two degrees of freedom: it is quite free to rotate axially, and can permit up to 10° of motion during flexion or extension of the head. In normal movements of the upper cervical spine, there appears to be relatively little translatory motion between the C1 and C2 vertebrae (cf. Jofe et al., 1983). Nevertheless, some motion can occur, and this complicates the nature of rotatory movements. Kapandji (1974) states that the atlas moves 2–3 mm downward in the vertical plane during axial rotation at the atlantoaxial junction.

The flexibility of the neck is further increased by movements across the lower cervical vertebrae. These vertebrae together appear to permit as much as 60° or more of flexion–extension (Table 1.1). In addition, the lower cervical column can undergo a more complicated, mixed movement that combines rotation with lateral flexion. As a consequence, the vertebrae are inclined laterally by about 25° when the lower cervical column is rotated to its maximum extent (Kapandji, 1974).

The data presented in Table 1.1 point to several important features of vertebral organization that must be considered when trying to analyze movements of the head and neck. First, head and neck movements in any direction can have widely distributed effects and can involve most joints of the cervical column. Moreover, the cooperation between different joints may be essential if certain types of movements are to be made. For example, a large, pure axial rotation of both the head and neck can occur only if the movements of the upper two vertebrae compensate for the lateral inclination that always takes place during rotation at lower cervical levels.

The need for interrelated movements along the whole cervical column poses intriguing questions about the synergies between long muscles that span several joints and short muscles that cross only one or two. The studies so far described have defined only the maximum extent of motion at different joints. They do not provide information about the use made of these same joints during a more varied range of voluntary movements, particularly movements that do not require a maximum amount of joint excursion. It is possible that motion at some joints could be constrained or prevented by contraction of appropriate intervertebral muscles. Without further information about the effect of muscle contractions on joint mobility, it is difficult to predict whether a small change in head position will be made by moving all of the neck joints just a little or by concentrating the movement at only one or two joints.

Table 1.1 suggests that much lateral flexion as well as much flexion–extension take place across lower cervical vertebrae in the human neck. Furthermore, preliminary fluoroscopic investigations suggest that the cervicothoracic junction may be even more flexible in the quadruped than in the human (Graf et al., 1986) (Fig. 1.4). For some head on body movements, the cervicothoracic region is the main site at which joint movement takes place. Until recently, muscles crossing suboccipital joints have been considered to be the prime movers of the head. However, muscles that operate across cervicothoracic joints must also play an important role in head movement by altering the position of the cervical column with respect to the rest of the body.

MUSCLE STRUCTURE

Movement of the skull and cervical column is controlled by an elaborate musculature whose basic organization follows a similar plan in bipedal humans and most laboratory quadrupeds. The most comprehensive descriptions of neck muscle structure are those for humans and the cat, but descriptions of varying thoroughness are also available for the monkey (Hartman and Straus, 1961; Szebenyi, 1969), rat (Greene, 1968; Hebel and Stromberg, 1976), rabbit (Craigie, 1960; Barone et al., 1973), and dog (Evans and Christensen, 1979). Neck muscles are characteristically arranged in layered groupings. An outermost shell of long muscles connects the skull to the shoulder girdle. Beneath this outer shell a second set of layered muscles links the skull with the vertebral column. Most deeply is found a third set of muscles that closely invests and interlinks the vertebrae of the cervical and thoracic region. A summary of neck muscle organization is given here only for humans and the cat. For additional information, the reader is directed to more detailed anatomical texts (*cat,* Elliott, 1963; Crouch, 1969; *human,* Lockhart et al., 1959; Friedman, 1970; Warwick and Williams, 1973; Kapandji, 1974; Pernkopf, 1980; Hiatt and Gartner, 1982).

Muscles That Link the Skull with the Shoulder Girdle

Two large muscles run between the skull and the shoulder girdle in humans (Fig. 1.5A). *Sternocleidomastoideus* originates as two separate heads from the clavicle and the sternum, respectively. The two heads mesh to form a single wide strap that runs obliquely to insert onto the mastoid process and lateral half of the occiput. *Trapezius* is a triangular, sheetlike muscle that overlies the dorsal neck and back. The rostral part of trapezius originates from the medial part of the occiput

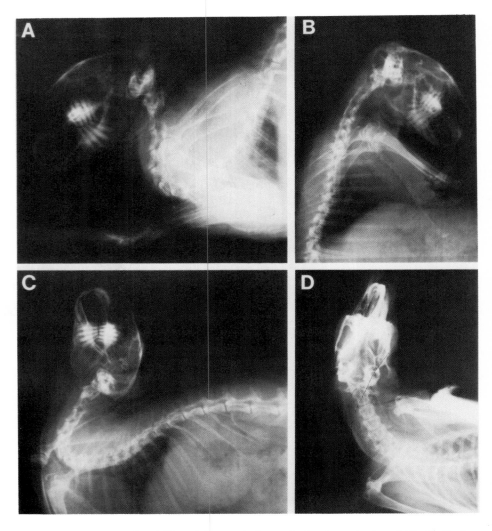

Figure 1.4.   Range of mobility of the cervical vertebral column in the rabbit. Radiophotographs of the alert and anesthetized animal show the animal in (A) resting position, (B) maximal ventriflexion, (C) maximal dorsiflexion, and (D) maximal lateral flexion. (Source: Graf, Vidal, and Evinger, unpublished.)

and the nuchal midline. It wraps in a shawl-like fashion to insert onto the clavicle. More caudal parts of trapezius originate from a midline raphe linking the spinous processes of cervical and thoracic vertebrae. Its muscle fibers run laterally to insert on the scapula.

In the cat, five separate muscles belong to the trapezius and sternocleidomastoideus muscle complex (Fig. 1.5B and C). Two muscles, sternomastoideus and cleidomastoideus, are homologous to the single sternocleidomastoideus found

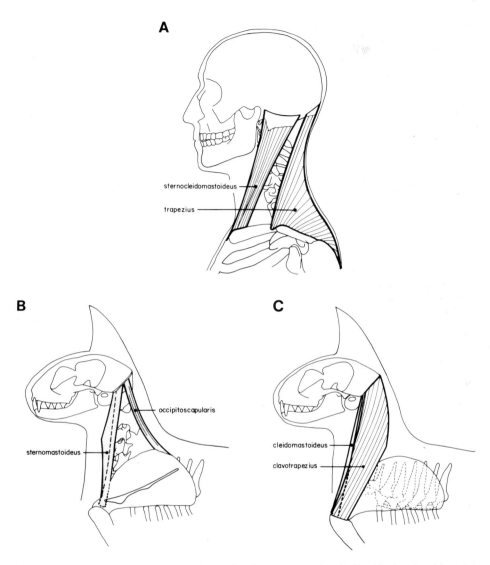

Figure 1.5.   Anatomical features of muscles that connect the skull with the shoulder girdle. Only two large muscles are recognized in the human (A), whereas the cat has four
muscles (B and C).

in humans. *Sternomastoideus* forms a wide triangular sheet that overlies the ventral neck. Its cranial part originates from the ventral midline of the neck and runs
rostrolaterally to insert onto the mastoid process and a conjoined aponeurosis that
runs beneath the parotid gland. The caudal part of sternomastoideus originates
from the manubrium and inserts onto the lateral part of the lambdoidal crest.
Cleidomastoideus runs ventrally to sternomastoideus (Fig. 1.5C). It originates from

the clavicle and from a lateral tendinous raphe called the cleidohumeral ligament, which joins cleidomastoideus in series to the forelimb muscle clavobrachialis. Cleidomastoideus inserts onto the mastoid process.

Trapezius has three separate heads. The most rostral head, *clavotrapezius*, originates from the lambdoidal crest and nuchal midline. It wraps ventrally around the neck to insert onto the clavicle and the cleidohumeral ligament (Fig. 1.5C). The more caudal heads, *acromiotrapezius* and *spinotrapezius*, have a wide origin along the dorsal midline of the back and insert onto the scapula. Of these three muscle heads, only clavotrapezius has an anatomical attachment appropriate for a direct role in head movement.

The cat has an additional muscle, *occipitoscapularis*, that is not found in humans. Occipitoscapularis forms a long, parallel-fibered strap that links the scapula to the lambdoidal crest of the skull (Fig. 1.5B). Elliott (1963) suggests that occipitoscapularis may be anatomically equivalent to part of the rhomboideus muscle in humans. At first glance, this suggestion seems farfetched, because few similarities are apparent between the anatomy of cat occipitoscapularis and human rhomboideus. However, some other primate species have a straplike muscle, called rhomboideus capitis, that spans between the skull and the scapula and resembles occipitoscapularis in its structure (Hartman and Straus, 1961). This muscle is not present in the human and certain other anthropoids.

The sternocleidomastoid and trapezius muscle groupings in both humans and the cat have their motor axons in the spinal portion of the spinal accessory nerve (cranial nerve XI). In contrast to the cranial origin of motor axons, sensory axons supplying trapezius and sternomastoideus run in separate nerve bundles that enter dorsal roots in segments C1–C5. The innervation of occipitoscapularis does not follow the same pattern as the other skull-to-shoulder muscles. Instead, its motor and sensory axons run mainly in the dorsal and ventral roots of C4.

Muscles That Link the Skull with the Vertebral Column

The skull is linked to the vertebral column by a number of muscles that can be distinguished by the adjective "capitis" in their names. The muscles can be divided into three sets: a superficial set of dorsal muscles that crosses several vertebral joints, a deeper set of suboccipital muscles that links the skull with the atlas and axis, and a set of ventral neck muscles that links the skull with the ventral surface of the vertebral column.

Long, Dorsal Muscles

In man, three long dorsal muscles run in differing orientations between the skull and the vertebral column (Fig. 1.6A). (1) *Splenius capitis* runs rostrolaterally from an extended origin along the nuchal and thoracic midline to insert in a line extending across the lateral part of the occiput and onto the mastoid process. (2) *Longissimus capitis* originates from the articular processes of lower cervical vertebrae and the transverse processes of upper thoracic vertebrae. It runs alongside the lateral margin of the vertebral column to insert onto the mastoid process, lateral to the attachment of splenius capitis. (3) *Semispinalis capitis* has a complex origin from articular processes in the lower cervical region and transverse pro-

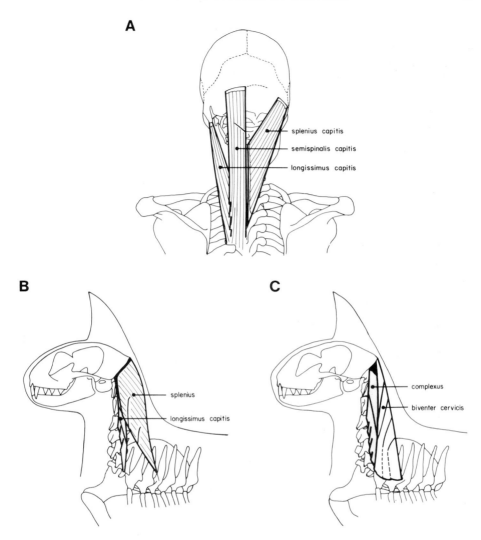

Figure 1.6. Long dorsal muscles connecting the skull with the vertebral column in the human (A) and cat (B and C).

cesses of the thoracic column. It runs parallel to the vertebral column immediately deep to splenius capitis and inserts onto the medial part of the occiput. It is divided into two serial parts by an incomplete band of collagenous tissue called a tendinous inscription that is variable in its form from one muscle specimen to another.

The long dorsal muscles of the cat neck follow a similar plan. Most comparable are the more superficial muscles splenius and longissimus capitis (Fig. 1.6B). *Splenius* in the cat originates from the entire length of the dorsal midline raphe and inserts along the length of the lambdoidal crest. Much of the lateral muscle attaches onto a unipinnate tendon that runs along the lateral margin of splenius and inserts onto the mastoid process. Thus, most fibers in splenius apply their forces onto the lateral part of the skull. *Longissimus capitis* lies on the lateral border of splenius. It originates from the articular processes of lower cervical vertebrae and inserts in a unipinnate fashion onto a tendon that attaches to the mastoid process.

The long neck muscles beneath splenius do not bear such a strong similarity to their counterparts in humans, although they have a close resemblance to equivalent muscles in subhuman primates such as the rhesus monkey (Hartman and Straus, 1961). In the cat, two muscles, biventer cervicis and complexus, run parallel to the vertebral column (Fig. 1.6C). *Biventer cervicis* has a complex multiple origin from articular and spinous processes of vertebrae C5–T2 and runs rostrally to a narrow insertion on the midline of the lambdoidal crest. *Complexus* lies more laterally alongside biventer cervicis. It originates from the articular processes of vertebrae C3–C6 and inserts along the lateral two-thirds of the lambdoidal crest.

The large size and ready accessibility of the long dorsal neck muscles have made these muscles a favorite target for experimental study. Detailed investigations of histochemistry, motor-unit architecture, and innervation have shown that dorsal neck muscles are structurally complex. Each muscle is divided by tendinous inscriptions into serially linked compartments that are supplied by nerves from different spinal segments (Armstrong et al., 1982; Richmond et al., 1985b). The intramuscular patterns of compartmentalization are unique to each muscle. For example, biventer cervicis is composed of five discrete compartments each containing a different population of motor units. The compartments are joined end-to-end by tendinous inscriptions through which no muscle fibers pass (Armstrong et al., 1982). Splenius is also divided into serial compartments of motor units, but the different sets of motor units are separated by tendinous inscriptions only in lateral splenius. In medial splenius, in-series compartments are also present, but the borders between the compartments are not discrete and the fibers of adjacent compartments interdigitate within shared muscle fascicles (Richmond et al., 1985b). The serial organization of compartments has significant implications for the physiological control of long neck muscles, because effective shortening and external tension development can be achieved only if different muscle parts contract in a coordinated fashion.

The in-series organization of segmentally innervated muscle compartments represents one level of complexity in the fiber organization of long neck muscles. However, recent glycogen-depletion studies suggest that yet another level of topographical specialization may exist within individual muscle compartments. When single motor units in biventer cervicis were depleted of glycogen by intracellular stimulation of their motoneurons, motor territories were found to be restricted to a narrow subvolume of muscle constituting only one-third to one-fifth of the cross-sectional area of a single compartment (Fig. 1.7). The extent and shape of the motor-unit territory were related to the fiber organization within each muscle compartment. Some motor units confined their constituent fibers to a subvolume of longer muscle fascicles that formed a "slip" arising from an articular process, whereas others occupied a medial subvolume of shorter fascicles running between two closely approximated inscriptions. This anatomical observation suggests that a single motor unit may be highly specialized and consist of a fairly homogeneous

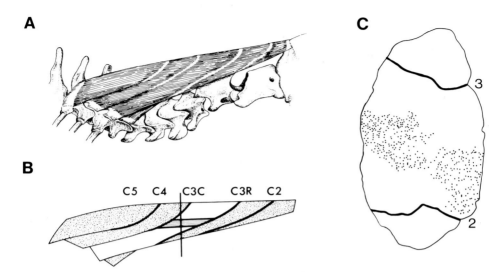

Figure 1.7.   Organization of motor units in biventer cervicis (BC). (A) Dorsal view of BC. (B) Line drawing showing the location of a single motor unit (striped band) marked by glycogen-depletion methods following intracellular impalement and stimulation of its motoneuron in the C3 segment. The unshaded part of the muscle represents the compartment supplied by the entire caudal branch of the C3 segment. This compartment is arranged in series with other compartments that are separated by tendinous inscriptions and supplied by other spinal nerves (C2, C3 rostral, C4, C5). (C) Camera lucida drawing of a muscle cross-section taken at the level of the vertical line in (B). Depleted fibers are shown as dots, distributed in a narrow band running from the dorsal to the ventral surface of the muscle. Tendinous inscriptions are shown as black lines above and below the depleted zone.

subpopulation of muscle fibers with similar length–tension properties and similar sites of force transmission. However, the properties of the motor unit will depend on the concurrent activity in other, dissimilar motor units arranged in parallel or in series. Thus, motor commands to inscripted neck muscles must be carefully balanced to ensure an appropriate matching of contractile performance in different muscle regions.

Suboccipital Muscles

The human neck contains four muscles that lie deep to the long dorsal muscles and serve to link the skull with the dorsal surfaces of the atlas and axis (Fig. 1.8A). *Rectus capitis posterior major* originates from the spinous process of the axis. It widens as it runs rostrolaterally to insert along the inferior nuchal line of the skull. *Rectus capitis posterior minor* has a shorter and more medially directed course, from the posterior arch of the atlas to the medial part of the occiput along the inferior nuchal line. *Obliquus capitis superior* is located laterally to the paired recti muscles. It runs between the transverse process of the atlas and the lateral part of the occiput. *Obliquus capitis inferior*, the fourth muscle conventionally

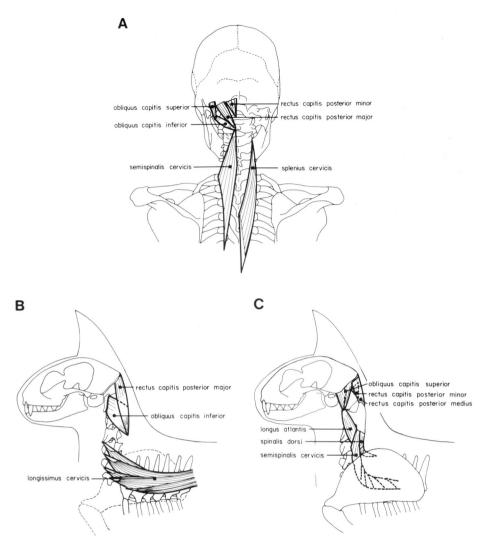

Figure 1.8. Suboccipital muscles and selected intervertebral muscles in the human (A) and cat (B and C).

included in the suboccipital muscle grouping, differs from the others in that it has no attachment to the skull. Instead it runs from the lateral aspect of the spinous process of the axis to insert onto the transverse process of the atlas.

Suboccipital muscles have a similar pattern of organization in the cat. However, the morphology of cervical vertebrae is different in the cat and the architectural features of suboccipital muscles vary accordingly (Fig. 1.8B and C). The rectus capitis posterior muscle grouping has three members instead of two. *Rectus capitis posterior major* originates from the length of the spinous process of C2.

It is angled less obliquely than its counterpart in humans and inserts on the medial part of the lambdoidal crest. More deeply, *rectus capitis posterior medius* runs from the rostral tip of the axial spinous process to insert onto the occipital bone beneath the attachment of rectus capitis major. *Rectus capitis posterior minor* lies deep to the other rectus posterior muscles. It originates on the medial part of the dorsal arch of the atlas and runs only a short distance to form a small triangular muscle overlying the posterior atlantooccipital membrane. The three rectus muscles are closely applied to one another and can be difficult to dissect apart.

Two obliquus muscles are present in the cat. *Obliquus capitis superior* (lateralis) originates from the ventrolateral border of the transverse process of the atlas and inserts onto the mastoid process and the lateral part of the occiput. *Obliquus capitis inferior* (caudalis) is a dense, thick muscle that originates from the whole lateral surface of the axial spinous process and inserts onto the dorsal surface of the transverse process of the atlas. The suboccipital muscles in both humans and the cat are supplied by nerves from the first and second cervical segments.

Ventral Muscles

Only three ventral muscles run between the skull and vertebral column in humans. *Rectus capitis anterior major* (also called *longus capitis*) originates from the transverse processes of C3 to C6 and inserts onto the base of the occiput. *Rectus capitis anterior minor* is more laterally placed and connects the lateral part of the atlas to the base of the occiput. *Rectus capitis lateralis* is found most deeply and laterally. It originates from the transverse process of the atlas and inserts onto the jugular process of the occiput.

In the cat, the same three muscles are present. *Rectus capitis anterior major* (or *longus capitis*) originates as a series of separate bundles from the transverse processes of vertebrae C2–C6. The bundles merge rostrally and attach onto the skull at a site medial and caudal to the tympanic bulla. *Rectus capitis anterior minor* lies deep to rectus anterior major and spans the space between the body of the atlas and the base of the occiput. *Rectus capitis lateralis* originates from the ventral surface of the C1 transverse process. It inserts onto the lateral part of the occiput just ventral to the attachment of obliquus capitis superior, against which it is closely applied.

Muscles That Interlink Vertebrae

The long dorsal muscles that insert onto the skull appear to be specialized elements of a more extensive axial muscle system that runs the length of the vertebral column. Thus, it is not surprising that the "capitis" muscles are often matched by corresponding "cervicis" muscles that have similar fiber orientations but insert on cervical vertebrae rather than the skull. In humans, three large intervertebral muscles correspond with splenius capitis, longissimus capitis, and semispinalis capitis, respectively. *Splenius cervicis* is located caudolaterally to splenius capitis. Its fibers run in the same oblique direction as splenius capitis but they link the spines of vertebrae T3–T6 with the transverse processes of the upper cervical vertebrae (Fig. 1.8A). *Longissimus cervicis* runs along the lateral margin of the vertebral column to join the transverse processes of T1–T5 with those of C2–C6 (not illustrated). *Semispinalis cervicis* runs obliquely between the transverse processes of T1–T6 and the spines of C2–C5 (Fig. 1.8A).

Beneath the longer intervertebral muscles, a deeply placed network of shorter muscles connects adjacent vertebrae. These muscles have complex architectural configurations. Fiber bundles composing *interspinales* muscles run between the neighboring spinous processes of cervical vertebrae. The *multifidus spinae* muscles lie more laterally; their fiber bundles are oriented obliquely to link the articular processes of lower cervical vertebrae with the spinous processes of more rostral vertebrae. The *rotatores spinae* originate on transverse processes and run rostrally to insert on the spinous processes of neighboring vertebrae. The fiber bundles of rotatores and multifidis muscles are closely associated and can be difficult to distinguish in some regions. *Intertransversarii* muscles run between the transverse processes of adjacent vertebrae. Finally, *longus cervicis* runs on the ventral surface of the vertebral column. Its fibers are directed in a variety of oblique angles between the vertebral bodies and transverse processes of lower cervical and thoracic vertebrae.

In addition to muscles interlinking vertebrae, there are scalenus muscles that link the vertebral column with the rib cage. Fiber bundles composing *scalenus anterior* originate from transverse processes of C3–C6 and insert onto the first rib. Those composing *scalenus medius* originate from more dorsal sites on the transverse processes of C2–C7 and have a more lateral insertion onto the first rib. *Scalenus posterior* is the smallest of the muscle set and is often fused to the dorsolateral margin of scalenus medius. Its fibers originate from the transverse processes of C4–C6 and insert onto the second rib.

The neck of the cat like that of humans has both long and short intervertebral muscles (Fig. 1.8B and C). The longer and more superficial muscles include longissimus cervicis and scalenus. *Longissimus cervicis* is the rostral subdivision of longissimus dorsi, a very long muscle that overlies the dorsal surface of the vertebral column for most of its length. In the neck, longissimus cervicis is composed of many thick bundles of obliquely directed fibers that originate from the spinous and articular processes of lower cervical and thoracic vertebrae and run rostrally to insert onto cervical transverse processes (Fig. 1.8B). *Scalenus* in the cat is a large, sheetlike muscle with extensive origins from the rib cage and from the transverse processes of the first thoracic and lower cervical vertebrae. The muscle has an extended insertion onto the transverse processes of all cervical vertebrae.

The short muscles investing cat vertebrae have an organization similar to those of humans (Fig. 1.8C). Most dorsally, spinous processes of vertebrae caudal to C2 are linked by short, inscripted bundles of fibers that collectively make up the *spinalis dorsi* muscle. More laterally is *semispinalis cervicis*, whose fibers originate from the articular processes of lower cervical vertebrae and insert onto the spinous processes of more rostral vertebrae, especially the spinous process of the axis. *Longus atlantis* is located rostrally and laterally to semispinalis cervicis. It originates from the lateral aspect and transverse process of the third cervical vertebra. Its fibers run alongside the axis and insert onto the wing of the atlas. The lateral aspect of the vertebral column is also invested by *intertransversarii* muscles that interconnect transverse processes of closely approximated vertebrae (not illustrated).

On the ventral surface of the vertebral column, the paired *longus colli* muscles (also called *centrotransversarii* muscles) lie between the transverse processes of cervical vertebrae. Fiber bundles arise from the transverse processes and lateral parts of the vertebral centra. They angle medially in complex multipinnate formations to insert on the midline of more rostral vertebral bodies up to and including the atlas.

OTHER "NECK" MUSCLES

The neck muscles described above have often been considered as the complete set of neck muscles playing a role in head movement. However, head movement depends not only on motion at upper cervical joints but also on the posture of the neck determined by the relative positions of lower cervical and upper thoracic vertebrae. As a consequence, additional muscles that act exclusively across the cervicothoracic column may in the future have to be recognized as part of the effector apparatus for head movement. Not only may these muscles actively contribute to head–neck movement, but their various activities may establish the posture that will define the axes of motion for more rostral muscle groups. Particular attention must be paid both to muscles that span the cervicothoracic junction and to muscles that run between the scapula and the cervical vertebral column. Muscles that connect the scapula to the vertebral column have not been considered above. In humans, they include the rhomboideus muscle complex (including rhomboideus major and minor) and levator scapulae. In cat they include muscles such as rhomboideus, levator scapulae, and levator scapulae ventralis.

FUNCTIONAL BEHAVIOR OF NECK MUSCLES

Descriptions of muscle anatomy typically are extrapolated to provide speculations about the physiological capabilities of individual muscles. A knowledge of muscle shape, attachment, and fiber architecture has often been used to predict the mechanical actions of an individual muscle, and this prediction is usually placed as a postscript to the anatomical descriptions that appear in most textbooks of anatomy. For neck muscles, these predictions are often quite arbitrary. Long multiarticular muscles are generally assigned actions of turning, extending, or ventriflexing the head and neck. Shorter muscles close to the vertebral column are considered to "stabilize" the vertebral column. Their functional behavior is less commonly discussed and frequently dismissed as relatively unimportant in the control of head movement (Jeffreys, 1980, Hiatt and Gartner, 1982).

More recently, experiments have been performed to investigate the functional properties and roles of neck muscles in a more systematic manner. One direction of research has been to define more precisely the physical organization of neck muscles. Information from such studies has revealed considerable heterogeneity in the lengths, cross-sectional areas, tendon arrangements, and fiber-type compositions of different neck muscles (cf. Richmond and Abrahams, 1975a) (Table 1.2). These specializations presumably adapt individual muscles to participate most

Table 1.2. Neck muscles of the cat[a]

Muscle	Origin	Insertion	Innervation	Slow fiber content (%)	Functional CSA (cm²)	Likely human homolog
Skull → shoulder girdle						
Sternomastoideus	Manubrium and ventral midline of the neck	Lateral part of lambdoidal crest and mastoid process	Motor: cranial XI Sensory: C1–C3	< 15	0.41	Part of sternocleidomastoideus
Cleidomastoideus	Clavicle and cleidohumeral ligament	Mastoid process	Motor: cranial XI Sensory: C2–C3	5–25	0.12	Part of sternocleidomastoideus
Clavotrapezius	Lambdoidal crest and nuchal midline	Clavicle and cleidohumeral ligament	Motor: cranial XI Sensory: C2–C4	<15 (a)	0.36	Part of trapezius
Occipitoscapularis	Lambdoidal crest	Scapula	C4	57 (b)	0.08	None
Vertebral column → skull						
Splenius	Dorsal midline of neck	Lambdoidal crest and mastoid process	C1–C4	25 (b)	0.78	Splenius capitis
Longissimus capitis	Articular processes, C3–C7	Mastoid process	C2–C4	15–30 (b)	0.14	Longissimus capitis
Biventer cervicis	Articular and spinous processes, C5–T3	Lambdoidal crest	C2–C5	50 (b)	0.57	Part of semispinalis capitis
Complexus	Articular processes, C3–C6	Lambdoidal crest	C1–C3	40 (b)	0.48	Part of semispinalis capitis
Rectus capitis posterior major	Spinous process of axis	Lambdoidal crest	C1	25 (b)	0.14	Rectus capitis posterior major
Rectus capitis posterior medius	Spinous process of axis	Occipital bone of skull	C1	30–45	0.19	Part of rectus capitis posterior major
Rectus capitis posterior minor	Dorsal arch of atlas	Occipital bone of skull	C1	50–75	0.07	Rectus capitis posterior minor

Muscle	Attachment	Attachment				
Obliquus capitis inferior	Spinous process of axis	Transverse process of atlas	C1(?), C2	0–60	1.48	Obliquus capitis inferior
Obliquus capitis superior	Transverse process of atlas	Mastoid process, lateral occiput	C1	NYA[b]	NYA	Obliquus capitis superior
Rectus capitis anterior major	Transverse processes, C2–C6	Base of occiput	C2	10–50	NYA	Rectus capitis anterior major
Rectus capitis anterior minor	Ventral aspect of atlas	Base of occiput	NYA	NYA	NYA	Rectus capitis anterior minor
Rectus capitis lateralis	Transverse process of C1	Lateral part of occiput	NYA	NYA	NYA	Rectus capitis lateralis
Intervertebral muscles						
Spinalis dorsi	Spinous processes of vertebrae caudal to C3	More rostral spinous processes	C3–C7(?)[c]	NYA	NYA	Interspinalis
Semispinalis cervicis	Articular processes of lower cervical vertebrae	Spinous processes of cervical vertebrae, especially C2	C3–C7(?)	NYA	NYA	Multifidus spinae, semispinalis cervicis
Longus atlantis	Lateral part of C3 vertebra	Transverse process of axis	C2, C3(?)	20–70	0.37[d]	Intertransversarii
Intertransversarii	Transverse processes of vertebrae	More rostral transverse processes	C3–C7(?)	NYA	NYA	Intertransversarii
Longissimus cervicis (rostral)	Spinous and articular processes, lower cervical and thoracic vertebrae	Cervical transverse processes	NYA	15–50	NYA	Longissimus cervicis
Longus colli	Transverse processes and lateral parts of vertebrae	Ventral midline of vertebral bodies	C2–C7(?)	NYA	NYA	Longus cervicis

[a] Information on muscle structure is based on descriptions by Crouch (1969) and Elliott (1963), and has been supplemented by laboratory dissections. Some measures of slow-fiber content have been published previously: (a) Keane, 1981 and (b) Richmond and Abrahams, 1975a. Other measures are new data, based on counts from three adult cats. In some instances, a range of values is reported because muscles exhibit a nonuniform distribution of fiber types. Values for functional cross-sectional area (functional CSA) are averaged from at least three cats weighing 3.2–3.4 kg.

[b] NYA, Not yet analyzed.

[c] (?), Needs experimental confirmation.

[d] Approximate measure only.

effectively in tonic or phasic tasks or to work across particular joints with different lever arms.

A detailed knowledge of muscle structure can bring us closer to understanding the physical adaptations and constraints that will affect the physiological behavior of muscles. However, this information is often insufficient to identify the functional role of a muscle, because patterns of muscle recruitment will depend on a number of other factors, such as the concurrent operation of other muscles or the positions and degrees of freedom of the joints across which the muscle must act. In the neck, most muscles are attached at both ends to bones that move, so that their action will depend on the stability of the muscle origin and insertion at any given time. For example, occipitoscapularis originates on the scapula and inserts on the skull, and thus has the potential to contribute either to head or shoulder movement. Its use in head movement will depend on the position and stability of the scapula. Conversely, its successful use to move the shoulder would require the synergistic recruitment of cervical muscles to stabilize the skull. A further complication is added because many neck muscles cross several vertebral joints. The movement produced by these multiarticular muscles will depend on the initial position of each joint and the degree to which the joints are free to move in each of one or more planes. Thus, patterns of muscle synergy during normal head movements are complex.

To obtain more direct information about the ways in which neck muscles are recruited during normal behavior, electromyographic (EMG) recording methods have been used to monitor muscle activity during head movements in alert, chronically instrumented cats or in humans whose muscle activity is recorded with surface electrodes. The earliest EMG studies focused on the behavior of a small number of dorsal neck muscles whose activity could be evoked or modified during head turns elicited by visual or vestibular stimuli (*cat*, Guitton et al., 1980; Vidal et al., 1982, 1983; Wilson et al., 1983; Darlot et al., 1985; *human*, Zangemeister et al., 1982b). Particular attention was paid to a cohort of muscles including splenius, longissimus capitis, obliquus capitis superior and inferior, and sternomastoideus, which appeared to participate in lateral head turning. More recently, simultaneous recordings have been made from a larger number of neck muscles (Peterson et al., 1985a; Richmond et al., 1985a; Roucoux et al., 1985). Preliminary results from the more extended studies suggest that patterns of neck muscle recruitment cannot be predicted simply. When the animal voluntarily holds its head stationary, EMG activity can be detected in only a few neck muscles including biventer cervicis, semispinalis cervicis, and occipitoscapularis (Richmond et al., 1985a; Roucoux et al., 1985). These muscles are characterized by their relatively high proportions of type SO muscle fibers. When the head moves, additional neck muscles are recruited in synergistic "teams" whose membership depends on several factors: the direction and speed of the movement, the initial position of the head, the presence and magnitude of loading on the head, and the joints around which the movement is made (Richmond et al., 1985a).

Although the specific patterns of muscle recruitment depend on the trajectory of the movement, all movements appeared to involve concurrent activity in long muscles crossing several joints and in smaller intervertebral muscles. An unexpected finding in comparisons of EMG records from many neck muscles is the extent to which EMG activity is synchronized from one muscle to another during some types of head movements. It is commonly accepted that the motor units in mammalian muscles fire asynchronously, presumably to smooth the development and transmission of contractile force (Burke, 1985). However, motor units in neck muscles often fire in rhythmic bursts, at a fairly constant frequency of 25–30 Hz. The timing of spike bursts in one neck muscle is synchronized with similar spike bursts in many, if not all, of the other concurrently active neck muscles. Synchronization can be detected most clearly by using cross-correlational methods to compare the temporal relationships between pairs of EMG records (Loeb et al., 1987). The presence of synchronization suggests that the control mechanisms underlying motoneuron recruitment in neck segments may be quite different from those in lumbosacral segments in which most studies of motoneuron connectivity have so far been conducted. Studies of electromyographic activity will undoubtedly provide a powerful method for the future study of neck muscle behavior. Such approaches will take on particular value when the biomechanical events occurring during the head movement can be analyzed simultaneously, using quantitative methods to monitor changes in the positions of joints or the lengths of muscles and their substituent compartments.

SUMMARY

Head movements are made by changing the alignments of the cervical vertebrae that link the skull with the body. The bones composing the cervical vertebrae have specialized structures and articular arrangements. Thus, individual joints differ in their abilities to move and these specializations have a significant affect on the way that head movements can be executed in any particular plane. There is a remarkable underlying similarity in the basic arrangements of bones and muscles in humans and in most laboratory quadrupeds, although differences can be identified in the detailed organization of the cervical column from one mammalian species to another. In all these species, the skull is commonly held at the top of a vertically oriented cervical column. The posture of the head and neck is controlled by more than 20 pairs of muscles that are arranged in layered groupings. The outermost layers of muscle span from the skull to the shoulder girdle, the middle layers span from the skull to the vertebral column, and the deepest layers run between vertebrae. Together these muscles are responsible for a diverse range of head and neck movements. Both anatomical and physiological observations suggest that several neck muscles can share a similar pulling direction, but the ways in which these muscles are coordinated to execute a single head movement is not yet clear. Electromyographic studies have shown that most head movements are made using several muscles. However, the particular role played by a single muscle cannot be predicted simply from its pulling direction; it also depends on its biomechanical properties, its fiber-type composition, and its relationships with different cervical joints.

2

Biomechanical Modeling of the Human Head and Neck

J. WINTERS

As is apparent from the previous chapter, the biomechanics of the head–neck system, which includes the head, the cervical axial skeleton, and the muscles within the head–neck region, is very complex. It is impossible to model this system totally, in part because of its sheer complexity and in part because of the lack of quantitative data on material properties, geometries, and boundary conditions of individual tissues. However, for the analysis of most of the tasks performed by this system, the idealized "perfect" model, including a complete biomechanical modeling of all aspects of the system, would in fact not be the "best" model. This is particularly true when considering the control of neurally initiated head movements. For instance, a group studying the vestibuloocular reflex need not model every muscle, ligament, vertebra, and disk in the neck. In general, the "best" model is the *simplest* model that can *adequately* represent the head–neck system for the task, or set of tasks, at hand. However, too simple a model comes at a great cost: potential misinformation.

The goals of this chapter are (1) to develop the basic mechanical principles of large-scale inertial systems and of the individual tissues (particularly muscle) that make up the system, (2) to review the existing work on biomechanical modeling of the human head–neck system, putting special effort into placing the very different types of models into perspective; and (3) to provide an intuitive "feel" for the role played by the biomechanical system so as to help put the movement data to be presented in later chapters into perspective, particularly for those who are less mechanically inclined.

BIOMECHANICAL TOOLS FOR ANALYSIS

The basic tools for biomechanical analysis and modeling are simply those of mechanics: statics (consideration of forces in equilibrium, with no motion occurring), kinematics (analysis of motion without regard to the forces causing motion), dynamics or kinetics (analysis of both motion and forces causing motion), and deformable solids (material properties of tissues). In addition, it is important to consider the mechanical properties of the skeletal muscles themselves, which have advantageous design features and nonlinearities not seen in human-made motors.

Static and Quasi-Static Analysis

As shown schematically in Figure 2.1, the head can be viewed as an inverted pendulum that is connected to what is essentially a tilted beam with complex mechanical properties (the cervical vertebral column). The basic bone-on-bone compressive connection between the occipital condyles and the atlantoaxial complex is supported and stabilized via tensile loading of both the ligamentous tissues surrounding this attachment and the many muscles that attach onto the skull. Of special importance are the following two observations: (1) the *mass* (approx. 4–5 kg) and subsequent *inertia* (approx. 0.02 kg-m^2 axial rotation, 0.03–0.04 kg-m^2 frontal and lateral flexion) of the head are large relative to those of the muscles and the neck; and (2) the cervical vertebral column can be bent fairly easily, because of the significant compliance of the vertebral disks and, to a lesser extent, other perivertebral soft tissues, for a significant operating range in every direction of rotation (e.g., Goel et al., 1984). Consequently, if all head–neck muscles were to relax, the head would fall due to gravitational forces. Since the *center of mass* of the head is anterior to the vertebral column, the head would fall forward by rotating about an *axis of rotation* that is somewhere between the first cervical and the first thoracic vertebrae, varying with increased rotation. The axis of rotation would be higher when most of the bending occurs between the skull and C2 as opposed to lower spinal levels such as between C4 and C6.

In an alert individual, under no loading from the environment (other than that due to gravity), the orientation of the head depends on the relative degree of activity in the individual muscles. Larger muscles with large *lever arms* have the greatest effect on determining head orientation since they can generate greater torque (M_t) for head rotation. This can be seen by a simple static analysis:

$$M_t = R_a\mathbf{F_m} = R_a(\sigma A_{pcs}) \tag{1}$$

where $\mathbf{F_m}$ is the muscle force, σ is the contractile stress of the muscle tissue, which can range from zero (relaxed muscle) up to 0.2 to 0.6 MPa (20–60 N/cm^2), R_a is the lever (or moment) arm (i.e., the distance between the muscle line of action and the axis of rotation), and A_{pcs} is the "physiological" cross-sectional area, that for parallel-fibered muscle is the muscle cross-section and for pennate muscle is often approximated as "[(mass)/(density × thickness)] × sin(2 × pennation angle)" (Alexander and Vernon, 1975).

There are a number of massive muscles within the human head–neck complex that have especially large cross-sectional areas (over 4 cm^2) and significant lever arms (over 2 cm) and thus are of greatest importance in generating torque (sternocleidomastoideus, splenius capitis, semispinalis capitis, longissimus capitis, and trapezius). The effect of each of these muscles in terms of head movement is a function of their developed torque (force applied relative to the instantaneous axis of rotation). For instance, strong activity in the sternocleidomastoideus causes head flexion, whereas strong activity in the semispinalis or trapezius causes head extension. If the sternocleidomastoideus on one side and the splenius on the other

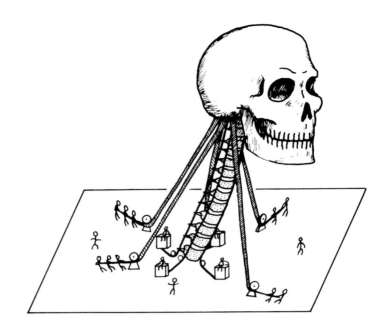

A

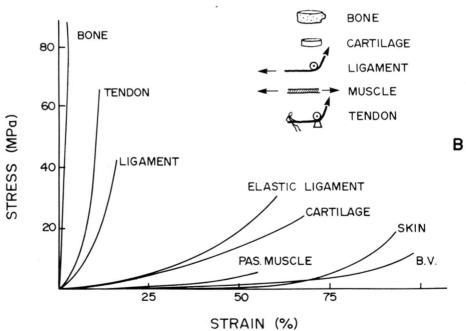

B

contract more strongly, then the head tends to rotate horizontally about its long axis (prove this to yourself). The final orthogonal direction of head rotation, i.e., lateral (sideways) flexion, would occur if all of these muscles were contracting only on one side. If the muscles on the other side of the neck were also active at similar levels, then there would be no visible movement of the head since the applied torques would all balance. (The subject would then, of course, be ever so slightly shorter due to axial compression of the intervertebral disks, although only a model including elastic disks would show this.) Of course, movements in directions outside of these three classical orthogonal planes can also be made by appropriately adjusting the activities of various muscles.

The above intuitive analysis is in fact quite soundly based and represents actual behavior of the head–neck system to a first approximation for both static and quasi-static situations. This simple analysis, however, does not necessarily provide the actual axis about which the head is rotating, nor describe translation (sliding motion) of the head. It also does not take into account two sets of muscles with potentially significant actions. These are (1) the short yet fairly thick muscles that connect the upper cervical vertebrae with the skull (e.g., various recti and oblique muscles discussed in Chapter 1), and (2) the muscles that connect the various torso regions with the transverse (side) or spinous (back) aspects of the cervical vertebrae (e.g., the various scalenus muscles). These muscles influence the subtle details of neck orientation and axis of rotation. For instance, a common movement such as anterior translation (forward sliding) of the head is accomplished by using a multitude of muscles, some located internally near the head–cervical junction, that cause mild head extension (e.g., longus capitis), other internal muscles that cause neck frontal flexion (e.g., scalenus), and some external muscles (sternocleidomastoideus causing forward movement, large back muscle complex helping to stabilize movement).

This analysis helps to show that even static models for the head–neck system can be complex. Nevertheless, it suggests that approximations can be made that simplify the analysis to the most relevant muscles.

In general, the typical values for the peak voluntary static torques that can be generated in three primary directions are about 40 N-m for head extension and

Figure 2.1. (A) Schematic showing the basic structural arrangement of the mechanically relevant head and neck tissues, with only a few representative muscles and ligaments shown and without ribs attached to the lower vertebrae. The bone and cartilage tissue can resist either tensile or compressive loading, while the ligamentous and muscle tissues load only in tension. Muscle can also generate tension as a function of "activity," as suggested here. Notice that the head, which is much heavier than the neck, requires a continuous extensor torque for there to be static equilibrium in the position shown. (B) Typical stress (force per unit area) versus strain (percentage change in length) behavior of a number of relevant biological connective tissues, extended relative to their approximate physiological (*in situ*) "rest length." Notice that with increasing tissue extension, the slope of the curve increases and thus the tissue becomes stiffer. The dashed line represents peak muscle contractile stress. PAS. MUSCLE, passive muscle; B.V., blood vessel.

lateral flexion, 20 N-m for head flexion, and about 10–15 N-m for axial rotation (e.g., Mertz and Patrick, 1971; Patrick and Chou, 1976).

Head–Neck Kinematics and Dynamics

The variables of interest for kinematic analysis are the translational and angular position $(\mathbf{x}, \boldsymbol{\theta})$, velocity $(\mathbf{v}, \boldsymbol{\omega})$, and acceleration $(\mathbf{a}, \boldsymbol{\alpha})$. These quantities are related as follows:

$$\frac{d^2\mathbf{x}}{dt^2} = \frac{d\mathbf{v}}{dt} = \mathbf{a}; \quad \frac{d^2\boldsymbol{\theta}}{dt^2} = \frac{d\boldsymbol{\omega}}{dt} = \boldsymbol{\alpha} \qquad (\mathbf{x} = \boldsymbol{\theta} \times \mathbf{r}; \quad \mathbf{v} = \boldsymbol{\omega} \times \mathbf{r}; \quad \mathbf{a} = \boldsymbol{\alpha} \times \mathbf{r}) \quad (2)$$

where $\mathbf{r}$ is the vector directed from an axis of rotation (e.g., muscle lever arm). Measurement of these variables has been accomplished by a number of methods, including photographic filming at medium or high speed (e.g., 1000 frames per second by Winters and Goldsmith, 1983), light-weight goniometer–potentiometer arrangements mechanically coupled to the head (e.g., Hannaford et al., 1984 for multiple head rotations, ongoing work by this author for both head rotations and translations), or video-based three-dimensional motion analysis systems (ongoing work by X author). Other techniques, such as imaging methods (e.g., X ray), have so far been used primarily for static analysis. Dynamic analysis, which extends a kinematic analysis by also considering the forces ($\mathbf{F}$) causing translational motion or the torques ($\mathbf{M}$) causing rotational motion, has its foundation in Newtonian mechanics:

$$\Sigma \mathbf{F} = m\mathbf{a}; \qquad \Sigma \mathbf{M} = I\boldsymbol{\alpha} \qquad\qquad (3)$$

where m is mass and I is inertia. The right sides of the actual dynamic equations are considerably more complex unless the head is assumed to be a sphere rotating about its centroid. In general, the applied forces and torques represented by the left side of these system equations cannot be measured directly without affecting the very system being measured, and thus models combining kinematic information with EMG and/or known external loads can often be used to estimate indirectly the system dynamics (e.g., Hannaford et al., 1984). Typically, for analysis of the head–neck system, all bones are considered as "rigid bodies," i.e., they do not deform. The resulting "equations of motion" for each of the rigid bodies of the head–neck system can be very complex, and head–neck dynamic analysis invariably requires extensive computer simulation.

The majority of quantitative data for voluntary head movements is for maximally rapid ("time optimal") movements constrained to axial (horizontal) rotation. For such movements, peak angular velocities on the order of 10 rad/sec are obtained within about 100 msec from the initiation of movement, with the time of peak velocity being a function of the magnitude of the movement (Zangemeister et al., 1981a, b; Hannaford et al., 1983, 1984). Hannaford et al. (1983) present some data on maximal oblique head movements under inertial, viscous, and elastic external loads. Their results suggest that horizontal and vertical movement kinematics are coupled—reasonable given that many of the same muscles are involved in both types of movement. Much less quantitative kinematic information is available for the more moderate range of speeds that are typically seen in every-day life. However, a survey of many sources suggests that bending in flexion–extension is fairly uniform at all speeds of movement, with the atlantooccipital joint bending up to about 20° and joints between C2 and T2 about 50° in either direction. The first 50% of axial head rotation is primarily executed about the median atlantoaxial joint, whereas additional bending causes uniform cervical rotation (Lysell, 1969; Norkin and Levangie, 1983). Finally, lateral flexion occurs by a coupling of lateral bending with axial rotation.

Experimental kinematic analyses of the head–neck system are especially common for *impact* and *whiplash* studies, with data available for humans, animals, and artificial replicas (e.g., reviews in Goldsmith, 1972, and Sances et al., 1981). The axis of rotation of the head depends on the direction of primary motion and on the type of impact. Peak accelerations usually occur within the period of the actual impact or shortly thereafter, whereas peak velocities occur about 10–50 msec later. Peak displacements typically occur between 100 and 300 msec after impact. Rear impacts are unusual in that they cause significant initial translation, and consequently rotation starts later (Winters and Goldsmith, 1983). Injury criteria and safety standards have been formulated by correlating translational and rotational acceleration trajectories with brain tissue damage, resulting in theories on injury mechanisms based on internal pressure gradients and shear strains, respectively (see Goldsmith, 1972, or Ommaya and Gennarelli, 1976).

Dynamic analysis of the head–neck system is extremely difficult. There is a variety of data on head–neck dynamics for fairly significant impulsive loading to human volunteers (e.g., Ewing and Thomas, 1972). A wide range of analytical and computer models of the head and head–neck system exist and will be considered in a later section. Suffice it to say that these efforts provide strong evidence that the viscoelastic properties of neck soft tissues significantly affect transient head–neck dynamics; however, interpretation tends to be limited by an inadequate modeling of muscle dynamics.

"Solids" Analysis: Tissue Material Properties

The overall mechanical properties of a given biological tissue depend, in an often complex manner, on the *materials* from which it is made and the *geometry* of both the tissue and the surrounding environment (Yamada, 1970). The mechanical properties of specific head tissues, reviewed by Goldsmith (1972), will not be discussed here since it is the neck tissues that are involved in head motion. For present purposes, four types of tissues can be distinguished. The first, *bone*, can be viewed as a rigid body. This is because the strain in bone, which is up to 2% for loads approaching failure in both tension and compression (e.g., Yamada, 1970), is very small relative to that for all other tissues.

The second is *soft connective tissues*, which have a significant compliance and have a tendency to become *stiffer with increasing extension*, as can be seen in Figure 2.1B. In general, vertebral ligaments composed mostly of collagen fibers (the majority) are stiffer, reaching peak tensile strains of 10–20% (Tkaczuk, 1968, for longitudinal ligament; Walters and Morris, 1973, for interspinous ligament), whereas those with a high percentage of elastin fibers, such as the flavum and nuchae, tend to be very compliant, reaching peak strains of approximately 50% (Nachemson and Evans, 1968). These data can be extended to the cervical region to obtain approximate ligamentous force–extension data (e.g., Winters and Goldsmith, 1983). Tendons have properties similar to the stiffer ligaments.

The third type of "tissue" is that of the intervertebral disk, which includes cartilage ("annulus fibrosis") that surrounds a fluid-type substance called nucleus pulposus. This viscoelastic material serves as an elastic "shock absorber" which can reach extension or compression strains of up to about 50% when resisting high tension or compression loads, respectively (Kulak et al., 1976; Myers and Mow, 1983).

The fourth tissue of interest, *muscle*, will be discussed later. As seen in Figure 2-1B, *skin* and *blood vessels* are much more compliant. Since these tissues essentially lie in parallel with the much stiffer ligamentous tissue and are not rigidly mounted to a solid foundation such as bone, it is estimated that their mechanical role, plus that of the *trachea* (Powell, 1975) and its surrounding tissues, is negligible. The *thyrohyoid* and *facial* muscles appear to play an insignificant role as long as the jaw is relaxed.

Mechanically, the *intact spinal column* can flex, extend, and axially rotate fairly easily but can bend laterally only by a moderate amount. Although a good deal of all head–neck rotations are due to the rotation of joints between the skull and C2, the entire cervical column, as well as the upper thoracic column, does in fact rotate significantly in all directions during normal movements. The ligaments that surround the column (anterior and posterior longitudinal, flavum, supraspinous and interspinous, transverse), together with the intervertebral disks and the vertebral facets, are primarily responsible for the passive resistance to bending. In each direction, the system becomes progressively stiffer with increasing bending. Peak normal head rotations range from 50 to 80°, with lateral flexion the least and extension the most. Macroscopically, the vertebra–disk–vertebra unit, with attached soft tissue, can be fairly well represented as an orthotropic viscoelastic beam (e.g., Terry and Roberts, 1968; Orne and Liu, 1971). Additional information on the mechanical contributions of the individual components, obtained by mechanical loading after selective dissection, is presented in Panjabi et al. (1975) and Goel et al. (1984) for the cervical region and Panjabi et al. (1976) for the thoracic region. A good review of the biomechanics of the cervical spine is presented by White and Panjabi (1978).

Muscle: An Active Tissue

The basic mechanical properties of muscle are summarized by using the classical model of Hill (1938), in which the "contractile element" (CE) of muscle lies in series with what is essentially an elastic element (SE) and in parallel with a passive elastic element (PE), as shown in Figure 2.2. This model has since been supported by numerous groups, including those modeling human muscle–joint systems (e.g., Wilkie, 1950; Winters and Stark, 1985).

The *contractile element* has three properties of particular relevance. The first stems from the temporal dynamics of the neuromuscular activation–deactivation process, of which calcium activation–deactivation is the rate-limiting step. This

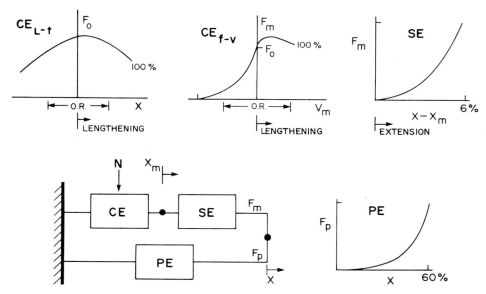

Figure 2.2. The classic three-element Hill model structure for muscle is presented in the lower left. The surrounding curves display the basic mechanical properties of each element. The contractile element (CE) includes two properties, the "length–tension" relation (upper left), which modifies the force $\mathbf{F_0}$ based on the ongoing length, and the "force–velocity" relation of the muscle "motor" (upper middle), which gives the force produced by the contractile machinery as a function of the ongoing CE velocity $\mathbf{V_m}$. The position X is measured relative to the normal *in situ* muscle length. The difference between the current $\mathbf{F_0}$ and $\mathbf{F_m}$ values is the force not passed. Both of the displayed CE curves are for the peak (100% effort) activation special case. The arrows under these curves define typical operating ranges (O.R.) possible when this element is part of a full muscle–joint system. The series element (SE) and the parallel element (PE) are shown as nonlinear springs that get stiffer with increased extension. Notice that $\mathbf{F_m}$ is the final force across both the CE and SE relations (due to series arrangement), whereas $\mathbf{F_m}$ and $\mathbf{F_p}$ add to give the total applied force that the muscle generates (property of parallel arrangement).

process appears to be adequately represented by time constants ranging from 5 to 20 msec for activation and 30 to 60 msec for deactivation, with the values depending on muscle size and fiber composition (Winters and Stark, 1985). The second property of the contractile element is its length dependency, as represented by the classic "length–tension" property of the contractile machinery (e.g., Gordon et al., 1966) in which there is an optimal region for muscle force generation, with muscle force diminishing for progressively shorter or longer lengths (Fig. 2.2, top left). For many muscles in the body, however, the *in situ* operating range is such that this effect is only moderate (Fig. 2.2). The third property is the well-known *"force–velocity"* relation of this "biological motor," which can be represented by "Hill's equation" for shortening muscle:

$$(\mathbf{F_{ce}} + a\mathbf{F_0})(\mathbf{v_{ce}} + a\mathbf{v_m}) = \text{constant} = \mathbf{F_0}(1 + a)a\mathbf{v_m} \tag{4}$$

which can be rearranged into a form which shows explicitly the force lost across a nonlinear viscous element b_h:

$$\mathbf{F}_{ce} = \mathbf{F}_o - (\mathbf{b}_h \mathbf{v}_{ce}); \qquad \mathbf{b}_h = \frac{\mathbf{F}_o(1 + a)}{a\mathbf{v}_m + \mathbf{v}_{ce}} \qquad (5)$$

where $\mathbf{F}_{ce}$ and $\mathbf{v}_{ce}$ are the force and the velocity of the contractile element, respectively; $\mathbf{F}_o$ is the output of the activation process, in force units; and a and $\mathbf{v}_m$ are constants, with a being unitless and ranging in value from about 0.1 (slow muscle) to 0.6 (fast muscle) and $\mathbf{v}_m$, the maximum unloaded contractile element velocity, ranging in value from about 2 muscle lengths per second (slow muscle) to about 10 muscle lengths per second (fast muscle). For lengthening muscle, an "inverted and skewed Hill's equation" (Winters and Stark, 1985) has been shown to approximate observed data for animals and humans. A typical force–velocity curve, for the maximum effort case, is displayed in Figure 2.2. Notice that since $\mathbf{F}_o$ changes with activation level there is actually an infinite number of curves. The "length–tension" relation can also be included into this curve by scaling $\mathbf{F}_o$ based on the current muscle length (Abbott and Wilkie, 1953).

The *series element*, which represents muscle and tendon elastic tissue in series with the contractile element, also plays an important role in muscle behavior. The resulting force–extension property is well approximated as having an exponential shape (Fig. 2.2). In general, the peak extension of this element is 5–6% (Winters and Stark, 1985). A simple consideration of neck-muscle lengths and lever arms suggests that the peak series extension for the angular systems of the head–neck structure are on the order of 20–40°, which is a significant amount. This suggests that the series element should have an impact on (1) any voluntary movement made at moderate-to-high speeds; (2) any movements with sudden changes in direction; or (3) any movements with external loadings. The consequences of these observations will be discussed later.

BIOMECHANICAL MODELING AND THE TYPE OF TASK OF INTEREST

There is tremendous variation in the types of biomechanical models that have so far been developed to approximate the human head–neck system. This is due to the fact that the choice of model depends on the type of task under consideration; for example, slow voluntary movements will be modeled differently than movements resulting from an impact to the head. To develop a perspective on past work, we must first identify the *types of tasks* that have been subject to modeling attempts. Movement of the head–neck structure can be produced by two methods (Fig. 2.3A). The first type of movement comes from neuromuscular activity and results from forces produced by muscles. The second type results from loading on the head, neck, or torso by an external source (e.g., impact to the head). As can be seen in Fig. 2.3A, these two types of inputs to the head–neck system will have different mechanical consequences if muscle is assumed to have significant contractile dynamics and/or series element extension (Fig. 2.2), and this helps explain why a number of different models need to be explored.

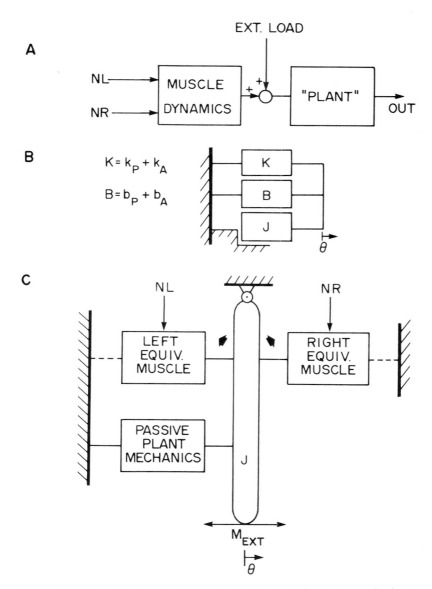

Figure 2.3. (A) Schematic showing the basic structural relation between the inputs and outputs for any muscle–joint system [notice that the external load (EXT. LOAD) occurs at a fundamentally different location than the neurocontroller inputs to left (NL) and right (NR) antagonistic muscles]. (B) Structure of the second-order model of the head–neck system, including lumped system inertia (J), viscosity [B, including both passive (constant b_P) and active (variable b_A) components], and elasticity [K, including both passive (constant k_P) and active (variable K_A) components]. (C) Structure of the antagonistic muscle–joint model of Stark's group. Each of the "equivalent" muscles has the basic structure shown in Figure 2.2. Notice that this model can be extended by allowing the "pendulum" to have additional degrees of freedom of motion and/or by coupling additional muscles to this structure.

There are essentially three different types of movement tasks that have been of interest in research on the head and neck. Not surprisingly, three general types of biomechanical models have been employed in direct correspondence to these types of tasks. These will be discussed below.

Whiplash-Impact Tasks: Detailed Passive Biomechanical Models

Human impact studies have already been reviewed briefly in the section on head–neck kinematics and dynamics. The head–neck models used for these studies (usually by mechanical engineers) are for tasks involving potentially injurious impact.

There are many passive analytical models of the head or the head and neck, and these are usually directed toward understanding the mechanical factors that may contribute to brain injury (see Ommaya and Gennarelli, 1976; Sances et al., 1981). For example, some analytical models have employed an elastic, isotropic beam to represent the neck and a fluid-filled rigid casing to represent the head (e.g., Landkof et al., 1976). Much less experimental information is available for the motion of the neck segments—this is where computer models become important. Simple mechanical "spring" necks had been developed by auto manufacturers for crash studies (Mertz, 1985). Dynamic and static data for more advanced multisegmental models of the neck have been obtained for artificial replica models (e.g., Winters and Goldsmith, 1983), lumped-parameter computer models (McKenzie and Williams, 1971; Orne and Liu, 1971; Reber and Goldsmith, 1979; Merrill et al., 1984), and finite element models (e.g., Khalil and Hubbard, 1977; Hosey and Liu, 1982). The head–neck system has also been modeled as part of complex full-body lumped-parameter systems (e.g., Huston and Passerello, 1978). Of most interest here are multielement models such as lumped-parameter models in which the head and the vertebral column are modeled as rigid bodies connected by viscous and elastic elements representing various soft tissues. These fairly complex models include many elements representing the mechanical properties of tissues such as the skull, vertebrae, disks, ligaments, or brain, and are used to determine the transient dynamics of the various tissues during external loadings that might be experienced by the head and neck during a crash. As mentioned previously, in general all such models do not include adequate active muscle contractile properties—a major limitation (Soechting and Paslay, 1973).

Low-Velocity Movement Tasks: Lower Order "Systems" Models

The second type of task involves slow-to-moderate voluntary movements (e.g., everyday eye–head movements) that are common for neurophysiological studies of the head–neck system and its coordination with eye movement (e.g., Gresty, 1974; Bizzi et al., 1976, 1978; Morasso et al., 1977; Zee, 1977; Lanman et al., 1978; Jones et al., 1982) and for studies of eye–head manual tracking tasks (e.g., Sugi and Wakakuwa, 1970; Chouet and Young, 1974; Shirachi et al., 1978). In such cases, the mechanical system simply follows neural signals with temporal dynamics that can be approximated by a pure time delay and a first- or second-order differential equation (Stark, 1968). For the majority of past neurophysiological studies in which head position is measured and then correlated to neural and/

or muscle electrical activity, a *first-order* biomechanical model was assumed, either implicitly or explicitly, of the form

$$T\dot{\theta}(t) + \theta(t) = GF(t) \tag{6}$$

where $\theta(t)$ is head position, $F(t)$ is some type of forcing function from the nervous system, T is the system time constant, and G is a "gain" factor that allows the units to match. For head rotations, T tends to be on the order of 0.1 to 1.0 sec, depending of course on the type of movement. If the movement time is large relative to T [i.e., the neural controller signal level $F(t)$ changes gradually and consequently $\theta(t)$ is small], then T might even be neglected and a static model results. Use of such an "intuitive" biomechanical model is often justified as long as only slow movements are involved or if only very crude head position information is required.

The next level of sophistication is the classic second-order lumped-parameter model, in angular units, with position as the output (Fig. 2.3B). A common form is

$$J\ddot{\theta}(t) + B\dot{\theta}(t) + K\theta(t) = \mathbf{M}(t) \tag{7}$$

or

$$\ddot{\theta}(t) + 2\xi\omega_n\dot{\theta}(t) + \omega_n^2\theta(t) = \mathbf{M}(t)/J \tag{8}$$

where J, B, K, ξ, ω_n, and $M(t)$ are the system inertia, viscosity, elasticity, damping ratio [$\xi = B/2(\sqrt{KJ})$], natural frequency ($\omega_n = \sqrt{K/J}$), and moment (torque) input, respectively. The behavior for this model can in general be overdamped ($\xi > 1$, nonoscillatory, smooth response), underdamped ($\xi < 1$, oscillatory response), or critically damped ($\xi = 1$). For the human head–neck system, the model tends to be slightly *overdamped*, with critically damped or underdamped input–output behavior possible with high levels of cocontraction or under unusual conditions such as forced external oscillation (Berthoz, 1973; Viviani and Berthoz, 1975). The primary advantage of this model is its simplicity and its intuitive feel. The disadvantage is that the model provides a structurally inadequate representation of muscle–joint systems. There are three basic reasons for this: (1) the model does not contain a series elastic element—any series element properties must somehow be lumped into a parallel element; (2) the model has only one input node, and thus cannot distinguish mathematically between an external load and a neural input, or between multiple neural inputs—all inputs simply sum at the same node and work through the same "plant"; and (3) fundamental phenomena such as cocontraction cannot be modeled without artificially manipulating the spring and dashpot parameter values. These problems can be seen explicitly in the work of Bizzi et al. (1976), in which the following equation was presented:

$$J\ddot{\theta} + (B_p + B_a)\dot{\theta} + (K_p + K_a)\theta = \mathbf{F}_e + \mathbf{N}_i \tag{9}$$

Notice that external loadings ($\mathbf{F}_e$) and neural inputs ($\mathbf{N}_i$) occur at the *same node* and that the spring and dashpot are artificially separated into two parameters—a "passive" and an "active" parameter. When these parameters are manipulated appropriately, this model can be made to fit experimental data. The same type of problem arises when trying to simulate frequency response data such as those of Viviani and Berthoz (1975). A mechanically sound model should not require such superficial parameter manipulation since, in the body, the same muscles are involved in all tasks, and these inherently nonlinear muscle properties never change. In summary, this type of model is not meant to simulate the head–neck biomechanical system, but rather to describe and catalog a group of input–output behaviors in a concise form (see Winters and Stark, 1987, for a complete treatment).

Fast Voluntary Movements: Antagonistic "Equivalent Muscle–Joint" Model

The third type of general task, which includes the second as a special case, is the modeling of stereotyped voluntary fast movements, such as those studied by Stark's group for horizontal (axial) head rotation under both unloaded (Zangemeister et al., 1981a,b) and loaded (Hannaford et al., 1983, 1984) conditions and for eye–head interaction (Zangemeister and Stark, 1982a; Winters et al., 1984). The previous arguments suggested that a second-order model was overly simplistic, and this has been shown to be true even for the interaction of fast and slow eye movements (Winters et al., 1984). However, a model using the Hill series structure for each of the involved muscles is too complex, especially given the limited data available on the properties of the tissues in the head–neck region and the complexity of the spinal column. Consequently, some type of compromise appears in order. Zangemeister et al. (1981b) proposed such a compromise by extending a sixth-order antagonistic muscle model structure used previously for eye movements (e.g., Cook and Stark, 1968) to horizontal (axial) head rotations. The same structural elements, including antagonistic muscles with contractile and series elements, were used; but the models differed in the parameter values that described the model elements. These values were estimated by fitting experimental data, primarily for fast head rotations, with the aid of sensitivity-analysis methods (Zangemeister et al., 1981c). Little effort is made to attribute the observed behavior to individual components. The initial model included the classic nonlinear "Hill equation" for CE torque velocity, a 50 msec time constant for the excitation–activation process, and linear series and parallel element elasticities. Although somewhat simplistic, this model has been used and extended by others (Hannaford et al., 1984; Winters and Stark, 1985; see also this volume, Chapter 19). Current versions include nonlinear parallel and series elasticities, both fit with exponential functions, with peak extensions being 20° for the series element and 80° for the parallel element (Winters and Stark, 1985). Because of the complexity of the head–neck system and the lack of good data for parameter estimation, the head–neck model is felt by this author to be inferior to similar models for eye and upper and lower limb muscle–joint systems also presented in Winters and Stark (1985). Nevertheless, this model appears to be the best currently available for studying voluntary head movements and appears to be the best place at which to start future work on head–neck movement biomechanics—particularly since there is a fairly good match between splenius EMG activity and the predicted controller signal for this model (Hannaford et al., 1984).

Probably the greatest advantage of this type of model is that it provides an "equivalent muscle," an "equivalent motoneuron," and an "equivalent joint." While admittedly a simplification, such an approach does have major advantages, particularly for nonbiomechanists such as neurophysiologists who are attempting to interpret neurological or behavioral phenomena by using physical data such as head orientation—the approximate contribution of biomechanical factors needs to be understood if correct interpretations are to be made. In addition, those studying peripheral sensory and motor systems need to have a solid understanding of the biomechanical system. A disadvantage of this model is that, unlike models for the upper and lower limbs (e.g., Winters and Stark, 1985; Hatze, 1978), the contributions made by the individual muscles have not yet been quantified, and probably cannot be quantified, until better information is obtained concerning the properties of the individual muscles and soft tissues surrounding the neck.

SUMMARY

One clear signal emerging from the above presentation is that there is in fact no unique and "better" way to model the head–neck system. The best model does indeed depend on the task(s) involved. Single-segment first- or second-order lag models are not as bad for the head–neck system as for some other systems because of the tendency for the head to be fairly smooth in its response. (For those primarily concerned with neural aspects of the head–neck system, such news comes as a mixed blessing.)

At the other extreme, a number of multisegment models using passive individual components were also reviewed. The lack of data on tissue properties and the complexity of the system unfortunately appear to limit the development of such models. For the present purposes, the more limiting factor of such models is the absence of attention to active muscle properties. However, an accurate lumped-parameter model that included, for example, 10 pairs of muscles which have both contractile and series elements would be over 40th-order and would include over 200 parameters for its development—a major undertaking that is possibly not worth the effort, particularly without a better knowledge of the mechanical properties of neck muscles.

For those interested in a reasonable, yet useful, general biomechanical model of the head–neck system for the study of the whole spectrum of normal head-movement tasks in all planes of motion and for a variety of speeds, an extension of the model of Stark's group, consisting of three types of elements, is suggested. The first element, which would represent the vertebral column down to the upper thoracic area including its soft connective tissues, would be a *flexible beam*. This beam should be modeled as a tilted (about 10°) and tapered (smaller cross-section near head) orthotropic viscoelastic beam, i.e., a beam that bends with both the applied force and the rate of change of force, with the ease of bending a function of the direction of bending. This beam would be attached to the second type of element—a large *rigid mass* representing the head. *"Equivalent" muscles* would be the third element, with each side of the head modeled by four muscles: (1) the "posterior" muscle, which would represent all of the posterior muscles (e.g., semispinalis capitis); (2) the "anterior-transverse" muscle, which would represent the sternocleidomastoideus complex; (3) the "posterior-transverse" muscle, which would include primarily the splenius muscle; and (4) a "lateral" muscle, representing primarily the longissimus capitis. Origins and insertions, axial rotations, and muscle pennations can be approximated easily so that the resulting peak static torques are compatible with the known torques generated by the human in various directions. The default values for peak CE velocity, CE shape parameter, peak series elastic extension, and series "shape" parameter (Winters and Stark, 1985) would be five muscle lengths per second, 0.30, 6%, and 3.0, respectively. Notice that all types of rotational movements could be performed with this model, and that the axis of rotation would change automatically with changing conditions. Translational (sliding) movements, which are typically of less importance and are fairly minor, would occur automatically. The result would be a model with eight neural controller locations and eight locations for sensory feedback that would have mechanical properties that were similar to those of the actual system while being fairly easy to understand conceptually. Furthermore, each of the eight controllers could be approximately measured by appropriate placement of surface EMG electrodes.

3

Cervical Motoneurons

P. K. ROSE and S. A. KEIRSTEAD

The study of the control of head movement has been dominated by two major lines of investigation. One approach has focused on the organization of neck muscles and their skeletal framework (see Chapters 1 and 2). These studies emphasize the important contribution of muscle biomechanics to the control of head movement. The other major type of investigation has focused on the nature of descending and segmental signals that impinge on neck motoneurons. This approach is perhaps best exemplified by the detailed studies of the many routes by which brainstem neurons project to the upper cervical spinal cord, and of the peripheral and central mechanisms that control the activity of brainstem neurons (see Chapters 12 and 13).

Neck motoneurons are strategically located between the peripheral motor apparatus and the central systems responsible for head movement, yet the contribution of neck motoneurons to the control of head movement has received relatively little attention. This is perhaps surprising because motoneurons must integrate the complex set of signals generated by segmental and descending systems. The action potentials generated by these cells will lead to muscle contraction. Although the final outcome of this muscle contraction is strongly affected by the biomechanics of the head-movement system, the control of motoneuron activity will also play an important role. The purpose of this chapter is to examine the morphological properties of neck motoneurons and their potential contribution to the control of head movement.

ORGANIZATION OF NECK MOTOR NUCLEI

Like motoneurons at other levels of the spinal cord, motoneurons in the upper cervical spinal cord are arranged in several nuclei. Each nucleus occupies a small subvolume of the ventral horn and contains motoneurons innervating a single neck muscle. The organization of neck motor nuclei has been studied in several species, but the most comprehensive descriptions of mammalian motoneurons come from experiments on the cat. The following review is based on the results of these experiments (for a description of neck motor nuclei in other species and possible species differences see Yeow and Peterson, 1986a, b).

The distribution of motoneurons innervating the dorsal neck muscles, splenius, biventer cervicis, complexus, and trapezius is summarized in Figure 3.1A. Most splenius motoneurons are found near the dorsal border of the ventromedial nucleus in a region corresponding to the ventral region of Lamina VIII and the dorsal region of Lamina IX (Richmond et al., 1978; Keirstead and Rose, 1983). Most motoneurons innervating biventer cervicis and complexus lie ventrally to those supplying splenius (Richmond et al., 1978; Rose, 1981). Trapezius motoneurons are confined to the spinal accessory nucleus (Holomanova et al., 1972; Rapoport, 1978; Keane and Richmond, 1981; Vanner and Rose, 1984). In spinal segments C2–C5, they form a continuous column in the lateral part of the ventral horn. In C1, the column shifts to the medial edge of the ventral horn (see, however, Rapoport, 1978); in the cervical enlargement, trapezius motoneurons occupy a central position within the ventral horn.

At present, little is known about the distribution of motoneurons innervating other neck muscles. However, there is one report describing the location of motoneurons innervating sternocleidomastoideus (Rapoport, 1978). These motoneurons are located in a small region of the medial part of Lamina VIII and may be intermingled with trapezius motoneurons. Bakker et al. (1984) have recently reported that most of the motoneurons innervating the suboccipital muscles, rectus capitis posterior major, medius, and minor and obliquus capitis caudalis, are found in the ventromedial nucleus of C1 and C2. Presumably, their motor nuclei overlap with motor nuclei of biventer cervicis and complexus, but the relative distribution of these motoneurons has not yet been explored using techniques such as double labeling.

Figure 3.1.   Organization of neck motor nuclei. (A) Transverse distribution of trapezius, splenius, biventer cervicis, and complexus motoneurons. All motoneurons were located in C3 and were antidromically identified and intracellularly stained with horseradish peroxidase. Each symbol represents a different group of motoneurons. Triangles, trapezius motoneurons; filled circles, splenius motoneurons; open circles, biventer cervicis and complexus motoneurons. SAN, Spinal accessory nucleus; VM, ventromedial nucleus; M, medial; L, lateral. (From Rose, 1981; Keirstead and Rose, 1983; Vanner and Rose, 1984). (B) Transverse distribution of biventer cervicis motoneurons retrogradely labeled with horseradish peroxidase. Cross-hatched zones indicate the location of labeled motoneurons. These were stained following exposure of the left biventer cervicis muscle to horseradish peroxidase. (Modified from Abrahams and Keane, 1984.) (C) Longitudinal distribution of clavotrapezius, spinotrapezius, and acromiotrapezius motoneurons. Horizontal view. Each symbol represents the location of an antidromically identified motoneuron intracellularly stained with horseradish peroxidase. Filled circles, clavotrapezius motoneurons; triangles, acromiotrapezius motoneurons; ×s, spinotrapezius motoneurons. (Based on data from Vanner and Rose, 1984.) (D) Longitudinal distribution of splenius motoneurons. Horizontal view. Each symbol represents the location of a splenius motoneuron antidromically identified and stained intracellularly with horseradish peroxidase. The different symbols represent motoneurons antidromically activated from different segmental nerves. Filled circles, C2; triangles, C3; ×s, C4. Electrophysiological experiments have shown that the caudal region of C3 contains splenius motoneurons whose axons travel in the C4 spinal nerve. (Based on data from Keirstead and Rose, 1983.)

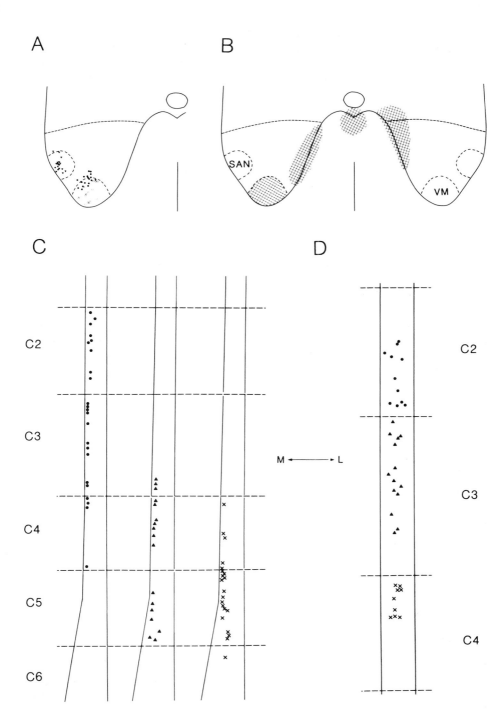

Motoneurons innervating biventer cervicis, complexus, and splenius have a further level of topographical organization within each of their nuclei. Indeed, a single motor nucleus is composed of several clearly delineated subnuclei (Fig. 3.1D). This feature was first recognized by Richmond et al. (1978) who reported that motoneurons innervating splenius and complexus are not confined to a single spinal segment as is common for motoneurons in the lumbosacral cord (for reviews of motor nuclei of hindlimb muscles see Burke and Rudomin, 1977; Burke 1981; Henneman and Mendell, 1981). Instead, dorsal neck motoneurons are distributed in several spinal segments. This arrangement is related to the multisegmental innervation of dorsal neck muscles. For example, splenius is innervated by four segmental nerves, C1 to C4 (Richmond and Abrahams, 1975a; Brink et al., 1981b; Richmond et al., 1985b). Using retrograde transport techniques, Richmond et al. (1978) found that motoneurons whose axons reached the splenius muscle via one of these segmental nerves are concentrated in the corresponding spinal segment. Motoneurons in adjacent spinal segments innervate splenius via adjacent segmental nerves. Thus, the motor nuclei of the dorsal neck muscles, splenius and complexus, are subdivided into several subnuclei, each subnucleus occupying a different segmental level and contributing axons to a different segmental nerve. This arrangement has been confirmed using electrophysiological techniques (Brink et al., 1981b) and intracellular staining techniques (Keirstead and Rose, 1983). Because each segmental nerve innervates a separate region of muscle and these regions are arranged in a serial fashion, the in-series organization of the motoneuron subnuclei corresponds to the peripheral organization of the muscle (Brink et al. 1981b; Richmond et al., 1985b).

Richmond et al. (1978) emphasized that the boundaries between adjacent subnuclei are poorly defined. They reported that some axons traveling in a single segmental nerve are supplied by a small number of motoneurons located rostrally or caudally to the corresponding spinal segment. In contrast, electrophysiological studies of splenius motoneurons suggest that there is a sharp boundary between adjacent subnuclei (Brink et al., 1981b; Keirstead and Rose, 1983). Abrahams and Keane (1984), using retrograde transport of horseradish peroxidase, have also reported that the rostral and caudal boundaries of motoneurons whose axons travel in the C3 segmental nerve and innervate biventer cervicis are sharply defined and correspond to the C2/C3 and C3/C4 segmental junctions. Thus, the overlap between adjacent subnuclei may be smaller than that originally described by Richmond et al. (1978). However, it should be noted that the degree of overlap has not been analyzed quantitatively and the electrophysiological studies were likely limited to a description of the distribution of α motoneurons, whereas the anatomical studies described the location of both α and γ motoneurons.

Recently, several studies of the organization of hindlimb motoneuron nuclei have demonstrated that the axons of motoneurons supplying a single muscle are arranged in several bundles that enter the muscle at different sites and innervate different compartments of the muscle (for example, see Weeks and English, 1985). Each bundle contains the axons of a population of motoneurons whose cell bodies occupy a fraction of the motor nucleus. This characteristic raises the possibility that the subnuclei of dorsal neck muscle motoneurons may be further divided according to the peripheral nerve branch by which the motoneuron axon reaches the muscle. As yet, this feature of neck motor nuclei has not been examined in detail. However, Richmond et al. (1978) have reported that biventer cervicis motoneurons whose axons travel in the caudal branch of the C3 segmental nerve occupy a small zone in the caudal half of C3. In contrast, motoneurons that innervate biventer cervicis via the rostral C3 branch are widely distributed throughout C3. It is also not known if motoneurons in a single subnucleus are evenly distributed along the entire rostrocaudal extent of the nucleus, as occurs in hindlimb motor nuclei, or if they are arranged in a series of clusters as in the phrenic motor nucleus (Berger et al., 1984).

The trapezius motor nucleus is also subdivided into several subnuclei (Keane and Richmond, 1981; Vanner and Rose, 1984). Each subnucleus contains motoneurons innervating one of the three heads of the trapezius muscle (Fig. 3.1C). The borders between adjacent subnuclei are not sharply defined, and motoneurons innervating acromiotrapezius are intermingled with clavotrapezius motoneurons in C3 and C4 and with spinotrapezius motoneurons in C4 and C5.

The arrangement of motoneurons innervating dorsal neck muscles is further complicated by the fact that motoneurons supplying a single muscle can be distributed widely in the ventral horn (Fig. 3.1B). Most motoneurons belonging to a single motor nucleus are concentrated in a circumscribed subvolume of the ventral horn, but some motoneurons lie well outside this subvolume. This feature was described originally by Richmond et al. (1978). More recently, Abrahams and Keane (1984) have reported that motoneurons traveling in the C3 segmental nerve of biventer cervicis appear to be arranged in four discrete regions of the C3 ventral horn. The ventromedial nucleus contains the largest number of motoneurons. These motoneurons range in diameter from 15 to 70 μm and presumably include both α and γ motoneurons. Motoneurons were also found along the medial wall of the ventral horn including the adjacent white matter, on the midline just ventral to the central canal, and in the contralateral ventral horn in the medial part of the Lamina VIII. Since these motoneurons rarely have a diameter of greater than 40 μm, Abrahams and Keane (1984) suggested that these subsets of biventer cervicis motoneurons may correspond to different types of γ motoneurons.

The motor nuclei of other dorsal neck muscles have not yet been described in similar detail. Bakker et al. (1984) have reported that motoneurons innervating suboccipital muscles are also found in different regions of the ventral horn in C2. The ventromedial nucleus contains the majority of motoneurons. However, small numbers of motoneurons are also found near the spinal accessory nucleus and adjacent white matter as well as in the medial part of Lamina VIII. The somata of motoneurons lying in the medial part of Lamina VIII are similar in size to those in the ventromedial nucleus, whereas the motoneurons in other regions have smaller somata.

Whether motoneurons lying outside the main nucleus have unique physiological features is not yet known. However, Rose and Richmond (1981) have described the dendritic morphology of a motoneuron with a small soma located in the medial part of Lamina VIII. This motoneuron, unlike other neck motoneurons, has a profuse collection of dendrites crossing the ventral commissure and terminating in the contralateral spinal cord. It is therefore possible that small motoneurons lying outside the main motor nuclei will receive different segmental and descending connections because of their different locations and dendritic distributions. The observation by Bakker et al. (1984) that large motoneurons innervating the suboccipital muscles are found in two separate areas, the ventromedial nucleus and a medial zone of Lamina VIII, may derive from the fact that the motor nuclei of four suboccipital muscles were labeled simultaneously. However, it is not possible to discount an alternative explanation—that motoneurons innervating extrafusal muscle fibers of a single suboccipital muscle are arranged in two separate zones of the ventral horn (cf. Yeow and Peterson, 1986b).

DISTRIBUTION OF DENDRITES FROM NECK MOTONEURONS

The description of neck motoneuron morphology has a curious history. The first study of neck motoneurons was published in 1909 by Ramón y Cajal, who used Golgi's silver staining technique to examine the structure of several motoneurons in the upper cervical spinal cord of fetal and newborn cats. Ramón y Cajal reported that dendritic trees of motoneurons in the spinal accessory nucleus are confined to a region along the lateral wall of the ventral horn. He also noted that many dendrites of these motoneurons project rostrally and caudally. Motoneurons lying more deeply in the ventral horn have dendrites that project dorsally, medially, and laterally. Most of the dendrites of these cells are confined to the gray matter in contrast to the rich projections of white-matter dendrites originating from motoneurons in the spinal accessory nucleus. It is remarkable that this description remained the sole study of neck motoneuron structure for over 70 years. Indeed, there has been only one further description of neck motoneuron morphology using the Golgi technique (Rose and Richmond, 1981). Our present understanding of neck motoneuron morphology is based largely on a series of studies by Rose and his colleagues (Rose, 1981, 1982; Rose and Richmond, 1981; Keirstead and Rose, 1983; Vanner and Rose, 1984; Rose et al., 1985) in which motoneurons in adult cats were identified electrophysiologically and stained with horseradish peroxidase. The dendritic tree was visualized by reconstructing all of the stained dendrites in serial histological sections. The following description of neck motoneuron morphology is based on these studies.

Motoneurons innervating the dorsal neck muscles, biventer cervicis, complexus, and splenius, have been examined. In addition, the morphology of motoneurons innervating the three heads of the trapezius muscle, clavotrapezius, acromiotrapezius, and spinotrapezius, have been described. All of these motoneurons share one outstanding feature—their dendritic trees are large and elaborate. Unlike the motoneurons described by Ramón y Cajal (1909), in which dendrites were confined to a relatively small fraction of the ventral horn, motoneurons stained intracellularly with horseradish peroxidase have dendrites that project throughout much of the ventral horn and the surrounding white matter. These differences may be a consequence of several factors, including the age of the animal, the use of single versus serial histological sections, and study of unidentified versus electrophysiologically identified motoneurons. Many dendrites of intracellullarly stained motoneurons are oriented longitudinally and span a distance of 1 to 2 mm in the longitudinal plane. Some dendritic trees, particularly those of trapezius motoneurons, have a length of 4 mm. The total combined length of all dendritic branches has been measured for 10 motoneurons and ranges from 66,660 to 95,390 µm. The total dendritic surface area (based on three trapezius motoneurons) is 415,000 to 488,000 µm². This area is 70 to 100 times larger than the surface area of the somatic region. Less than 20% of the dendritic surface area lies within 300 µm of the cell body and approximately 25% of the surface area is found more than 1000 µm from the cell body.

In spite of the complexity of the dendritic structure of neck motoneurons, dendrites are arranged in well-ordered patterns. Dendrites of motoneurons in a single motor nucleus have a stereotyped distribution (or distributions, see the description of trapezius motoneurons below). For example, many dendrites of biventer cervicis and complexus motoneurons project dorsolaterally and dorsomedially along the lateral and medial borders of the ventral horn (Fig. 3.2A). Thus, in the transverse plane, they appear to form a "V" with the apex at the base of the ventral horn. Other dendrites follow a rostral or caudal path and interdigitate to form a rich collection of dendrites in the motor nucleus. Splenius motoneurons are easily distinguished from biventer cervicis and complexus motoneurons on the basis of their dendritic structure (Fig. 3.2B). Splenius motoneurons have dorsolaterally and medially directed dendrites similar to biventer cervicis and complexus motoneurons, but dendrites of splenius motoneurons also project laterally and ventrally. Dendrites of splenius motoneurons also travel rostrally and caudally, but many of these dendrites are located dorsally to the ventromedial nucleus and are shorter than the rostrally and caudally directed dendrites of biventer cervicis and complexus motoneurons. Motoneurons innervating the trapezius muscle lie laterally and dorsally to splenius motoneurons. Dendritic trees of trapezius motoneurons throughout most of C2, C3, and C4 have a fusiform appearance

Figure 3.2.   Reconstructions of the dendritic trees of a complexus (A) and splenius (B) motoneuron. Both motoneurons were found in C3. (From Rose, 1981; Keirstead and Rose, 1983.)

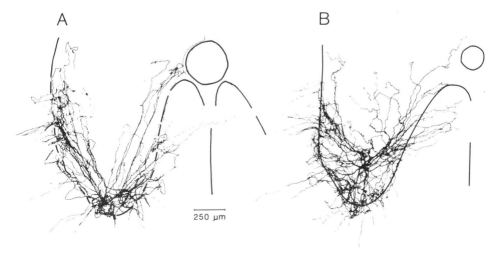

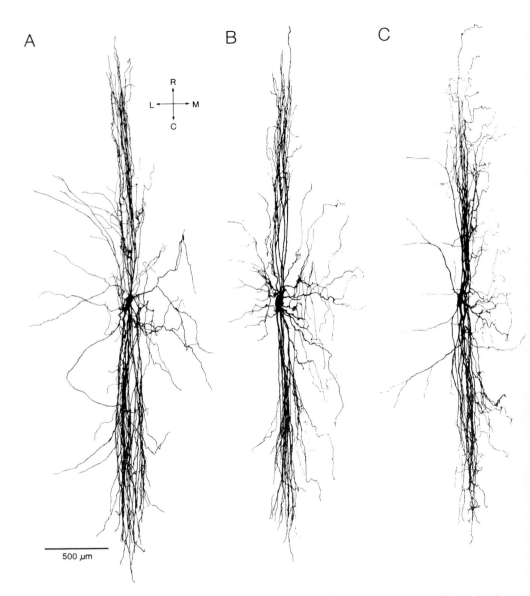

Figure 3.3.   Dendritic morphology of clavotrapezius (A), acromiotrapezius (B), and spinotrapezius (C) motoneurons located in C3 and C4. Horizontal view. R, Rostral; C, caudal; M, medial; L, lateral. (From Vanner and Rose, 1984.)

(Figs. 3.3 and 3.4B). The majority of dendrites are oriented in a rostrocaudal direction and form a compact bundle that is largely confined to the spinal accessory nucleus. Dendrites also project dorsally along the gray–white border and terminate in the lateral parts of Lamina VI and VII. Others dendrites are directed ventromedially and medially from the cell body where they spread throughout much of the ventral horn.

Three features of the dendritic distribution of neck motoneurons deserve special comment. First, the methods used to classify dendritic trees are qualitative. Although all motoneurons assigned to a single class of dendritic structure have many common characteristics, the dendritic distributions of all motoneurons in a single class are not identical. This problem is best illustrated by motoneurons whose somata lie near the borders of adjacent motor nuclei. For example, a splen-

Figure 3.4. Dendritic morphology of clavotrapezius motoneurons located in caudal C1 (A) and C3 (B). Upper figures, horizontal view. R, Rostral; C, caudal; M, medial; L, lateral. Lower figures, stick-figure representations of the above dendritic trees rotated into the transverse plane. The filled circles represent the location of the cell bodies. (From Vanner and Rose, 1984.)

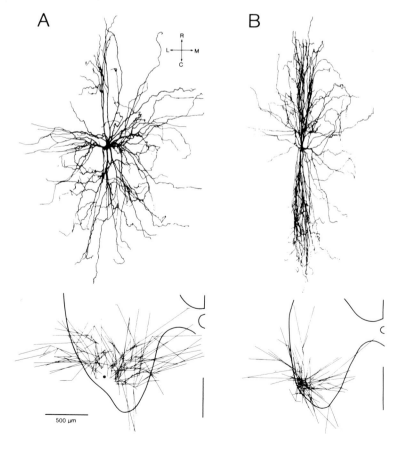

ius motoneuron, lying on the lateral edge of the splenius motor nucleus just adjacent to the spinal accessory nucleus, has been described, and this motoneuron shares some of the features characteristic of trapezius motoneurons. This splenius motoneuron, unlike its more medial counterparts, has an unusually rich collection of rostrally and caudally directed dendrites (a prominent feature of trapezius motoneurons). Dendritic distribution may therefore depend not only on the motor nucleus in which the motoneuron is located, but also, to some degree, on the location of its cell body within the motor nucleus and the characteristics of the dendritic trees of motoneurons in adjacent motor nuclei. The second feature of dendritic distribution that merits special attention is the similarity of the dendritic structure of motoneurons innervating different muscles. For example, biventer cervicis and complexus motoneurons have the same dendritic structure. Motoneurons in C3, C4, and C5 that innervate clavotrapezius, acromiotrapezius, or spinotrapezius have the identical dendritic morphology (Fig. 3.3). Thus, neck motoneuron dendritic structure may not be associated closely with the mechanical action of the muscles that they innervate. Finally, some neck muscles, such as clavotrapezius and spinotrapezius, are innervated by two types of motoneurons and each has a different dendritic structure. These differences in dendritic structure are related to the segmental position of the motoneuron. For example, clavotrapezius motoneurons located in the rostral part of the trapezius motor nucleus, near the junction of C1 and C2, have a stellate dendritic tree with most dendrites projecting dorsally to the cell body (Fig. 3.4). In contrast, the dendritic trees of clavotrapezius motoneurons located in C2, C3, and C4 extend primarily in a rostrocaudal direction.

The dendritic tree of each neck motoneuron is composed of several components. Each component consists of the branches originating from a primary dendrite of the motoneuron. An analysis of the distribution of the branches emerging from primary dendrites of biventer cervicis and complexus motoneurons further illustrates the highly organized structure of the dendritic trees of neck motoneurons. Branches from a single primary dendrite are arranged in several different patterns (Fig. 3.5). In some instances, they project to a small fraction of the territory occupied by the complete dendritic tree. In others, branches of a single primary dendrite can spread throughout the region occupied by the complete dendritic tree. Thus, the total dendritic tree can be subdivided into several classes of primary dendrites, each class defined by the distribution of its branches. The frequency and characteristics of these dendrites show little variation from motoneuron to motoneuron.

The subdivision of the neck motoneuron dendritic tree into a collection of smaller trees, each with its own unique distribution, may also be related to quantitative characteristics of the dendritic trees. Only a weak relationship exists between the diameter of the primary dendrite and either the total dendritic length or total surface area of all of its branches (unlike the close relationships seen in hindlimb motoneurons, see, for example, Ulfhake and Kellerth, 1983). However, if the relationship between dendrite diameter and the total dendritic length or total surface area is examined for second order dendrites that contribute branches to the same region of the dendritic tree, then the relationship is much stronger. Moreover, the nature of the relationship depends on the direction in which the dendrites

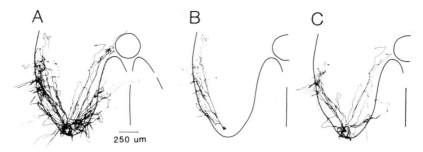

Figure 3.5. Distribution of dendritic branches originating from single primary dendrites of a complexus motoneuron. (A) Complete reconstruction of the dendritic tree. (B) An example of a primary dendrite whose branches projected dorsolaterally to the cell body. (C) An example of a primary dendrite whose branches projected dorsolaterally, caudally, and dorsomedially from the cell body. The caudally projecting dendrites were largely confined to the ventromedial nucleus. (From Rose, 1982.)

project. Thus, although the rules governing the geometry of neck motoneuron dendritic trees appear to be complex, the quantitative geometry of the dendritic tree, like its distribution, is not randomly organized.

FUNCTIONAL CONSIDERATIONS

In comparison to other motor systems, the study of the control of head movement is still in its infancy. Nevertheless, it is possible to identify several features of neck motor nuclei and motoneuron morphology that may have important implications for the control of head movement.

Neck motor nuclei are divided into several subnuclei. Each subnucleus contains motoneurons that innervate a different compartment of the muscle, and these compartments are organized in a serial fashion (Brink et al., 1981b; Armstrong et al., 1982; Richmond et al., 1985b). Contraction of a single compartment is unlikely to generate significant force at the origin or insertion due to the large series elastic component of the neighboring inactive regions. Thus, activity of motoneurons in each subnucleus must be closely co-ordinated. Indeed, there is evidence that compartments of dorsal neck muscles are cocontracted when they are recruited during normal head movements (Wilson et al., 1983; Loeb and Richmond, 1986). However, the mechanism underlying this coordination is unknown. It cannot be attributed to segmental monosynaptic connections from muscle spindle primary afferents because these are not distributed uniformly in the motor nucleus (Brink et al., 1981b; Rose and Keirstead, 1986). The distribution of descending systems to different subnuclei has not been examined systematically. Recent experiments have demonstrated that the problem of coordination of motoneurons in different subnuclei may be more acute than originally realized. Loeb et al. (1987) have found a very close coupling between the activity of motor units in different compartments of dorsal neck muscles. Thus, it appears that the activity of individual motoneurons lying in different subnuclei is coordinated in a very precise fashion.

Although it is clear that there is order in the apparent chaos of neck motoneuron dendritic trees, the significance of this order is not immediately obvious. Earlier attempts to understand the functional significance of dendritic trees in hindlimb motoneurons led to the proposal that each dendritic projection is positioned to receive contacts from afferents of different origins (Ramón y Cajal, 1909). It is unlikely that such a simple scheme can explain the complex structure of neck motoneuron dendrites. At least for biventer cervicis and complexus motoneurons, afferents of different origin may terminate on similar regions of the dendritic tree. For example, the lateral vestibular spinal tract and the medullary reticular spinal tract both terminate in the ventromedial nucleus and could contact the rostrally and caudally directed dendrites (Holstege and Kuypers, 1982). Nevertheless, this proposal emphasizes the potential contribution of dendritic structure to the regional organization of terminals on the dendritic surface. The functional consequences, for example, the degree of nonlinear summation of postsynaptic potentials, will depend on the specific pattern of terminal distribution.

SUMMARY

Motoneurons innervating neck muscles are arranged in several nuclei in the upper cervical spinal cord. Each nucleus forms a column that occupies a small subvolume of the ventral horn. Most large motoneurons supplying a single muscle are restricted to one nucleus. These nuclei are subdivided into several subnuclei which contain motoneurons whose axons supply different segmental nerves and innervate different regions of the muscle. Since these regions are arranged in a serial fashion, the series-elastic component of inactive compartments will dissipate the force developed in active compartments. Consequently, the activity of motoneurons in each subnucleus must be closely coupled. The central mechanisms responsible for this coordination are, as yet, unknown.

Most of the surface area available for synaptic contacts is located on the dendritic tree of neck motoneurons. Dendrites of each motoneuron extend throughout much of the ventral horn, including the surrounding white matter. While the dendritic trees are complex, they are organized in several orderly patterns. The particular pattern of dendritic distribution appears to depend primarily on the column in which the motoneuron's cell body is located. Since motoneurons in a single column may innervate a single neck muscle, there is a close relationship between the distribution of neck motoneuron dendrites and the muscle innervated by the motoneuron. The highly organized distribution of neck motoneuron dendrites may play an important role in the integration of segmental and descending signals reaching neck motoneurons.

4

The Sensorium: Receptors of Neck Muscles and Joints

F. J. R. RICHMOND, D. A. BAKKER, and M. J. STACEY

In most considerations of head movement, attention is usually focused on the *motor* behavior of the muscles and joints, which together develop and transmit the forces that alter head position. However, neck muscles and joints can also be regarded in a second way, as the repositories for dense arrays of receptors that provide information about head position and movement. This chapter reviews the growing body of information now available on the organization of proprioceptors in the neck. It suggests that the proprioceptive apparatus of the neck has specializations not commonly seen in other motor systems, and that these features may have important implications for the way in which nuchal sensory input is used by the nervous system.

HISTORICAL BACKGROUND

For more than 100 years, we have known that sensory receptors in the neck play a special role in the control of posture and movement. As early as 1845, Longet reported that surgical damage of neck muscles in a wide range of species led to generalized but transient motor disturbances characterized by an ataxia similar to that which followed cerebellectomy. A similar deficit in motor function was observed by Magendie (as reported by Bernard, 1865) during experiments in which neck muscles were incised to permit the aspiration of cerebrospinal fluid at the base of the occiput. The apparent disequilibrium caused by this surgical intervention was initially thought to be caused by the removal of cerebrospinal fluid, but was later found to occur in animals that underwent the surgical procedures alone. Since that time, many experimental studies on animals have extended the observations of Longet and Magendie by describing in detail the broad-based stance and staggering, crab-like gait that follow nuchal deafferentation produced by a range of procedures (Biemond, 1939, 1940; Cohen, 1961; Abrahams and Falchetto, 1969; Biemond and De Jong, 1969; Igarashi et al., 1969; Hinoki et al., 1975; Richmond et al., 1976; De Jong et al., 1977; Manzoni et al., 1979). In general, the degree of motor impairment was found to depend on the extent of sensory damage. It was most severe following section of several cervical dorsal roots.

Motor disturbances can also be observed in human patients who have suffered damage to the neck. Case studies in the clinical literature describe the syndrome, "cervical vertigo" (Weeks and Travell, 1955; Cope and Ryan, 1959) or "cervical nystagmus" (Biemond and De Jong, 1969), that is characterized by symptoms of gait disturbance, dizziness, and nystagmus. In these patients, symptoms often followed an episode of neck muscle strain, and could be relieved by injecting local anesthetic into neck muscles or by applying a cervical collar. Symptoms of disequilibrium can also be produced experimentally in humans by injecting neck muscles with local anesthetic (De Jong et al., 1977) or by vibrating neck musculature (Lund, 1980). One subject described the sensations as "a strong sense of falling or tilting like the pull of a magnet" (De Jong et al., 1977).

Nuchal sensory input also contributes to the development of postural reflexes. In the early 1900s, Magnus and de Kleijn reported that rotation of the head of a decerebrate animal led to asymmetric alterations in body posture and extensor tone (Magnus, 1926). These "tonic neck reflexes" were not dependent on vestibular input, but could be abolished by cutting nerves that traveled in the upper cervical roots. Tonic neck reflexes acting in concert with tonic labyrinthine reflexes are thought to have an important role in postural stabilization (Lindsay et al., 1976). This system of reflexes is explored more thoroughly in Chapters 8 and 9 of this volume.

What are the receptors that play such a significant role in postural processes? Until recently, it has been generally assumed that the receptors were located in the cervical joints. This view largely stemmed from observations by McCouch et al. (1951) who showed that tonic neck reflexes were not abolished following denervation or section of neck muscles but were lost when dorsal root ganglia were excised. McCouch and his colleagues (1951) were careful to point out that the sensory contributions could not be unequivocally assigned to joint receptors because "dissection of the ligaments discloses the presence of an appreciable number of muscle fibers so intimately applied to them as to escape separation." Nevertheless, the overgenerous interpretation of these experiments led to the common textbook view that joint receptors played the preeminent role in reflexes initiated from the neck (Mountcastle, 1980; Kelly, 1985) and relatively little attention was paid to the potential participation of other receptor forms.

It has only been in the last 15 years that proprioceptors in the neck have been subjected to systematic examination. In part, these analyses were spurred by the rediscovery that postural disturbances could be observed even when damage was confined to neck muscles or neck muscle nerves (Cohen, 1961; Abrahams and Falchetto, 1969; Biemond and de Jong, 1969). In addition, it was stimulated by histological studies that described large receptor populations in both neck muscles (Cooper and Daniel, 1963; Richmond and Abrahams, 1975b; Richmond and Abrahams, 1979b) and neck joints (Wyke, 1967). Given the wealth and variety of proprioceptors that have been reported in different tissues of the neck, it would seem oversimplistic to expect that only one receptor type should have the key role. Instead, it is likely that receptors in a variety of tissues will contribute to reflexes and other types of motor behavior. Understanding the uses of sensory information first depends upon understanding the distribution and behavior of receptors throughout both the muscles and the joints of the neck.

MUSCLE RECEPTORS

Most muscles contain at least four types of receptors: muscle spindles, Golgi tendon organs, Paciniform corpuscles, and free nerve endings. Of these, muscle spindles and Golgi tendon organs have long been thought to signal changes in muscle length or force development. However, free nerve endings and Paciniform corpuscles may also play a role in proprioception.

The Muscle Spindle

Overview

The *muscle spindle* is a sensory receptor that provides the nervous system with information about muscle length and length change (cf. Matthews, 1972; Hulliger, 1984). It consists of a bundle of small (intrafusal) fibers that lie in parallel with the ordinary (extrafusal) fibers of the muscle. The middle third of the intrafusal bundle is enclosed in a capsule that is swollen in its central (equatorial) region to form a fluid-filled space. In the equatorial region, the intrafusal muscle fibers are always innervated by a primary sensory ending and usually by at least one secondary ending. These endings have different response properties which result from different terminal arrangements on the intrafusal fibers.

The intrafusal fiber bundle is an essential part of the transductive apparatus, with at least three features that are important in shaping the specialized responses of primary and secondary endings.

1. Intrafusal fibers vary in their morphology, enzyme profiles, and physiological properties. Most cat and primate spindles contain at least three types of intrafusal fibers, identified by functional and anatomical criteria, and called dynamic bag$_1$, static bag$_2$, and chain fibers (chain fibers may be further subclassified according to their lengths and more subtle differences in enzyme profiles) (cf. Boyd and Gladden, 1985) (Fig. 4.1). Primary axons branch to terminate on every intrafusal fiber in the spindle (Banks et al., 1982). Thus, impulses in the primary axon result from a complex addition of signals generated in several different terminals, whose individual properties depend on the intrafusal fiber with which it is associated. A large part of the terminal contact area from the primary ending is distributed to the dynamic bag$_1$ fiber (Banks et al., 1982). This fiber appears to be responsible for the marked velocity-sensitive response of the primary ending (Boyd, 1976; Boyd and Smith, 1985). In contrast, the secondary axon distributes most of its terminals onto chain fibers (Banks et al., 1982). Impulse rates in secondary endings quite accurately reflect muscle length alone, with a much smaller dynamic component (cf. Matthews, 1972).

2. Intrafusal fibers change structurally at different points along their length. Primary endings are located on the central, or equatorial portion of the intrafusal fiber bundle, where muscle fibers contain many centrally situated nuclei. Sec-

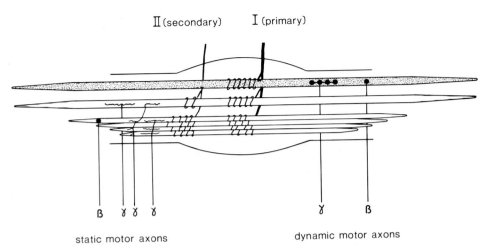

Figure 4.1.   Schematic drawing of a muscle spindle showing its typical sensory and motor innervation. A typical spindle is usually supplied by two types of afferent fibers, a thicker primary axon that has terminals in the equator, and a variable number of secondary axons terminating in juxtaequatorial regions. Motor innervation is supplied both by static fusimotor axons (β and γ) that typically end on bag$_2$ and chain fibers and by dynamic fusimotor axons (β and γ) on bag$_1$ fibers. Different types of motor endings are normally intermixed in a single polar region, in contrast to the pattern shown for illustrative purposes in this line drawing. The bag$_1$ fiber is on top and is coarsely stippled; the bag$_2$ fiber is lightly stippled; chain fibers are unstippled.

ondary endings are found in the more musclelike juxtaequatorial regions. The viscoelastic properties of the various fiber regions differ when observed directly (Poppele and Quick, 1985), and this may be a significant factor affecting the way in which stretch is transmitted to the sensory endings.

3.   Motor axons innervate the polar ends of intrafusal muscle fibers. By causing these regions to become stiff or to contract, activity in motor axons can change the sensitivity of sensory endings that are located in the equatorial zone of the intrafusal fiber. This "fusimotor" control is complex. In the cat, up to six different populations of motor axons supply a typical spindle. Two varieties of axons are supplied by motoneurons that also innervate extrafusal fibers (skeletofusimotor or β axons) and these innervate the bag$_1$ and long chain fibers, respectively (Fig. 4.1). A population of dynamic fusimotor (γ) axons supply only the bag$_1$ fiber, and up to three different populations of static fusimotor (γ) axons may supply the bag$_2$ and chain fibers (Boyd and Gladden, 1985). Because most axons innervate only one or two types of intrafusal fiber, they will alter the sensitivity of terminal ramifications on one type of intrafusal fiber but will not change the output from terminals on the other intrafusal fibers. The fusimotor system therefore has an enormous potential to modify selectively the several different aspects of sensory transduction in the spindle.

To date, most studies of spindle morphology and distribution have been conducted in the large hindlimb muscles of cats or rats. Most of these muscles contain low densities of morphologically similar spindles. In the cat, a typical hindlimb spindle exists as a single isolated capsule containing a single nuclear bag$_1$ fiber, a single nuclear bag$_2$ fiber, and a collection of four to six nuclear chain fibers (Fig. 4.1). However, spindles can exhibit a range of structural variations both within a single muscle and, more strikingly, across groups of different muscles. Intrafusal fiber content can range from 1 to more than 20 fibers (Eldred et al., 1974; Richmond and Abrahams, 1975b). In addition, muscle spindles do not always exist singly, but can be associated with one another in a number of different ways. These include (1) *paired associations* in which two or more spindles lie side-by-side, (2) *parallel associations* in which two or more intrafusal fiber bundles are contained within a common capsule for some part of their length, and (3) *tandem associations* in which two or more spindle units are linked in series by a common intrafusal fiber that runs through each spindle unit in succession (cf. Richmond and Abrahams, 1975b). Some muscle spindles are found in close association with other types of receptors including Paciniform corpuscles (Richmond and Bakker, 1982) or Golgi tendon organs (Marchand et al., 1971). These complex forms are relatively uncommon in most large limb muscles and have not attracted much attention in considerations of spindle function. However, complexes of receptors are much more common in neck muscles and their presence poses important questions about their functional significance.

Distribution of Spindles in Neck Muscles

Frequency of occurrence. Neck muscles are exceptionally rich in muscle spindles. In studies on the human fetus, Voss (1937, 1958) noted the remarkable variation in muscle–spindle density from one muscle to another, and showed that muscles of the digits and the neck contained the highest densities of spindles. These observations were later extended by Cooper and Daniel (1956, 1963). Cooper (1966) remarked on the "bewildering number of spindles" in suboccipital muscles of the human neck. It is not only in humans that neck muscles are rich in spindles. Neck muscles in the cat and rat also contain a wealth of spindles (rat, Thompson, 1970; cat, Richmond and Abrahams, 1975b; Richmond and Bakker, 1982; Bakker and Richmond, 1982). In the cat, the highest spindle densities were found in the intervertebral musculature, but large numbers of spindles were also present in most of the long dorsal neck muscles that attach to the skull (Table 4.1).

Morphology and distribution. In neck muscles, complexity of spindle form is the rule. The majority of spindles in cat dorsal neck muscles, suboccipital muscles, and intervertebral muscles are found as part of receptor complexes. In the long dorsal muscles, spindle complexes commonly consist of two to five spindle units linked to one another in paired and tandem configurations (Richmond and Abrahams, 1975b) (Figs. 4.2 and 4.3). In intervertebral muscles, complexes may contain as many as 12 units, linked in chainlike arrays, that often span the entire length of the muscle (Bakker and Richmond, 1982). Many spindle complexes in neck muscles attach at one or both ends to a tendon or tendinous inscription, where they are often associated with a Golgi tendon organ. Single spindles ac-

Table 4.1. Numbers and Densities of Muscle Spindles in Some Cat and Human Muscles

Muscle	Weight (g)	Mean spindle Content	Density	Source
Cat				
Medial gastrocnemius	7.3	62	9	Chin et al. (1962)
Soleus	2.5	56	23	Chin et al. (1962)
Fifth interosseus (hindlimb)	0.3	29	88	Ip (1961)
Clavotrapezius	8.0	254	32	Keane (1981)
Splenius	2.9	170	59	Richmond and Abrahams (1975b)
Biventer cervicis	1.7	140	82	Richmond and Abrahams (1975b)
Intertransverse (C3–C4)	0.6	176	293	Bakker and Richmond (1982)
Human				
Triceps brachii	364	520	1.4	Körner (1960)
Opponens pollicis	2.5	44	17.3	Schulze (1955)
First lumbrical (foot)	1.7	36	21.0	Voss (1937)
Trapezius	201.2	437	2.2	Voss (1956)
Rectus capitis posterior major	4.0	122	30.5	Voss (1958)
Obliquus capitis superior	3.3	141	42.7	Voss (1958)

count for only 30–50% of receptors in most neck muscles. The exceptions are muscles that link the skull to the shoulder girdle (e.g., occipitoscapularis, trapezius) in which more than 65% of spindles exist as single receptors (Richmond and Abrahams, 1975b; Keane, 1981). Spindle complexes with similar features have also been described in neck muscles of humans (Cooper and Daniel, 1963; Bakker and Richmond, 1981).

The functional significance of spindle complexes is far from clear. However, some insight into the potential behavior of one type of spindle complex has come from anatomical and histochemical studies of a specialized spindle form called the tandem spindle. Tandem spindles in human neck muscles were described as early as 1956 by Cooper and Daniel (1956, 1963), who noted that encapsulations varied in their size and that "the spindle farthest from the belly of the muscle is often very small" (Cooper and Daniel, 1963). Since that time, studies in cat neck and limb muscles have shown that most tandem spindles contain two morphologically different types of encapsulation that are linked in series by a long, continuous bag_2 fiber (Banks et al., 1982; Richmond et al., 1986). One type of encapsulation resembles the conventional single spindle in its size and intrafusal fiber content. The other type is smaller and contains only a few intrafusal fibers, including the bag_2 fiber that it shares with the other member(s) of the tandem array and its own small complement of nuclear chain fibers (Fig. 4.3). Notably absent from the smaller encapsulation is the bag_1 fiber. The two basic types of encapsulation have been called b_1b_2c and b_2c spindle units, respectively (Banks et al., 1982).

The b_1b_2c and b_2c units in neck and other muscles have significant differences

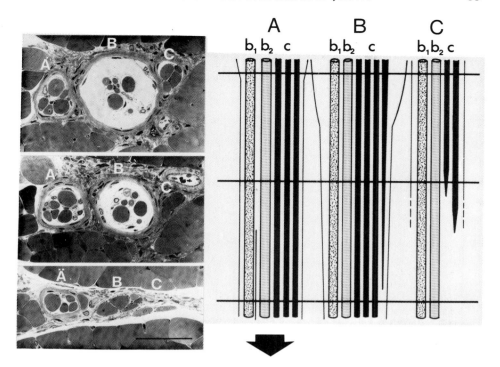

Figure 4.2. A reconstructed segment of a spindle complex in cat neck muscle. The photomicrographs (left) show the structural features of three paired muscle spindles (A, B, C) at different cross-sectional levels. Spindle (A) is a tandem spindle, sectioned at its site of transition from a b_1b_2c unit to a b_2c unit (at the end marked by an arrow). Each spindle contains a bag$_1$ (b_1) and bag$_2$ (b_2) fiber, and a collection of chain (c) fibers. Bar = 50 μm.

in their innervation (Banks et al., 1982; Richmond et al., 1986) (Fig. 4.3). The b_1b_2c unit has a rich supply of afferent and efferent fibers. Within the capsule there is a single primary ending, one to five secondary endings, and a collection of motor endings similar to that found in single spindles of cat hindlimb muscles. The b_2c unit has a sparse nerve supply that usually consists of a single primary ending and one to four motor axons ending in trail ramifications. The b_2c unit not only has no bag$_1$ fiber, it has none of the motor endings normally supplied to the bag$_1$ fiber by fusimotor and skeletofusimotor axons. In the conventional spindle, the bag$_1$ fiber is known to play a major role in the production of the velocity-sensitive response in the primary ending (Boyd, 1981). Without a bag$_1$ fiber, the b_2c afferent axon would be expected to have a reduced dynamic response. Furthermore, the differences between the signals of the b_2c afferent axon and the b_1b_2c primary axon will be exaggerated during stimulation of dynamic fusimotor systems, because the firing of the former should not be influenced by this stimulation, whereas that of the latter should be markedly enhanced during muscle stretch.

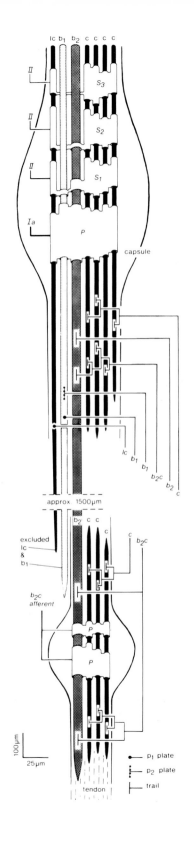

Physiology. Neck muscle spindles have been studied in much less detail than hindlimb spindles in the cat. In a study by Richmond and Abrahams (1979a), single fiber recording was used to analyze the discharge of neck muscle spindles in response to controlled muscle stretch in the anesthetized, paralyzed cat. These experiments showed that many spindle afferents had response patterns similar to those of primary and secondary axons elsewhere. However, there were a number of significant differences between the properties of neck and hindlimb spindles. First, spindle afferent fibers from neck muscles could not be classified as primary or secondary axons by their conduction velocities as is customary in studies of cat hindlimb spindles. Primary and secondary endings from neck muscles both had relatively low conduction velocities in the wide range of 20–90 m/sec. Primary axons usually had faster conduction velocities than secondary axons but there was a significant overlap in their ranges. Second, not all afferent fibers from neck spindles had the properties of typical primary or secondary axons. Instead, several axons had "intermediate" response patterns that did not fit the usual classification, which is based on a combination of physiological criteria including dynamic index, firing patterns during ramp stretch, and firing-rate variability (Richmond and Abrahams, 1979a). These properties would be consistent with anatomical evidence suggesting that some spindle units in neck muscles have a transductive apparatus that is different from that of the typical primary or secondary ending. Unfortunately, the physiological studies were carried out at a time when b_2c units in tandem spindles had not yet been recognized as morphologically distinct entities. Thus, the opportunity was not taken to develop specific tests that might identify and uniquely characterize a third receptor type.

The Golgi Tendon Organ

Overview
The Golgi tendon organ (GTO) is an encapsulated receptor that lies in-series with extrafusal fibers at the musculotendinous junction (cf. Proske, 1981). The capsule of the GTO encases bundles of collagen strands that serve as attachments for a collection of 5–20 neighboring muscle fibers. The GTO is generally supplied by a single sensory nerve fiber (the Ib fiber) that divides into several branches (Fig.

Figure 4.3.   Innervation of a tandem spindle from cat neck muscle. Two types of encapsulations are linked by a long bag_2 fiber running through each capsule in succession. The b_1b_2c encapsulation is larger and is supplied by many more afferent and efferent axons. In this specimen, sensory innervation is provided by a single primary ending (P) and three secondary (S_1, S_2, S_3) endings. Motor innervation to the proximal pole of the encapsulation is provided by six motor axons; additional axons supplied the distal pole (not illustrated). The smaller b_2c unit is supplied by only one afferent axon and two motor axons. The b_2c unit excludes the bag_1 and long chain fiber of the adjacent encapsulation. Note that the b_2c unit is supplied only by trail endings, whereas motor axons supplying the b_1b_2c unit end either in plates or trails as they do in single spindles. b_1, bag_1 fiber; b_2, bag_2 fiber; c, chain fiber; lc, long chain fiber.

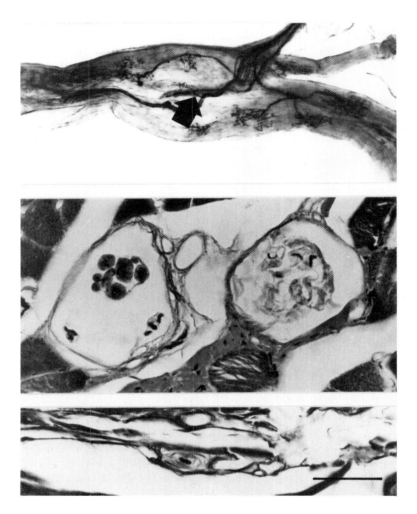

Figure 4.4.   Photomicrographs of muscle receptors. Top: Longitudinal view of a gold-toned GTO. The Ib fiber serving the GTO divides into several smaller branches as it enters the capsule from the top (right) of the photomicrograph. The Ib fiber is accompanied by an axon of smaller caliber that supplies a Paciniform corpuscle within the capsule of the GTO (marked by an arrow). Middle: Cross-section through a dyad between a muscle spindle and a GTO stained by the Holmes' method. The muscle spindle (left) contains several intrafusal fibers whereas the GTO is filled with collagen fibrils. Bottom: Paciniform corpuscle in the outer layers of a cervical joint capsule. Holmes' method for axons. Bar = 50 μm.

4.4). Each branch supplies a series of fine unmyelinated endings that are interwoven between collagen bundles inside the receptor (Bridgman, 1968; Zelena and Soukup, 1983). GTOs are usually silent in the passive, nonstretched muscle. When the muscle contracts, its GTOs fire at frequencies that increase in proportion to increasing muscle tension. A single GTO can be exquisitely sensitive to the contraction of even a single motor unit provided that one of the fibers from the motor unit inserts into the GTO (Houk and Henneman, 1967; Stuart et al., 1972; Binder, 1981). The GTO is typically much less sensitive to passive muscle stretch, although most GTOs will discharge if the muscle is stretched substantially (cf. Proske, 1981).

GTOs in Neck Muscles

Neck muscles appear to be a rich source of GTOs, but descriptions of their distribution in most neck muscles are quite incomplete. In dorsal neck muscles, GTOs are found at the ends of the muscle and along the tendinous inscriptions that serve as intramuscular sites of fiber attachment. The most systematic studies of GTO distribution have been conducted recently in biventer cervicis (BC) (F. J. R. Richmond, unpublished observations), which contains more than 120 GTOs. The majority of these receptors are located in the rostral half of BC where they are quite evenly distributed on the aponeurosis of insertion and on both sides of the tendinous inscriptions. Large numbers of GTOs are also distributed in a nonuniform pattern throughout intervertebral and suboccipital muscles of the neck. They are common along internal aponeuroses and are also found at some sites at which muscles attach onto vertebral processes (Richmond and Bakker, 1982).

A striking observation in both dorsal and deep neck muscles is the consistent association between GTOs and muscle spindles. Most GTOs in neck muscles are located in spindle-rich muscle regions and 25–50% of GTOs lie alongside one or more spindles (in a "dyad" configuration, Marchand et al., 1971) (Fig. 4.4). In the past, there has been a tendency to view GTOs and muscle spindles as independent, unrelated receptors. However, in neck muscles, spindles and GTOs are often clustered together in complicated receptor arrays. In intervertebral muscles, receptor arrays can contain up to a dozen spindles as well as one or more GTOs. These receptor groupings must be supplied by more than a dozen sensory fibers and thus have the potential to provide considerable information about length and tension in a restricted region of muscle. It remains to be explored whether the peripheral association between receptors is matched by a central association or convergence between the various afferent inputs supplying the same receptor complex.

The GTOs in neck muscles are morphologically similar to GTOs elsewhere, and it is logical to expect that their physiological properties will also be similar. This supposition is supported by physiological observations that neck muscle GTOs discharge on the rising slope of a twitch contraction and can be made to fire tonically by stretching the muscle to its longest lengths (Richmond and Abrahams, 1979a). However, the functional properties of GTOs in the neck have not yet been studied systematically. In particular, it is not clear how GTOs in different muscle regions will be affected by the complicated muscle fiber architecture of compartmentalized neck muscles.

Paciniform Corpuscles

Paciniform corpuscles are small (approximately $15–30 \times 60–500$ μm) cylindrical encapsulations that ensheath the end of a sensory nerve fiber in a series of thin, flattened lamellae (Stacey, 1969; Barker, 1974) (Fig. 4.4). The Paciniform corpuscle thus has the appearance of a Pacinian corpuscle that has been stripped of its multilayered outer coating. Unlike GTOs and spindles that always lie within the substance of the muscle, Paciniform corpuscles can also be found in joint capsules, near blood vessels, or between layers of fascia. It is likely that these receptors are part of a receptor family that is distributed in many different tissues. In the neck, Paciniform corpuscles are often found in deep muscle and connective tissue regions close to cervical joints (Richmond and Bakker, 1982). In addition, many Paciniform corpuscles are embedded in certain pinnate intervertebral muscles such as semispinalis cervicis and longus colli, where they lie close to internal tendinous attachments.

The receptor properties of Paciniform corpuscles are still poorly understood. Most commonly they are considered to be joint receptors, whose rapidly adapting responses have the potential to provide information about the initiation and possibly the speed or acceleration of joint movement (Boyd, 1954; Burgess and Clark, 1969). However, Paciniform corpuscles in muscle may have a specialized role because of their placement near contracting muscle fibers. It is not a simple task to study the physiology of these intramuscular Paciniform corpuscles using conventional methods of single-fiber recording. Much guesswork is needed to sort the putative responses of Paciniform corpuscles from those of free nerve endings. Furthermore, it is impossible to standardize natural stimuli for receptors that in some cases may be situated near the muscle surface, while in other cases are located deeply within the muscle mass where their sensitivities may be influenced by changes in muscle tone. However, Paciniform corpuscles tend to be served by axons of relatively fine caliber, in the Group II and Group III range. Many Group III fibers from skeletal muscle have mechanoreceptive properties (Paintal, 1960; Bessou and Laporte, 1961) and more recent studies conducted in the hindlimb muscles of the cat suggest that Group III fibers may be subclassed into several types (e.g., Mense and Meyer, 1985; Mense, 1986). Whether this reflects intrinsic specializations in the properties of the receptors or simply differences in their placement is not known. Approximately 25% of neck muscle afferents from BC conduct in the Group III range, and these are found consistently to supply mechanoreceptors (Abrahams et al., 1984a). It remains to be ascertained whether these mechanoreceptors are in fact Paciniform corpuscles. We might predict that Paciniform corpuscles will fire at onset of muscle contraction or during an abrupt change in muscle force in the course of normal movement. How their activity contributes to proprioception, kinesthesia, or motor processing is not yet known.

Free Nerve Endings

Free nerve endings were until recently the least understood receptors of skeletal muscle but were commonly viewed as "pressure–pain" receptors (Paintal, 1960) with a nociceptive function. In the last few years, they have been subjected to close scrutiny as part of studies of Group III and IV fibers in cat limb muscles (Mense and Meyer, 1985). A high proportion of afferent fibers in the Group III and IV range is now known to respond to mechanical stimuli or to muscle contraction, suggesting that free nerve endings may be able to contribute information about nonnoxious events. Afferents in the Group III and IV range may also be temperature sensitive and they can have a number of chemical specificities (see Mense and Meyer, 1985, for discussion). In addition, morphological studies have divided "free" nerve endings into a number of types according to their structural features and their locations in different target tissues (Andres et al., 1985). It is likely that the response features of the free nerve ending may depend on the nature of the tissue with which the receptor is associated as well as the specialized sensitivities of the ending itself.

Free nerve endings appear to be distributed widely throughout all types of muscle and connective tissues (Stacey, 1969; Andres et al., 1985). However, free nerve endings are difficult to study morphologically not only because they lack a clearly identifiable terminal structure at the light microscopic level, but also because, in nonsympathectomized preparations, they can be confused with autonomic axons. As a result, the numbers and distribution of free nerve endings cannot be quantified by the approaches so far used to examine other populations of muscle receptors.

JOINT RECEPTORS AROUND VERTEBRAE

Joint capsules around cervical vertebrae contain Paciniform corpuscles and free nerve endings (Wyke, 1967; Richmond and Bakker, 1982). In addition, Wyke (1979) has described a third receptor, called a Type I receptor, that is distributed in superficial layers of fibrous joint capsules around cervical vertebrae. The nerve axon that supplies this receptor divides into three to six branches, each ending in a thinly encapsulated corpuscle measuring about 100–400 μm in diameter. The receptor is reported to behave as a slowly adapting mechanoreceptor that responds to mechanical deformations of the surrounding fibrous capsule (Wyke, 1979). In both their morphology and function, Type I endings appear to correspond with Ruffini endings described in other cat joints (Boyd, 1954; Skoglund, 1956; Polacek, 1966). Wyke (1967) states that Type I receptors are particularly common in cervical joints. However, no quantitative information is yet available concerning their distribution. In a systematic study based on the analysis of serially sectioned, decalcified necks, Richmond and Bakker (1982) could not identify Type I endings and suggested that other methods might be needed to study their incidence and distribution.

SUMMARY

The proprioceptive system available to monitor head movement is composed of a diverse population of receptors arranged in complex but nevertheless predictable patterns. Most neck muscles contain unusually large numbers of muscle spindles;

these are commonly arranged in groupings and exhibit a range of structural forms. Neck muscles also contain substantial numbers of Golgi tendon organs, Paciniform corpuscles, and free nerve endings. Cervical joints are also sites in which receptors can be found, but the organization and physiology of cervical joint receptors have been studied less thoroughly. Together, muscle and joint receptors have the potential to provide an enormous volume of sensory information that could be used to build a detailed topographical and functional map of peripheral events underlying head movement.

In the past, there has been a tendency to view priorioceptors as a series of separate, functionally isolated receptors. However, the complicated receptor arrangements in the periphery, and in particular the physical associations between different types of receptors, lead us to question whether signals from different types of proprioceptors may be functionally coupled or used in a complementary fashion by the nervous system. Perhaps the receptor population should not be viewed as a series of "private lines." Instead it may provide a detailed matrix of input in which receptor position as well as receptor function play a significant part in producing a detailed three-dimensional picture of events that occur throughout the neck during head movement.

5

Central Projections from Nuchal Afferent Systems

D. A. BAKKER and V. C. ABRAHAMS

The experiments of Sherrington (1910) and Magnus (1926) showed that postural reflexes arise from receptors located in neck structures whose axons entered the upper cervical cord. These experiments were the initial stimulus for many anatomical studies whose aim has been to identify the central pathways and structures served by input from the upper cervical cord. Since that time, it has become understood that neck receptors play a more general role in postural regulation. Furthermore, it has been established that both large and small dorsal neck muscles contain an extraordinary concentration of receptors. These observations have aroused interest in the central mechanisms that may originate with or utilize the neck afferent system and have made it important to understand the central connections made by the sensory apparatus of the neck. The purpose of this chapter is to provide an overview of the knowledge so far obtained. The order in which the material is presented is largely historical. The presentation of the material has been divided into sections based on the experimental techniques that were used. Anatomical studies on spinal and supraspinal structures have been divided and the literature on spinal projections has been dealt with first. Anatomical studies using degeneration techniques have been considered separately from studies based on axonal transport and, in turn, they have been separated from studies that have utilized electrophysiological techniques.

SPINAL PROJECTIONS FROM UPPER CERVICAL DORSAL ROOTS

Anatomical Studies Using Degeneration Techniques

The initial degeneration studies used the Marchi technique and were based on experiments in which dorsal roots C1 to C3 were sectioned in a variety of species (cat, Ranson et al., 1932; Corbin and Hinsey, 1935; monkey, Ferraro and Barrera, 1935; Corbin et al., 1937; Walker and Weaver, 1942; rabbit, Yee and Corbin, 1939). With the improvement in degeneration techniques introduced by Nauta and Gygax (1954) and improved by Fink and Heimer (1967) further experiments were performed to study degeneration in both unmyelinated and myelinated axons (cat, Escolar, 1948; Imai and Kusama, 1969; Kerr, 1971, 1972; Wiksten and Grant, 1983; dog, Petras, 1966; monkey, Shriver et al., 1968).

The data obtained from all these experiments are relatively consistent. Fibers that enter the upper cervical cord travel both rostrally and caudally in the dorsal columns. The caudal projections are not extensive and in experiments in which single dorsal roots were cut, caudally coursing axons were usually found to terminate one to two segments below the level of the root entrance (Ranson et al., 1932; Corbin and Hinsey, 1935; Shriver et al., 1968; Imai and Kusama, 1969), although Liu (1956) reported that some fibers traveled caudally for four to five segments. Many axons entered the spinal cord and terminated in the dorsal horn. Close to the segment of entry, collaterals of dorsal column fibers could be seen in abundance entering the spinal gray matter through the medial aspect of the base of the dorsal horn. Some fibers terminated within Laminae III and IV, and degenerating terminals were also seen in the substantia gelatinosa. Consistent with the long-established pattern seen in the lumbosacral cord, Escolar (1948) reported that fine myelinated and unmyelinated fibers from the C2 and C3 dorsal roots entered the tract of Lissauer. These fibers then terminated in the substantia gelatinosa as far rostrally as the pyramidal decussation but no farther caudally than the third spinal segment. Many workers have pointed out that there are special characteristics in the distribution of fibers entering the cord at C1. Afferent fibers originating in the C1 root (a root characterized by the absence of cutaneous input) projected only sparsely to the substantia gelatinosa and nucleus proprius (Shriver et al., 1968; Imai and Kusama, 1969; Kerr, 1971, 1972) and, in some instances, no dorsal horn projections were reported (Escolar, 1948). Fibers in the dorsal column pathway traveled rostrally to the region of spinomedullary transition.

Degenerating fibers from upper cervical dorsal roots were most prominent in the intermediate spinal cord in a medial area of Lamina VII. Densest degeneration was reported around a group of cells located laterally to the central canal, which was considered in earliest studies to be the spinal portion of the intermediate nucleus of Cajal (Ranson et al., 1932; Corbin et al., 1937; Yee and Corbin, 1939; Escolar, 1948; Torvik, 1956; Kerr, 1971, 1972). In later studies this same group of cells was called the central cervical nucleus (Shriver et al., 1968; Imai and Kusama, 1969; Wiksten and Grant, 1983). Cells from this nucleus are now known to provide mossy-fiber projections to the cerebellum (e.g., Wiksten and Grant, 1983). Degenerating terminals were also seen in the intermediomedial nucleus, located lateral to the central canal, in medial and central portions of Laminae V and VI, and in the ventral horn (Yee and Corbin, 1939; Liu, 1956; Shriver et al., 1968; Kerr, 1971). Occasional degenerating fibers were frequently observed coursing through the posterior commissure to the contralateral spinal cord. Degeneration was at its most prominent in the segment at which dorsal root transection or ganglionectomy took place and was less dense in adjacent segments.

Anatomical Studies Using Axon Transport Methodology

Although occasional degeneration studies utilized transganglionic degeneration (Grant and Ygge, 1981), most descriptions of afferent pathways prior to 1975 relied on separation of axons from their cell bodies by dorsal root section or extirpation of dorsal root ganglia. These methods lead to anatomical descriptions based on segmental anatomy. They do not permit the analysis of pathways followed by afferent fibers traveling in a single nerve or serving individual structures. Major advances in pathway tracing have come from the development of new tracer techniques based on the transport capacity of individual nerves and on the ability to inject tracers into single axons. These techniques now permit the identification of pathways that are functionally organized. One commonly used tracer is horseradish peroxidase (HRP) which migrates extensively into cell processes when injected intracellularly or intraaxonally (Brown et al., 1976). HRP and its lectin conjugates such as wheat germ agglutinin (WGA/HRP) are also transported in significant amounts into both the dorsal root ganglia and the central processes of sensory axons (Grant et al., 1979; Mesulam and Brushart, 1979). Thus when a tracer is injected intraaxonally it provides a picture of the central course of a single afferent axon and its collateral fibers and the anatomy can be correlated with the function of the receptor giving rise to that axon. When taken up by a peripheral nerve, the tracer can be used to provide maps of the central organization of afferent pathways from a single organ or parts of that organ.

HRP injected intraaxonally has provided detailed information about the organization of single large-diameter afferents from identified receptors in neck muscles (Hirai et al., 1984b; Rose and Keirstead, 1986). These experiments immediately proved the long-held suspicion that muscle afferent axons, unlike cutaneous axons, had no terminations in the more superficial parts of the dorsal horn. However, boutons were present in and around the central cervical nucleus (CCN), reinforcing the notion that this precerebellar nucleus has an important role in processing proprioceptive information. Terminations were also distributed throughout the ventral horn, particularly the medial and ventral regions that are known to contain the cell bodies of neck muscle motoneurons (See Chapter 3).

More generalized pictures of the organization of central afferent pathways were obtained from experiments in which whole nerve bundles were exposed to tracer (Figs. 5.1 and 5.2). In cat and rat, afferent fibers from neck muscles terminated primarily around the large multipolar cells of the CCN and neighboring cells in Lamina VII (Mysicka and Zenker, 1981; Ammann et al., 1983; Abrahams et al., 1984b; Bakker et al., 1984). Experiments on cats also suggested that the density of the HRP reaction product in the CCN was most intense when HRP was transported from nerves supplying intervertebral muscles (Bakker et al., 1984). It was considerably less intense following exposure of nerves supplying the superficial neck muscles, biventer cervicis and complexus (Abrahams et al., 1984b). These results suggest that receptors in deep neck muscles may have a more powerful influence on cells of the CCN than do receptors in superficial neck muscles, a suggestion which is also implicit in the results of electrophysiological studies (Hirai et al., 1978, 1984b; Abrahams et al., 1979). Recent experiments (Edney and Porter, 1986) suggest that the conclusions may not be true for the cynomolgus monkey. In that species the injection of HRP and WGA/HRP into suboccipital muscles led to only sparse labeling in the CCN in C1.

HRP transported by neck muscle nerves in the cat was also found in areas located dorsally, medially, and ventrolaterally to the CCN (Abrahams et al., 1984b;

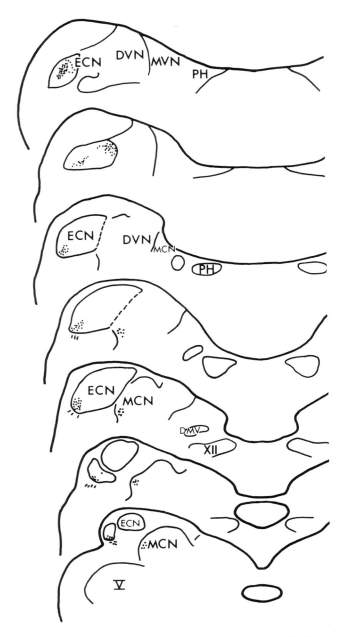

Figure 5.1.   Diagram of sections through the medulla to show distribution of HRP reaction product in ECN and MCN following exposure of BC/CM nerves to HRP. Rostral, top; caudal, bottom. DVN, Descending vestibular nucleus; ECN, external cuneate nucleus; MVN, medial vestibular nucleus; MCN, main cuneate nucleus; PH, nucleus praepositus hyoglossi; V, spinal nucleus of V; XII, hypoglossal nucleus. (Reproduced from Abrahams et al., 1984b, with permission.)

Bakker et al., 1984). In some cases, labeled axons could be traced into the posterior commissure and into the ipsilateral ventral horn (Abrahams et al., 1984b; Bakker et al., 1984). The extent of primary afferent projections from muscle into the ventral horn could not be determined in these experiments because of the simultaneous and intense staining of retrogradely labeled motoneuron dendrites.

Thus, despite the extraordinary concentration of receptors in neck muscle, particularly in the suboccipital muscles, frankly unusual aspects of the spinal projections from these receptors are seen neither in the distribution of their terminations nor in the density of their terminations. There is, in general, parallelism between the patterns of sensory projections from neck structures and those from dorsal root fibers entering lower in the spinal cord.

What also became apparent from axon transport experiments was that as elsewhere in the cord, the central course of afferent fibers from the skin of the neck was markedly different from that of muscle afferent fibers (Abrahams et al., 1984b). Exposure of cutaneous nerves to HRP resulted in dense accumulations of reaction product in Laminae I and II and in contiguous regions of Lamina III and lateral Lamina IV (Abrahams et al., 1984b). The presence of reaction product in Laminae I and II in the cat was in sharp contrast to the picture following muscle nerve exposure when virtually no reaction product could be detected in Lamina II of the substantia gelatinosa. Some reaction product was present in Lamina I after superficial neck muscle nerves were exposed to HRP (Abrahams et al., 1984b), but not when deep neck muscle nerves were exposed to HRP (Bakker et al., 1984). A number of studies in which afferent fiber projections from forelimb and hindlimb muscles were examined in the cat and rat have also noted the absence of muscle projections to the substantia gelatinosa (Craig and Mense, 1983; Nyberg and Blomqvist, 1984; Abrahams and Swett, 1986). The only exceptions so far reported are in the experiments of Mysicka and Zenker (1981) who described weak labeling in the substantia gelatinosa following application of HRP to the sternomastoid nerve of the rat and in the experiments of Edney and Porter (1986) on the monkey. These latter workers report sparse labeling in the substantia gelatinosa in two of four monkeys after injection of label into suboccipital muscles.

The absence of a projection from muscle afferent fibers to the substantia gelatinosa is part of a broader picture which suggests that the major sensory input to the substantia gelatinosa is from receptors in skin. As with muscle afferent fibers, visceral afferent fibers do not project to the substantia gelatinosa (pelvic nerve, Morgan et al., 1981; Nadelhaft et al., 1983; splanchic nerve, Cervero and Connell, 1983, 1984). The presumption has always been that many small myelinated fibers and unmyelinated fibers are nociceptive in function. Virtually all small fibers entering the spinal cord were believed to terminate in or close to the substantia gelatinosa and the substantia gelatinosa in turn was viewed as a critical physiological structure in the regulation of nociceptive input to higher central nervous system (CNS) levels. If the small fibers from muscle and viscera do not terminate in the substantia gelatinosa, control of their afferent information flow must lie elsewhere in structures outside the substantia gelatinosa. Thus, it may be inappropriate for strategies for the control of chronic pain originating in neck or other skeletal muscles to be based on the known physiology of the substantia gelatinosa.

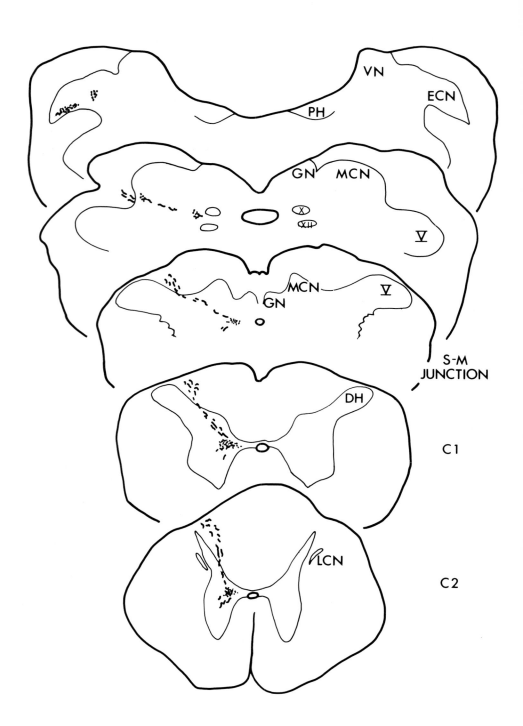

MEDULLARY PROJECTIONS FROM UPPER CERVICAL ROOTS

Anatomical Studies Using Degeneration Techniques

Degeneration experiments designed to investigate the medullary projections from upper cervical segments have been performed by Ranson et al. (1932), Corbin and Hinsey (1935), Ferraro and Barrera (1935), Corbin et al. (1937), Walker and Weaver (1942), Escolar (1948), Liu (1956), Torvik (1956), Shriver et al. (1968), Imai and Kusama (1969), and Kerr (1971, 1972). Virtually all degeneration experiments find that fibers from the spinal cord ascend into the medulla in a bundle situated between the main cuneate nucleus (MCN) and the spinal nucleus of V. Fibers turned from this bundle and coursed ventromedially to terminate in the region of the intermediate nucleus of Cajal (inC). Degeneration was present in the inC from the caudal pole of the hypoglossal nucleus to the level of the pyramidal decussation. Fiber degeneration was also present in a number of other medullary sites: the hypoglossal nucleus, the nucleus of the solitary tract, restricted ventrolateral regions of the MCN, the supraspinal nucleus at caudal medullary levels, the descending vestibular nucleus, and cell group x of the vestibular complex. All reports agree that the most consistent and intense degeneration was present within the external cuneate nucleus (ECN). In all species examined, but particularly in the monkey and cat, the conclusion was consistently made from degeneration experiments that the projection pattern within the ECN was segmentally organized.

Anatomical Studies Using Axon Transport Methodology

Axon transport methodology is particularly important in permitting an analysis of the input to the CNS from individual muscles. Consistently, neck muscle afferent fibers were traced supraspinally mainly to three regions in the medulla, the ECN, the inC, and the MCN. The major medullary target for afferent fibers from all neck muscles was the ECN, which, like the CCN, supplies mossy-fibers to the cerebellum (Mysicka and Zenker, 1981; Ammann et al., 1983; Abrahams et al., 1984b; Bakker et al., 1984, 1985; Nyberg and Blomqvist, 1984; Edney and Porter, 1986). These more recent experiments did not support the earlier evidence from degeneration experiments that the ECN is segmentally organized. Rather they point to a musculotopic organization in which each muscle is represented

---

Figure 5.2. Line drawings of transverse sections through the cervical spinal cord and medulla which illustrate the central projections of afferent fibers supplying suboccipital muscles. The courses of labeled axons are shown as black lines whereas the sites of termination are shown as dots. Drawings from top to bottom represent progressively more caudal sections. PH, Nucleus prepositus hypoglossi; GN, nucleus gracilis; MCN, main cuneate nucleus; ECN, external cuneate nucleus; V, spinal nucleus of V; S–M junction, spinomedullary junction; VN, vestibular nuclei, X, dorsal motor nucleus of the vagus; XII, hypoglossal nucleus; DH, dorsal horn; LCN, lateral cervical nucleus. (Reproduced from Bakker et al., 1984, with permission.)

within its own volume of the ECN. However, the pattern of musculotopic organization is not a simple one. Terminations from cat neck muscles served by C1, C2, and C3 dorsal roots were found throughout the entire rostrocaudal extent of the ECN (Abrahams et al., 1984b; Bakker et al., 1984, 1985; Nyberg and Blomqvist, 1984). The density of HRP reaction product was not the same in all regions and was often greatest in the rostral one-third of the ECN (Abrahams et al., 1984b; Bakker et al., 1984, 1985). The projection picture is made even more complicated by the observation that in the rostral half of the ECN, afferent terminations from biventer cervicis and complexus occupied two separate zones, one in the ventrolateral part of ECN that was a continuation of a termination zone in the caudal ECN and a second zone located on the medial border of the ECN (Abrahams et al., 1984b). There is also some overlap in projections and, in the rostral tip of the ECN, deep and dorsal neck muscle afferent projections shared a common territory in the central region of the nucleus. However, in contrast, in the caudal half of the ECN, the projection from deep neck muscles (Bakker et al., 1984, 1985) was separated from that of large dorsal neck muscles. The parts of the ECN occupied by neck muscles, both deep and superficial, were always separate from the ECN territory occupied by muscle afferent projections from shoulder and forelimb muscles (Nyberg and Blomqvist, 1984; Bakker et al., 1985; Abrahams and Swett, 1986).

HRP from neck muscles was occasionally seen in a small zone located medial to the ECN (Abrahams et al., 1984b; Bakker et al., 1984, 1985). This territory is occupied by vestibular and associated nuclei. However, the cytoarchitectonic evidence did not permit the projection to be assigned to a specific cell group such as the descending vestibular nucleus or other cell groups such as group x and group f, which lie adjacent to the ECN and to which neck muscle afferents are believed to project. Another projection site, the inC, showed the presence of reaction product only when deep neck muscles were exposed to HRP (Mysicka and Zenker, 1981; Ammann et al., 1983; Bakker et al., 1984). The HRP reaction product seen in the inC was continuous with the deposits in the CCN of the upper cervical spinal cord and faithfully replicated the pattern seen in degeneration experiments (Ranson et al., 1932; Corbin et al., 1937; Yee and Corbin, 1939; Escolar, 1948; Torvik, 1956; Shriver et al., 1968).

The MCN has long been known to receive muscle afferent input and a sparse projection to confined ventrolateral regions of the MCN could be demonstrated. When the nerves of superficial muscles were exposed to HRP, the projection was located close to the area receiving cutaneous input from the neck. The projection extended throughout the length of the nucleus (Abrahams et al., 1984b). However, labeling from deep neck muscles was found only in a small deep region at the level of the obex (Bakker et al., 1984).

As expected, medullary projections from afferent fibers supplying the skin of the neck were mostly confined to the MCN and fitted with existing plans of somatotopy (Abrahams et al., 1984b). Many labeled cutaneous afferent fibers were traced from the dorsal columns into a dense mass of HRP reaction product which occupied the most ventrolateral part of the MCN and formed a column extending throughout the length of the nucleus. In addition, some labeled fibers from the dorsal columns contributed to an intense particulate deposit of reaction product which occupied a circumscribed isthmus of gray matter lying between the dorsal horn of the medulla and the MCN (Abrahams et al., 1984b). Echoing the long-held notion of the functional and anatomical contiguity between the upper cervical cord and lower medulla, fibers from cutaneous nerves also projected to the medulla in the tract of Lissauer to terminate in the substantia gelatinosa of the dorsal horn of the medulla and among isthmus cells close to the medullary surface.

As with the projections to the spinal cord the significance of the very high receptor content in neck muscle is not expressed in some unique organization of afferent pathways to the medulla although the dense projections in the ECN are striking. The extensive representation of neck muscles in the ECN may bear a relation to the fact that there are large numbers of receptors in neck muscle. Physiological analysis of forelimb input to the ECN (Rosén and Sjölund, 1973b) has shown that there is a minimum of convergence between receptors originating in individual forelimb muscles. If this principle is extended and there is minimum convergence between input from individual receptors in all muscles projecting to the ECN, then the volume of individual muscle representation within the ECN would be a reflection of muscle receptor content. This then would explain the large volume of the ECN occupied by neck muscles. However, it does not by itself explain the role played by such dense projections of neck muscle afferents in the precerebellar nuclei in which they are so strongly represented.

ELECTROPHYSIOLOGICAL STUDIES OF NECK AFFERENT INPUT

Spinal Projections

The electrophysiological analysis of cervical spinal projections has been based on a variety of stimulation procedures including electrical stimulation of branches of the cervical dorsal rami, dorsal root ganglia, and regions close to cervical joints (Berthoz and Llinás, 1974; Wilson et al., 1976; Anderson, 1977; Coulter et al., 1977; Kenins et al., 1978; Hirai et al., 1978; Abrahams et al., 1979; Rapoport, 1979; Brink et al., 1980, 1981a, b; Murakami and Kato, 1983) and on vibration and controlled movement of neck muscles and joints (Campbell et al., 1974; Ezure et al., 1978; Manzoni et al., 1979; Denoth et al., 1979a, b; Boyle and Pompeiano, 1980a, c; Kubin et al., 1981a, b; Chan et al., 1982; Dykes et al., 1982; Mergner et al., 1982, 1983). The results of these studies complement the anatomical studies and compound the evidence that nuchal afferent fibers have a set of circumscribed targets in the spinal cord and medulla. In the spinal cord, short-latency unit responses were recorded in Laminae IV and V, in the intermediate region and the ventral horn of the upper cervical cord (Abrahams et al., 1979). Single and multiunit discharges were readily recorded in the intermediate zone of the spinal gray matter in and around cells of the CCN (Hirai et al., 1978, 1984b; Abrahams et al., 1979). A particular aspect of the projections from the upper cervical roots is that they frequently project, both in the upper cervical cord and caudal medulla, onto cells that also receive input from trigeminal nerves (Kerr and Olafson, 1961;

Abrahams et al., 1979). The physiological evidence supports the anatomical findings from degeneration experiments that primary efferent fibers from neck structures and the trigeminal system have overlapping terminal fields (Kerr, 1971, 1972).

Intracellular recordings from neck motoneurons have repeatedly demonstrated monosynaptic connections from neck structures (Anderson, 1977; Ezure et al., 1978; Rapoport, 1979; Brink et al., 1981b; Rose and Keirstead, 1986). A unique characteristic of monosynaptic excitation in the upper cervical cord and one that functionally distinguishes this projection from the similar and much studied lumbosacral monosynaptic connection is the relatively weak EPSPs. Indeed, it has been possible to provoke motoneuron discharge at monosynaptic latencies only in a small proportion of neck motoneurons (Abrahams et al., 1975; Ezure et al., 1978; Rose and Keirstead, 1986). However, excitation of neck motoneurons by neck muscle afferents is readily evoked after longer latencies. This is due to the existence of extensive polysynaptic connections between neck motoneurons and cervical afferent fibers (Abrahams et al., 1975), connections that must include those that underlie the cervicocollic reflex (see Chapter 7).

It is not possible to consider head mechanisms in total isolation, for the movement of the head is seldom accomplished in the absence of other postural adjustments. Consistent with this is the finding that nuchal afferent input has an extensive spinal influence and can modify the excitability of both forelimb and hindlimb motoneurons. Electrical stimulation of nerves from neck extensor muscles has been shown to evoke a facilitation in flexor and extensor hindlimb motoneuron pools (Abrahams and Falchetto, 1969; Abrahams, 1971). Originally the spinospinal effects were thought to involve a long loop reflex through the cortex (Abrahams, 1971). This conclusion was not supported by later experiments in which the spinospinal effects were still present after chronic cortical lesions (Abrahams, 1972). Intracellular recordings from hindlimb motoneurons showed similar long-latency facilitatory effects following electrical stimulation of cutaneous or dorsal neck muscle nerves; these effects were abolished in spinalized cats (Kenins et al., 1978). However, propriospinal projections from the neck also exist, for a short-latency facilitation of hindlimb motoneurons can persist after high spinal transection (Kenins et al., 1978). In experiments in decerebrate cats in which neck receptors are activated by rotation of the body on the head, changes in reflex excitability in forelimb muscles are produced (see Chapter 8). These experiments emphasized the considerable ability of nuchal input to influence forelimb motoneuron excitability. More extensive experiments have shown that rotation of the neck while maintaining the head stationary always produced facilitation of monosynaptic reflex activity to ipsilateral extensor muscles and inhibitory effects in the monosynaptic reflex of ipsilateral antagonist flexor muscles (Wenzel and Thoden, 1977; Wenzel et al., 1978).

Medullary Projections

The anatomical findings suggest a considerable nuchal afferent input to the ECN that has been amply confirmed by electrophysiological experiments. Cells in the ECN can be excited by electrical stimulation of neck muscle nerves or by manipulation of neck muscles (Johnson et al., 1968; Campbell et al., 1974; Abrahams et al., 1979; Dykes et al., 1982; Murakami and Kato, 1983). The studies, which involved stimulation of single muscles or functionally related muscle groups, support the neuroanatomical evidence for a specific musculotopic organization of afferent input within the ECN for the cat (Rosén, 1969; Cooke et al., 1971; Rosén and Sjölund, 1973a, b; Dykes et al., 1982; Murakami and Kato, 1983), rat (Campbell et al., 1974), and raccoon (Johnson et al., 1968). In electrophysiological experiments, as has previously been discussed, convergence was rarely found in the ECN. Most cells that were tested for forelimb (Cooke et al., 1971) or neck (Murakami and Kato, 1983) input appeared to receive input from only a single neck or forelimb muscle nerve. Antidromic excitation showed that at least some of the nuchal input projected onto precerebellar neurons (Murakami and Kato, 1983). In addition to exciting cells in the ECN, electrical stimulation of dorsal neck nerves can evoke unit activity in the subnucleus caudalis of the spinal nucleus of V at caudal medullary levels (Abrahams et al., 1979; Amano et al., 1986), in the deep layers and ventral margin of the main cuneate nucleus, and within the inferior olive (Abrahams et al., 1979).

Since the early work of Magnus (1926) interactions between vestibular and neck reflexes have been regarded as important in the regulation of posture and movement. Evidence for the convergence of excitatory inputs from vestibular and cervical afferent fibers has been seen for unidentified neurons in the vestibular nuclei (Fredrickson et al., 1966; Rubin et al., 1975, 1977), for identifed vestibulospinal neurons (Boyle and Pompeiano, 1979a, b, 1980a, c, 1981a; Kasper and Thoden, 1981), and for vestibular neurons that project to the abducens nucleus (Hikosaka and Maeda, 1973). Furthermore, there are numerous studies showing that the discharge characteristics of vestibulospinal neurons in Deiter's nucleus are influenced by electrical stimulation of neck muscle nerves (Mori and Mikami, 1973; Brink et al., 1980, 1981a) as well as during neck rotation (Boyle and Pompeiano, 1979a, b, 1981a; Kasper and Thoden, 1981). Cell group x is also believed to be an important medullary target for nuchal input. Neuronal responses were recorded there following electrical stimulation of neck nerves (Wilson et al., 1976) and during neck rotation (Mergner et al., 1982). No evidence of convergent input in cell group x from other receptor systems was observed. Neurons of group x appear to serve as a primary relay for neck proprioceptive inputs to the cerebellum (Wilson et al., 1976; Mergner et al., 1982).

Nuchal input also projects to reticular nuclei and large numbers of neurons within both magnocellular and parvocellular regions of the lateral reticular nucleus change their firing rate following electrical stimulation of neck muscle nerves (Coulter et al., 1977) or sinusoidal rotation of the neck (Kubin et al., 1981a, b). In addition, clusters of neurons were found in the posteroventral regions of the nucleus prepositus hypoglossi that responded to "passive deflection" of neck vertebrae in alert cats (Gresty and Baker, 1976). These units were in close proximity to other units that responded to vestibular and visual stimulation and eye movement.

Cerebellar Projections

In common with most somatosensory systems there is a cerebellar projection from the neck. Berthoz and Llinás (1974) first demonstrated that electrical stimulation of neck afferent fibers in the C2 dorsal roots led to electrical activity in lobules V and VI of the anterior lobe of the cerebellum. The latencies of the observed cerebellar activity suggested that neck input reaches the cerebellum by way of both mossy and climbing fibers (Berthoz and Llinás, 1974). Nuchal projections to the cerebellum were also shown to converge in some areas with projections from other sensory systems including extraocular muscle nerves, trigeminal afferent fibers, and forelimb and hindlimb input (Berthoz and Llinás, 1974). Wilson et al. (1975a, b, 1976) demonstrated mossy-fiber and climbing-fiber inputs from neck afferents to the flocculus in experiments in which cervical dorsal rami and the C2 ganglion were electrically stimulated. A more extensive investigation suggested that the mossy-fiber input from neck relayed in cell group x (Wilson et al., 1976). Later experiments which involved activation of neck receptors by rotation of the body with respect to the head have provided further evidence for widespread influences of neck input in the cerebellum. Sinusoidal stimulation of neck receptors or electrical stimulation of neck muscle nerves influences activity of neurons located in the medial zone of the cerebellum, i.e., in the vermal cortex and the fastigial nucleus (Erway et al., 1978; Denoth et al., 1979a, b, 1980), in the intermediate zone of the cerebellum, i.e., the paravermal cortex and the interpositus nucleus (Boyle and Pompeiano, 1979a, 1980c), and in the cerebellar lateral zone and dentate nucleus (Chan et al., 1982). Many of these neurons responding to neck rotation were also influenced by macular labyrinthine receptors.

Forebrain Connections

Neck afferent input is also known to project to the cerebral cortex. Projection areas of low-threshold cutaneous afferent fibers were found in the anterior suprasylvian gyrus and sulcus, the anterior ectosylvian gyrus, and a small area near the postcruciate dimple (Landgren and Silfvenius, 1968). The projection areas of dorsal neck muscle nerves were found to overlap into regions supplied by cutaneous afferent projections in the anterior suprasylvian gyrus and sulcus and the postcruciate dimple (Landgren and Silfvenius, 1968). Neuronal responses to neck rotation have also been demonstrated within the anterior suprasylvian sulcus (Becker et al., 1979). Furthermore, evoked field and single-unit responses have been detected in frontal regions of the cerebral cortex following vibration or electrical stimulation of nerves supplying both large neck extensor muscles and small suboccipital muscles (Dubrovsky and Barbas, 1977; Barbas and Dubrovsky, 1981a, b). These latter studies demonstrated that 60% of the cells in the pericruciate presylvian and coronal regions of the frontal cortex received input from both extraocular and dorsal neck muscles (Barbas and Dubrovsky, 1981a).

The early presumption that the nuchal input to the superior colliculus originates in muscle (Abrahams and Rose, 1975) has not been supported by later work. Abrahams et al. (1984a) showed that there was a substantial content of cutaneous fibers in nerves entering neck muscle and later electrophysiological experiments have demonstrated a considerable nuchal input from cutaneous receptors (Abrahams and Clinton, 1986).

So far neither anatomical nor physiological experiments have explained the particular significance of the extraordinary concentrations of receptors in neck muscles. Everything that has been done has suggested that sensory properties and the general pattern of projection arising from these receptors are not unlike those seen at other spinal levels. There is a need for a cell-by-cell analysis based on existing anatomical data to establish the nature of information carried by the ascending pathways, and the way in which transformations and regulations of this information flow are achieved at the level of second and later order cells. The significance of the anatomical organization described here is to lay a secure basis for the further physiological analyses that are to be made.

SUMMARY

The central projections from sensory receptors in the neck have been studied anatomically with degeneration and transganglionic tracer techniques and physiologically with electrophysiological techniques. Major differences are seen in the patterns of projection from nerves supplying neck muscles compared to those supplying neck skin. At spinal levels, afferents from neck muscles terminate primarily in the intermediate levels of the cervical spinal cord, particularly in medial Lamina VII in and around the central cervical nucleus where they can excite precerebellar neurons. Neck muscle afferents also have collaterals in the ventral horn and some of these collaterals synapse onto neck motoneurons. However, neck muscle afferents do not appear to terminate in the substantia gelatinosa. In contrast, cutaneous afferent fibers have their densest terminations in the superficial layers of the cervical dorsal horn and have extensive terminations in Lamina III and lateral Lamina IV.

Cutaneous and muscle afferents project to several sites in the medulla. Cutaneous terminations are found primarily in the ventrolateral parts of the main cuneate nucleus. Terminations from muscle occupy a large part of the external cuneate nucleus in which some afferents make excitatory connections with precerebellar relay neurons. Smaller terminal zones from muscle are present in the ventrolateral part of the main cuneate nucleus, in the intermediate nucleus of Cajal, and in the region of the vestibular nuclei. The anatomically defined projections suggest that neck muscle afferents may project substantially to the cerebellum by both spinal and medullary relay systems. Electrophysiological studies have confirmed the presence of projections to sites identified by anatomical methods. In addition, they have provided information on multisynaptic pathways that project to reticular nuclei, vestibular nuclei, the superior colliculus, the cerebellum, and regions of the cerebral cortex.

6

Segmental Organization of the Upper Cervical Cord

E. E. BRINK

Movements of the head will result, ultimately, from interaction of a host of descending and spinal systems capable of influencing the activity of neck motoneurons. Several later chapters will consider the descending actions on neck muscles. It is the purpose of this chapter to describe spinal mechanisms that occur within the neck segments of the spinal cord and that may be expected to mediate head and neck movements. These include reflex actions from neck cutaneous and muscle afferents and local mechanisms that modulate reflex expression. The description is not exhaustive; some phenomena related to hindlimb motoneurons, for example, have yet to be studied within the neck segments. [For a general review of spinal neuronal systems, see Baldissera et al. (1981).] Furthermore, the description here is limited largely to phenomena elicited by electrical stimulation of peripheral nerves and studied by intracellular recording from motoneurons in the cat. Reflexes in neck muscles elicited by natural stimulation (i.e., the cervicocollic reflex, probably a stretch reflex) are discussed in the next chapter.

As Chapter 1 has shown, numerous muscles or muscle systems act on the head or neck. Neck muscles are rich in receptors detecting changes in length (spindles) and tension (Golgi tendon organs) (Richmond and Abrahams, 1975b; Richmond and Bakker, 1982). They are also innervated by numerous small-diameter, higher threshold Group III and IV afferents sensitive to strong pressure or noxious stimuli (see Chapter 4). With so many muscles and receptors, the variety and distribution of reflexes arising from neck muscle and cutaneous afferents are likely to be extensive. However, study has been limited so far to actions elicited from or in the most accessible muscles, and the actions to be described pertain to these muscles. These include biventer cervicis (Biv) and complexus (Comp), which elevate the head; splenius (Spl), which acts as a lateral flexor and, bilaterally, as a dorsal extensor; and sternocleidomastoideus (Scm), a ventriflexor and rotator (Reighard and Jennings, 1963; Crouch, 1969). Also included are three muscles whose described actions are on the scapula, but whose attachments to the head or upper cervical vertebrae make participation in head movements also likely. One muscle, occipitoscapularis (Ocspl), attaches to the skull and might be expected to act in lateral flexion and elevation. Indeed, occipitoscapularis is active together with dorsal neck muscles in evoked (Baker et al., 1985) and free (Richmond et al., 1985a) head movements. The remaining muscles are levator scapulae ventralis (LSV), which might be expected to act as a ventriflexor and rotator, and trapezius (rostral portion, clavotrapezius, Trap) which has been described as acting in head rotation and extension (Duchenne, 1867; Bizzi et al., 1971).

In the following discussion, ipsilateral actions are described first; actions on motoneurons located on the contralateral side of the spinal cord and innervating contralateral muscles are considered in a later, separate section.

MONOSYNAPTIC EXCITATION FROM MUSCLE AFFERENTS

For limb and many other kinds of motoneurons (listed in Jankowska and Odotula, 1980), stimulation of primary (Group Ia) spindle afferents leads to monosynaptic excitation of homonymous and synergist motoneurons. This monosynaptic pathway from low threshold, stretch-sensitive afferents is the simplest substrate for the reflex contraction of muscle upon stretch of the muscle (reviewed in Matthews, 1972; Baldissera et al., 1981).

Similarly, stimulation of homonymous muscle afferents produces excitatory postsynaptic potentials (EPSPs) in neck motoneurons (Fig. 6.1; Wilson and Maeda, 1974; Anderson, 1977; Rapoport, 1979; Brink et al., 1981b; E. Brink and I. Suzuki, unpublished). Central latencies of the EPSPs, measured from the time of arrival of the fastest conducting afferents at the spinal cord, range from 0.4 to 1.5 msec, mainly less than 0.9 msec; this permits time only for central conduction and one synaptic delay (Eccles et al., 1956; Munson and Sypert, 1979a, b).[1] As illustrated in Figure 6.1A, the EPSPs are elicited with weak electrical stimuli, at or near strengths necessary to activate the lowest threshold afferents. Amplitudes of the EPSPs grow rapidly with increasing stimulus strength, reaching maxima with stimuli of about two times threshold of the afferent volley or less. In these features, the EPSPs behave like EPSPs in hindlimb or other motoneurons (e.g., Eccles et al., 1957a, b; Sears, 1964): in the neck as elsewhere, the EPSPs are probably largely due to actions of Group I spindle afferents. That primary spindle afferents from neck muscles produce monosynaptic EPSPs in neck motoneurons has been demonstrated by spike-triggered averaging of effects from single identified afferents (Keirstead and Rose, 1984). It is not known whether Group II (secondary) spindle afferents from neck muscles also produce monosynaptic EPSPs, as those from hindlimb and other muscles may (Stauffer et al., 1976; Lündberg et al., 1977; Appenteng et al., 1978; Lüscher et al., 1980; Munson et al., 1980; Kirkwood et al., 1982). Neither is it known whether monosynaptic EPSPs may be evoked from the neck muscle spindle afferents that have intermediate properties (Richmond and Abrahams, 1979a).

Two features that may be expected to influence monosynaptic EPSPs in neck motoneurons are (1) the number of spindles in neck muscles, and (2) the segmented innervation of many neck muscles. The distribution of monosynaptic EPSPs across segments has been studied for biventer cervicis and splenius (Brink et al., 1981b), muscles typically innervated by three major nerves and four nerves, respectively. In fact, input is fairly restricted: motoneurons receive most of their

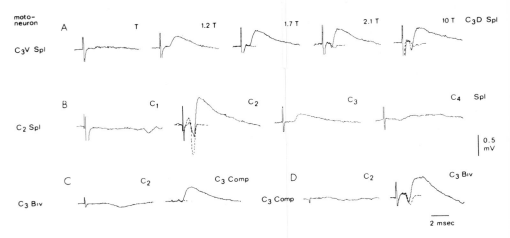

Figure 6.1.   Monosynaptic EPSPs in neck motoneurons. All records are computer averaged. Dotted lines represent extracellular fields recorded nearby. (A) Growth of the monosynaptic EPSP with increasing stimulus strength. EPSPs were evoked by stimulating muscle afferents in a dorsal branch of the C3 nerve to splenius and were recorded in a motoneuron
with its axon in another (ventral) branch of the C3 nerve. In this and subsequent figures,
stimulus strength is indicated relative to threshold (T, weakest stimulus) for eliciting an
afferent volley recorded from the cord dorsum. (B) Segmental distribution of the monosynaptic EPSP. Records are from a splenius motoneuron located at C2. Segmental nerves
to splenius were stimulated at strengths to obtain maximal EPSPs (2T for C2, >3T for
others). (C, D) Monosynaptic EPSPs between synergists. (C) Records from a C3 Biv
motoneuron on stimulating C2 and C3 nerves to Comp. (D) Records from a C3 Comp
motoneuron on stimulating nerves to Biv. Stimuli at strengths to obtain maximal EPSPs.

homonymous monosynaptic excitation from afferents of the same segment (Brink
et al., 1981b and unpublished). A smaller contribution comes from adjacent segments. Input from more distal segments diminishes in frequency of occurrence
and average amplitude and is, therefore, on average, rather trivial (less than 100
μV, E. E. Brink, K. Jinnai, and V. J. Wilson, unpublished). There is rostrocaudal
asymmetry in the extrasegmental input: afferents caudal to the recorded motoneuron are more effective than those rostral. This is illustrated in Figure 6.1B for
a splenius motoneuron. Typical for splenius, caudal afferents produce EPSPs,
whereas rostral afferents are wholly ineffective. The rostrocaudal asymmetry is
less pronounced for biventer cervicis: afferents of the rostral adjacent (but not
more distal) segment also produce small EPSPs. The biased distribution of monosynaptic input to neck motoneurons is reminiscent of that seen for some hindlimb
motoneurons in so far as largest actions are produced by the nerve branches containing the axon of the studied motoneuron (Hamm et al., 1985 for references).
However, the rostrocaudal asymmetry seen for neck muscles seems peculiar (so
far) to the neck muscles.

     Because monosynaptic input to neck motoneurons is distributed, estimates of
the total maximal EPSP from homonymous muscle afferents are obtained by sum-

ming effects from the individual segmental nerves. For biventer cervicis and splenius motoneurons, the resultant total EPSPs average about 1.2 mV (E. E. Brink, K. Jinnai, and V. T. Wilson, unpublished), with EPSPs from the segmental nerve containing the motoneuron's axon averaging about 0.9 to 1 mV. While the total values are roughly comparable to the sizes of maximal EPSPs in a few hindlimb motoneuron species, they are smaller than the values obtained for the majority of hindlimb (Eccles et al., 1957b; Eccles and Lundberg, 1958; Hamm et al., 1985) and forelimb (Fritz, 1981) motoneurons.[2]

Because of the high number of spindles in some neck muscles (Richmond and Abrahams, 1975b), the number per segmental nerve is likely to be roughly comparable to the total number of spindles in many of the hindlimb muscles studied (tabulated in Boyd and Davey, 1968, and in Botterman et al., 1978). Thus, smaller same-segment or total EPSPs are probably not due to fewer spindle afferents per se. Among other possibilities,[3] a partial explanation may be in the sparse connectivity of spindle afferents with neck motoneurons (Keirstead and Rose, 1984), compared to the high projection frequencies of spindle afferents to hindlimb motoneurons (Mendell and Henneman, 1971; Scott and Mendell, 1976; Watt et al., 1976; Nelson and Mendell, 1978; Munson and Sypert, 1979b). Lower projection frequency has also been adduced to explain the similarly small size of homonymous EPSPs in jaw elevator motoneurons (Appenteng et al., 1978).

The distribution of monosynaptic EPSPs across motoneuron species has been studied for only a small number of neck muscles, summarized in Table 6.1. The only synergistic connection so far described is that between biventer cervicis and complexus (Wilson and Maeda, 1974; Anderson, 1977). These are adjacent muscles with similar action; in some species, they are not separable as two distinct muscles (Vallois, 1922; Slijper, 1946). The spatial restriction and asymmetry of monosynaptic input described for a single motoneuron pool holds also for input between synergists (Fig. 6.1C; Brink et al., 1981b).

OTHER EFFECTS FROM MUSCLE AFFERENTS

For limb flexor and extensor motoneurons, stimulation of primary spindle (Group Ia) afferents leads not only to excitation of homonymous and synergist motoneurons but also to disynaptic reciprocal inhibition of antagonist motoneurons (reviewed in Baldissera et al., 1981). Among neck muscles, there is no such inhibition between the ventriflexor, sternocleidomastoideus, and the dorsal extensors, biventer cervicis and complexus (Rapoport, 1979). Whether there is any reciprocal inhibition at all among neck muscles remains to be determined. Possibly, given the complexity of head movements, in which muscles might act oppositely in one movement but together in others (for example, in up and down versus side to side or rotary movements, Basmajian and DeLuca, 1985), hard-wired reflex linkages may be a hindrance. Similar arguments may explain the lack of reciprocal inhibition between thigh abductors and adductors (Eccles and Lundberg, 1958) and between thoracic muscles with inspiratory and expiratory (as well as postural) actions (Sears, 1964).

Table 6.1. Distribution of Monosynaptic Excitation among Neck Motoneurons (Frequency of Occurrence)[a]

	Nerve stimulated							
Motoneuron	Biv	Comp	Spl	Ocspl[b]	C_2VR (Scm)[c]	C_3VR (Trap)[c]	Co[d] Biv, Comp, Spl	Co C_2–C_3 VR[c]
Biv	+[e]	12/14	0/16		}0/6	0/4	0/15	}0/9
Comp	12/13	+	3/18				0/16	
Spl	3/12	0/11	+				0/10	
Ocspl[b]		0/3		0/12	+			
Scm[c]		0/6			+		0/14	}0/2
Trap[c]						+		

[a]Most data from Anderson (1977, modified from Table 1 and text).
[b]From E. E. Brink and I. Suzuki (unpublished).
[c]From Rapoport (1979 and unpublished). VR, ventral rami.
[d]Co, Contralateral.
[e]+, Homonymous EPSP.

Neck muscles contain Golgi tendon organs, but the actions on neck motoneurons of afferents from these receptors, or of secondary or intermediary spindle afferents, have yet to be identified. However, when electrical stimulation of muscle nerves is used, strong stimuli (usually at least three times nerve threshold and more) lead to complex excitatory or inhibitory postsynaptic responses (Anderson, 1977; Gura and Limanskii, 1976; E. E. Brink and I. Suzuki, unpublished; E. E. Brink, K. Jinnai, and V. J. Wilson, unpublished) (examples are given in Fig. 6.2). Latencies, measured from the earliest sign of the afferent volley at the cord dorsum, indicate polysynaptic transmission (probably trisynaptic and longer, Eccles and Lundberg, 1959), although some of the increased latency is due to slower peripheral conduction of the responsible afferents. The potentials are facilitated by multiple stimuli (Fig. 6.2C), typical of transmission in polysynaptic pathways.

Because of overlap in thresholds for electrical activation of muscle afferents of different function (Eccles et al., 1957c; Jack, 1978; indicated for neck afferents by overlap of conduction velocities, Richmond and Abrahams, 1979a; Abrahams et al., 1984a) and because spatial and/or temporal facilitation will particularly influence the strength of stimuli needed to elicit a polysynaptic action, some caution is necessary in interpreting results of graded electrical stimulation in terms of the afferents responsible. Therefore, a conservative estimate is that the actions appearing in neck motoneurons with strong stimuli are largely due to the smaller caliber (Richmond et al., 1976), high threshold Group II and Group III afferents, as in hindlimb motoneurons (Eccles and Lundberg, 1959). These afferent classes include nociceptive afferents (reviewed in Boyd and Davey, 1968; McIntyre, 1974; Willis and Coggeshall, 1978). However, the possibility remains that Golgi tendon organ afferents, and even primary spindle afferents (through contributing to actions from tendon organs: Fetz et al., 1979; Jankowska and McCrea, 1983), produce similar actions or contribute to effects, as they do for hindlimb motoneurons (Eccles et al., 1957c; Eccles and Lundberg, 1959).

The responses to strong stimuli in neck motoneurons are qualitatively similar

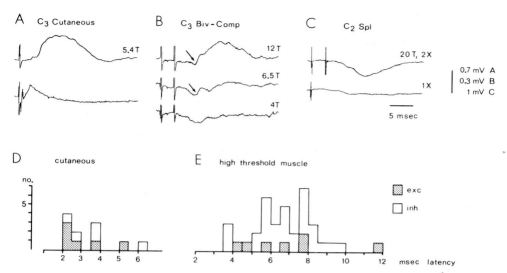

Figure 6.2.   Actions of cutaneous and high threshold muscle afferents in neck motoneu-rons. All traces in (A), (B), and (C) are computer-averaged intracellular recordings *except* the lower trace in (A), which is a recording from the cord dorsum. Amplitude calibrations apply to intracellular records only. Records in (A) and (B) were obtained from the same Ocspl motoneuron and in (C) from a C4 Spl motoneuron. In (B), a depolarizing potential (indicated by arrow) appears with strong stimulation and grows as stimulus strength is increased, and can be attributed to high threshold muscle afferents. The nature of the earlier inhibition was not fully investigated: it might be recurrent inhibition or (disynaptic or trisynaptic) inhibition from Group I afferents. In (C), strong stimulation produces a hyperpolarization barely detectable with a single stimulus. With double stimuli, the re-sponse to the second is enhanced. Another example of an inhibitory response is in Figure 1C, on stimulating C2 Comp afferents. (D) and (E) are histograms of latencies of exci-tatory (exc) and inhibitor (inh) potentials from cutaneous and high threshold muscle af-ferents. Central latencies were measured from the positive peak of the effective afferent volley [e.g., the first deflection after the stimulus artifact in the lower trace of (A); the later potential, after the triphasic afferent volley, reflects monosynaptic activation by cu-taneous afferents of interneurons in the upper dorsal horn]. In effect, most latencies were obtained from trials in which single stimuli were used. (E) does not include data from potentials of questionable origin (i.e., possible Group I effects and, particularly, disynaptic recurrent inhibition). Latencies reported by Gura and Limanskii (1976) for effects from muscle afferents are similar, ranging from 3.8 to 5.8 msec (excitation).

to those produced by high threshold (Group II and III) muscle afferents in hind-limb motoneurons (Eccles and Lundberg, 1959). For hindlimb motoneurons, al-though other actions may be evoked, the most typical pattern of response is ex-citation of flexors and inhibition of extensors, elicited by high threshold afferents of both flexors and extensors. Joint and cutaneous afferents evoke similar re-sponses. For this reason, these and high threshold muscle afferents have been called "flexor reflex afferents" (FRA, Eccles and Lundberg, 1959), that is, af-ferents that may elicit the flexion withdrawal reflex.[4] Data on the pattern of responses in neck motoneurons are limited (see Table 6.2). This information might help in classifying muscle function, similar to Sherrington's (1910) classification of hindlimb muscles as flexors or extensors according to their contraction or relaxation during the flexion reflex.

EFFECTS FROM CUTANEOUS AFFERENTS

Cutaneous afferents contribute to the FRA response, but, as probable for other elements of the FRA, also act on motoneurons through independent reflex paths (Baldissera et al., 1981). This is indicated, for limb motoneurons, in part by actions not conforming to the FRA pattern (for example, excitation of extensors, Hagbarth, 1952; Fleshman et al., 1984), and by disynaptic latencies of some cutaneous effects (Illert et al., 1976; Fleshman et al., 1984) compared to more commonly observed trisynaptic latencies (reviewed in Lundberg, 1975; Baldissera et al., 1981).

The responses seen in neck motoneurons on stimulating cutaneous afferents of the head and neck closely resemble cutaneous actions in hindlimb motoneurons (Eccles and Lundberg, 1959; Burke et al., 1970). The effects are large, complex (Fig. 6.2), and may consist of mixed excitation and inhibition (Anderson, 1977). Cutaneous actions are reliably evoked with single stimuli and appear with stimuli near threshold for the afferent volley (E. E. Brink and I. Suzuki, unpublished). Thus, reflex actions are produced by the lower threshold cutaneous afferents, primarily mechanosensitive, as well as by higher threshold afferents, including those conveying nociceptive information (summarized in Boyd and Davey, 1968; Willis and Coggeshall, 1978). This suggests a role of cutaneous reflexes in the ongoing feedback control of movement, as well as in protective maneuvers (Baldissera et al., 1981). Latencies of cutaneous actions in neck motoneurons (Fig. 6.2) are compatible with trisynaptic transmission.

Stimulation of cutaneous afferents that innervate dorsal aspects of the head and neck produces inhibition in the ipsilateral dorsal extensors biventer cervicis and complexus (Anderson, 1977), which would seem to conform to an FRA pattern. Excitation is produced in other species of motoneurons tested (Table 6.2). It has been suggested (Anderson, 1977) that the predominant excitation of splenius is related to the greater percentage of fast motor units in this muscle (Richmond and Abrahams, 1975a), since, within mixed extensor muscles of the hindlimb, cutaneous effects are predominantly excitatory in fast motor units and inhibitory in slow motor units (Burke et al., 1970).

In contrast to the differential cutaneous actions described above, stimulation of the lip or Gasserian ganglion (Alstermark et al., 1983c and unpublished), or of the infraorbitalis nerve (Abrahams and Richmond, 1977; Gura and Limanskii, 1976) leads to excitation of all muscles listed in Table 6.2. Latencies suggest disynaptic as well as longer pathways. Because low threshold as well as higher threshold afferents contribute, B. Alstermark et al. (unpublished) suggest that the response might be, in part, part of an orienting movement, rather than simply a reflex withdrawal from pain. Cutaneous afferents capable of influencing activity of neck motoneurons are not confined to the head and neck: long latency (about

Table 6.2. Effects from Cutaneous and High Threshold Muscle Afferents (Frequency of Occurrence)[a]

	Afferents stimulated							
	Ipsilateral				Contralateral			
	Cutaneous		High threshold muscle[c]		Cutaneous		High threshold muscle[d]	
Motoneuron	E[b]	I[b]	E	I	E	I	E	I
Biv	0/9	9/9		(3)	0/10	10/10	1/22	12/22
Comp	4/12[e]	8/12		(2)	2/10	8/10	2/26	13/26
Spl	6/7	1/7	(4)	(15)	3/9	6/9	3/18	4/18
Ocspl[f]	5/5	0/5	(1)	(3)				
SAN[g]	E		E					

[a]Most data from Anderson (1977, data modified from Tables 2 and 3).

[b]E, Excitation (predominantly); I, inhibition (predominantly).

[c]From E. E. Brink, K. Jinnai, and V. J. Wilson (unpublished) and E. E. Brink and I. Suzuki (unpublished).

[d]From Anderson (1977). Data from stimulating Spl or Compl combined. Data from Biv not included as this nerve may contain cutaneous afferents.

[e]Includes two examples of mixed excitation and inhibition.

[f]From E. E. Brink and I. Suzuki (unpublished).

[g]From Gura and Limanskii (1976). SAN, Spinal accessory nerve (includes Scm and Trap).

11 msec and longer) effects are produced on stimulation of afferents of the forelimb (Gura and Limanskii, 1976; E. E. Brink and I. Suzuki, unpublished). Certainly, the pattern of cutaneous actions in neck muscles, as in limb and other muscles, promises to be quite complex once a study of the effects from afferents of specified type and location is undertaken.

PRESYNAPTIC ACTIONS

In addition to evoking postsynaptic actions in target neurons, afferents also act presynaptically on the terminals of other afferents. The terminals are depolarized (primary afferent depolarization, effected by means of axoaxonic synapses); this results in less effective invasion by subsequent action potentials and, consequently, depression of transmission from the terminals (reviewed in Schmidt, 1971, 1973). By controlling transmission through first-order synapses in reflex as well as other pathways, presynaptic actions provide a means of controlling reflex expression.

The depolarization spreads electrotonically from the terminals back along the afferent fibers, and may be recorded from dorsal root filaments as the dorsal root potential (DRP). Presynaptic actions in the neck segments of the spinal cord have been detected by recording dorsal root potentials from filaments of the third and fourth cervical dorsal roots (E. E. Brink, unpublished).

In the neck, as in the limb segments of the spinal cord (Schmidt, 1971, 1973), both cutaneous and muscle afferents evoke dorsal root potentials (Fig. 6.3). DRPs evoked from cutaneous afferents of the head and neck are large; the depolarization is often sufficient to evoke action potentials (dorsal root reflexes) in the target afferent fibers (Fig. 6.3A). The DRPs are easily elicited with single stimuli. The potentials appear with weak electrical stimuli (Fig. 6.3A), activating only the lowest threshold afferents, and continue to grow with increasing stimulus strength, so that both low and higher threshold afferents contribute. Central latencies suggest trisynaptic (and longer) pathways, as in the hindlimb region (Schmidt, 1971, 1973; Jankowska et al., 1981).

DRPs evoked from neck muscle afferents are relatively small compared to those evoked from cutaneous afferents (compare Fig. 6.3A and 6.3B), and usually require temporal facilitation. The DRPs can be obtained with rather low-strength stimuli (less than or at two times nerve threshold, Fig. 6.3B and C), with thresholds for the potentials ranging down to 1 to 1.25 times nerve threshold. This suggests a contribution from the lowest threshold muscle afferents (Group I afferents from spindles and Golgi tendon organs). The DRPs increase sizably with increasing stimulus strength (Fig. 6.3C), indicating that higher threshold muscle afferents, in addition to Group I afferents, exert presynaptic actions.

In these basic features, the organization of presynaptic actions in the neck segments appears similar to that in segments controlling the limbs. In the hindlimb segments, the patterns of different afferent types giving and receiving primary afferent depolarization are very specific (Schmidt, 1971, 1973). For example, Ia (spindle) afferents depolarize only other Ia afferents and are depolarized only by Ia and Ib (Golgi tendon organ) muscle afferents. Additionally, in general, Group I muscle afferents from flexors are more effective than those from extensors. How presynaptic actions are distributed within the neck segments, whether there is differential effectiveness associated with muscle function, and how patterns of presynaptic actions align with patterns of reflex actions to control transmission through them (cf. Brink et al., 1984a) remain to be determined.

RECURRENT INHIBITION

Another common spinal mechanism for controlling motor output is recurrent inhibition of motoneurons (reviewed in Haase et al., 1975; Baldissera et al., 1981; tabulated in Jankowska and Odutola, 1980). By means of axon collaterals, motoneurons project to interneurons (Renshaw cells) within the ventral horn of the spinal cord; activity in motor axons excites the Renshaw cells which in turn inhibit homonymous, synergist, and other motoneurons. In this way, activity of the motoneurons is limited and stabilized; recurrent inhibition may also serve to limit spatially the spread of monosynaptic excitation among synergists (Brooks and Wilson, 1959).

Neck motoneurons, like motoneurons in many other segments of the spinal cord, are subject to recurrent inhibition. Neck motoneurons give off axon collaterals that show (presumptive) terminal swellings (Keirstead et al., 1982); recurrent inhibitory potentials have been recorded in neck motoneurons upon electrical stimulation of motor axons (Rapoport, 1979; Jankowska and Odutola, 1980; Brink and Suzuki, 1987). Examples of recurrent inhibitory postsynaptic potentials (IPSPs) in neck motoneurons are illustrated in Figure 6.4. The distribution of recurrent inhibition across species of motoneurons is summarized in Table 6.3. As for limb

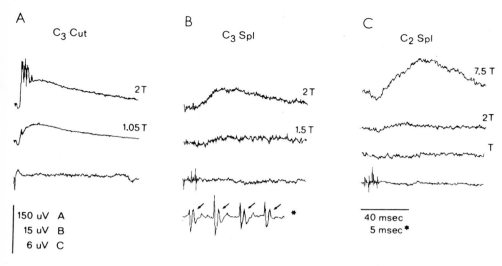

Figure 6.3.   Dorsal root potentials produced by neck cutaneous and muscle afferents. The potentials were recorded differentially from rostral C3 dorsal root filaments (interelectrode distances 3–4 mm): records in (A) and (B) are from the same experiment. All are averaged records. The lowest traces in (A), (B), and (C) are cord dorsum potentials: in (B), this has been also expanded (below) to show the afferent volleys (indicated by arrows) following the stimulus artifacts. Amplitude calibrations apply to DRPs only.

and other motoneurons, the inhibition of neck motoneurons is disynaptic, with central latencies ranging from 1.0 to 2.5 msec (median 1.4 msec, same segment, Brink and Suzuki, 1987). The distribution of recurrent inhibition is wide, extending beyond patterns of synergism (compare Tables 6.1 and 6.3), but is limited: there are pairs of muscles that have few or no recurrent inhibitory connections. Recurrent inhibition is obtained from motor axons of adjacent segments as well as from those of the same segment as the recorded motoneuron (Brink and Suzuki, 1987). It is likely that the spatial distribution is more extensive, as it is among thoracic respiratory motoneurons that have a similar pattern of segmented innervation (Kirkwood et al., 1981).

Additionally, neurons monosynaptically excited by stimulation of motor axons to neck muscles, and presumably mediating the recurrent inhibition, are frequently encountered in the neck segments of the spinal cord (Keirstead et al., 1982; Rapoport, 1979; Brink and Suzuki, 1987). All species of motor axons tested so far (listed in Table 6.3) have been effective. The response of a neuron located in the neck segments is illustrated in Figure 6.4D; like Renshaw cells in the hindlimb segments (Eccles et al., 1961b), the cell responds to a single stimulation of motor axons with a high frequency burst of action potentials. Also like Renshaw cells in the hindlimb region (Eccles et al., 1961b; Ryall, 1981), those in the neck region receive convergent excitation from several species of motoneurons (Brink and Suzuki, 1987). However, the input to Renshaw cells is spatially restricted (Eccles et al., 1961a; Ryall et al., 1971; Brink and Suzuki, 1987), presumably

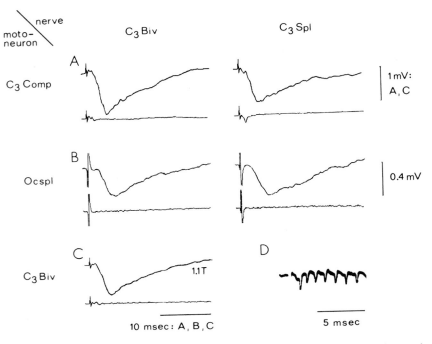

Figure 6.4.   Recurrent actions produced by antidromic volleys in nerves to neck muscles. In these experiments, dorsal roots were cut to prevent afferent input to the spinal cord (A, B, and C) Averaged records of recurrent inhibition in Comp and Biv motoneurons (located at C3) and an Ocspl motoneuron (located at C4) on stimulating motor axons of Biv or Spl. The lower traces are extracellular records. Stimuli were supramaximal for activating all α motor axons in all cases but for the example of homonymous recurrent inhibition (C). Here, the stimulus was just above the strength needed to activate the lowest threshold motor axons. (D) Response of a Renshaw cell located at C3 to (supramaximal) stimulation of C3 Biv motor axons. The first response is on the antidromic field potential. The trace is single-sweep recording photographed rom the oscilloscope, with negativity down.

due to the short length of the axon collaterals projecting to the Renshaw cells (Cullheim and Kellerth, 1978).

   If there is any difference so far apparent between recurrent inhibition in the neck versus the hindlimb segments, it is that the recurrent inhibitory potentials produced by individual segmental muscle nerves in neck motoneurons are, on average, relatively small compared to potentials in hindlimb motoneurons, and Renshall cell responses are correspondingly weaker (Brink and Suzuki, 1987, compared to Eccles et al., 1961a, b; Hultborn et al., 1971). However, when effects from the several segmental nerves to a single neck muscle are summed, the total recurrent IPSP produced by a single motoneuron pool may be quite sizable and more comparable to the potentials produced by hindlimb motor pools (Brink and Suzuki, 1987).[5] On the other hand, recurrent inhibition in neck motoneurons

Table 6.3. Distribution of Recurrent Inhibition (Frequency of Occurrence)[a]

Motoneuron	Nerve stimulated									
	Biv	Comp	Spl	Ocspl	LSV	Scm[b]	Trap[b]	Co[c] Biv, Comp, Spl[d]	Co Scm[b]	Co Trap[b]
Biv	+[e]	29/36	22/32	5/20	0/6	}0/3	0/5	0/33	}0/4	0/6
Comp	6/6	+	5/6	2/3	0/3			0/36		
Spl	8/16	3/14	+	2/8	1/9			0/26		
Ocspl	14/16	8/13	21/23	+	1/11					
LSV	0/8	0/4	6/11	0/6						
Scm[b]	0/1		0/1				0/4		}0/2	
Trap[b]	0/6		0/6				+			

[a]Most data from Brink and Suzuki (1987).

[b]From Rapoport (1979 and unpublished).

[c]Co, Contralateral.

[d]From Anderson (1977, modified from Table 3): no disynaptic inhibition (≤2.5 msec) with strong stimuli. Data from stimulating Biv, Comp, or Spl nerves combined.

[e]+, Homonymous recurrent IPSP.

appears to be stronger than that in respiratory motoneurons (Kirkwood et al, 1981; Lipski et al., 1985).[6]

CROSSED EFFECTS

Movements of the axial skeleton, including the neck and head, will necessarily involve action of both ipsilateral and contralateral muscles. For example, in moving the chin toward the shoulder, some ipsilateral muscles will contract and contralateral muscles will be stretched. In lifting the head, dorsal muscles will contract bilaterally. It is possible that crossed reflexes exist to support this close relationship between the bilateral axial muscles. Indeed, in contrast to the lack of crossed monosynaptic and disynaptic reflexes between the limb muscles, tail muscles are subject to crossed monosynaptic excitation (Curtis et al., 1958), crossed disynaptic reciprocal inhibition (Curtis et al., 1958; Lloyd and Wilson 1959; Jankowska et al., 1978), and crossed recurrent inhibition (Jankowska et al., 1978). On the other hand, dorsal back muscles show none of these crossed connections (Jankowska and Odutola, 1980, see also for table of effects on other muscles).

Information on crossed reflexes for neck muscles is summarized in Tables 6.1, 6.2, and 6.3. Although sampling is limited, there is thus far no evidence for crossed monosynaptic excitation (Table 6.1). Nor does there appear to be any crossed reciprocal inhibition between dorsal extensors (from Anderson, 1977, no disynaptic inhibition with strong stimuli) or between crossed muscles of antagonist function (Rapoport, 1979). Additionally, there is no evidence for crossed recurrent inhibition (Table 6.3). Thus, among the axial muscle systems, organization of the neck resembles that of the back. The tail is apparently unique with its tight coupling between crossed muscles.

There are a number of crossed polysynaptic reflexes between the limbs, originating from a variety of muscle and cutaneous afferents (Sherrington, 1909, 1910; Perl, 1958; Holmqvist, 1961; Harrison and Zytnicki, 1984, and see for references). These reflexes appear to assist in shifting support of body weight from one limb to the other. The best known is probably the crossed extensor reflex: stimuli that lead to the flexion reflex (lifting of the ipsilateral limb) also produce increased activity of extensor muscles in the contralateral limb. Given the different relationships between crossed muscles of the limbs versus those of the neck, it is not necessarily likely that the patterns of crossed reflexes seen for limbs will occur for neck muscles. Indeed, the pattern of crossed limb reflexes would be counterproductive for the neck: activity of contralateral (dorsal) extensors would counteract, rather than support, ipsilateral (ventral) flexion so that the head would not be able to move away from a noxious stimulus. Data support this idea: stimulating dorsal cutaneous afferents or high threshold muscle afferents mainly inhibits, rather than excites, the contralateral dorsal extensors (Table 6.2, from Anderson, 1977). In this case, effects on the ipsilateral and contralateral homologous muscles are parallel, rather than opposing as for the limbs. In other cases, depending on the direction of the withdrawal movement, different patterns of ipsilateral and contralateral reflexes might be anticipated.

SUMMARY

Muscles producing head and neck movements are subject to a variety of spinal muscle and cutaneous reflexes and are affected by several segmental mechanisms that control transmission in reflex pathways. In general, the basic organization of cervical segmental reflexes and mechanisms is similar to that in hindlimb segments, in which the phenomena have been studied most extensively. For example, the lengths of pathways, forms of the responses, and types of afferents responsible for the reflexes are similar in cervical and hindlimb segments. However, cervical organization has notable differences in the rostrocaudal asymmetry of input in the monosynaptic reflex, in the relatively small size of the total monosynaptic EPSPs, and in the apparent lack of (Ia) reciprocal inhibition. Other differences are also observed in the distribution of reflex actions: the pattern of crossed actions from cutaneous and high-threshold muscle afferents in the neck is distinct from that for limb afferents. Some of the variations in segmental organization that are observed at different levels of the spinal cord may represent specializations to subserve different repertoires of movements. In addition, some variations parallel, and may derive from, differences in the anatomical arrangement of muscles and their innervation, which is not necessarily distinct from functional variation. The study of distribution of reflex actions, of recurrent inhibition, and of presynaptic actions in the neck segments has been very limited and deserves further attention. A knowledge of segmental connectivity may provide insight into the degree of coupling, or functional relatedness, between different neck muscles, as it does for limb muscles (e.g., Baldissera et al., 1981). Basic data concerning the distribution of actions will undoubtedly reveal features of spinal organization unique to the neck segments and particularly suited to the mediation of head–neck movements.

Acknowledgments. The author wishes to thank Drs. M. Anderson, S. Rapoport, B. Alstermark, S. Sasaki, and M. Pinter for discussing aspects of this chapter, and for granting permission to use their published data in modified form, or to make use of unpublished results. Particular acknowledgment is owned Dr. S. Rapoport, who allowed the author to go through his original data.

Notes

1. Typical ranges of central latencies for effects classified as monosynaptic, disynaptic, or trisynaptic are as follows. Monosynaptic: 0.45–1.0 msec (EPSPs in motoneurons, Eccles et al., 1956). Disynaptic: 1.25–1.6 msec (Ia reciprocal inhibition, Eccles et al., 1956); 1.1 or 1.3 − 1.8 or about 2.2 msec (Ib or Group I IPSPs or EPSPs, Eccles et al., 1957c; Fetz et al., 1979). Trisynaptic: about 2.2 or 2.5 − 3.2 or 3.6 msec (Ib or Group I IPSPs or EPSPs, Eccles et al., 1957c; Fetz et al., 1979); 1.7–3.8 msec (primary afferent depolarization from cutaneous or Group I muscle afferents, Jankowska et al., 1981); 3 msec or more (high threshold muscle afferent actions in motoneurons, Eccles and Lundberg, 1959).

2. For comparison, the average amplitudes of EPSPs in 23 species of hindlimb motoneurons studied by Eccles et al. (1957b) and Eccles and Lundberg (1958) ranged from 1.6 to 6.2 mV with a median of 3.1 mV. The smallest EPSPs were in iliopsoas, semimembranosus, and anterior biceps (Eccles et al., 1957b; Eccles and Lundberg, 1958; Hamm et al., 1985).

3. Many factors, including methodological ones as well as ones of physiological interest, will influence amplitude of postsynaptic potentials. Thus, there may be a number of causes underlying differences in effects produced in different groups of motoneurons. The problem is compounded for disynaptic and polysynaptic effects, in which there are more possible sites for variability of circuitry and modulation of transmission. Any physiological difference is interesting as a likely example of neural organizational specialization (as mentioned in conclusions). In this text, because of the obvious difficulties in comparing strengths of effects, any comparison made is rough at best, with differences pointed out when such differences are quite sizable (e.g., note 2).

4. Stimulation of unmyelinated (C fiber, or Group IV) afferents also leads to, or at least contributes to, a long latency excitation of flexors in the hindlimb; the study of this has been hampered by difficulty in stimulating C fibers in isolation (reviewed by Matthews, 1972; McIntyre, 1974). The action of unmyelinated fibers in the neck segments has not been studied.

5. While recurrent IPSPs of several millivolts may be obtained in neck motoneurons, the average amplitudes of heteronymous potentials are about 200 to 400 µV (Brink and Suzuki, 1987). Although recurrent inhibition in hindlimb motoneurons is sometimes this size, values are often larger (Eccles et al., 1961b; Hultborn et al., 1971).

6. Potentials in both thoracic respiratory (Kirkwood et al., 1981) and diaphragmatic (Lipski et al., 1985) motoneurons are only about 100 µV.

7

Cervicocollic and Cervicoocular Reflexes

B. W. PETERSON

Movement of the head with respect to the body bends the neck and thus gives rise to changes in sensory discharge related to the lengthening and shortening of neck muscles or the deformation of tendons and ligaments. The altered sensory input in turn excites or inhibits muscle activity throughout the body. The most direct neck reflex is the cervicocollic reflex (CCR) in which neck bending acts back upon the neck muscles themselves. This reflex is similar to limb stretch reflexes in which muscle stretch initiates a negative feedback mechanism that causes the muscle to contract and thus to oppose the stretch. As with stretch reflexes in the limb, the CCR is mediated in part by monosynaptic pathways in which neck sensory fibers synapse directly with neck motoneurons (cf. Chapter 6). Less direct pathways link neck sensory input to extraocular motoneurons, constituting a cervicoocular reflex (COR), and to limb motoneurons, constituting a neck–limb reflex. As will be described below and in Chapter 8, these reflexes are more complex and variable than the CCR.

The previous chapter described electrophysiological studies of neural pathways involved in the CCR. Another approach to investigating this reflex is to analyze the changes in muscle electromyographic (EMG) activity that occur in response to imposed head-on-neck movement. Investigators taking this approach have adopted the techniques developed by engineers for the analysis of linear systems such as electronic circuits. This chapter will begin by using recent studies of the cervicocollic reflex to illustrate the linear systems analysis approach. Investigations of neural pathways responsible for the cervicocollic reflex will be examined next. A final section will describe the input–output properties and neural substrates of the cervicoocular reflex.

EVALUATION OF LINEARITY OF CERVICOCOLLIC REFLEX

The systems analysis techniques that will be described below can be applied only to systems whose behavior is approximately "linear." Two important properties characterize a linear system. First, if a sinusoidal input of only one frequency is applied to such a system, an undistorted sinusoidal output must be produced.

Fourier analysis is often used to detect the presence of distortion, which shows up as energy in the output signal at frequencies other than the frequency of the input.

Peterson et al. (1985b) tested the linearity of the decerebrate cat's CCR by applying sinusoidal horizontal rotations to the neck while recording EMG activity from several dorsal neck muscles. To avoid eliciting vestibular reflexes, sinusoidal horizontal rotations were applied by moving the animal's body while its head remained fixed in space. The inset records in Figure 7.1 show rectified EMG activity of the right complexus muscle averaged over multiple cycles of rotation at three amplitudes. The sinusoidal form of the EMG activity is one indication that the CCR is linear. The authors used the ratio of the second response harmonic (i.e., output at twice the input stimulus frequency) to the first harmonic as a measure of distortion. This ratio was typically much less than 0.5 unless the neck rotation was made so large that EMG activity ceased during part of the stimulation cycle. Such response saturation or rectification caused a rapid rise in second harmonic distortion. The signal-to-noise ratio, which is the ratio of the amplitude of the first harmonic signal to the root-mean-square amplitude of frequency components above the second harmonic, was typically greater than 1.0. Although such behavior would not constitute high-fidelity performance in an electronic circuit, it is typical of biological systems whose behavior is sufficiently linear that systems analysis techniques can be applied.

The second criterion for linear behavior is superposition: when presented with two signals in combination, the system's output should be the sum of its responses to the two signals applied alone. A corollary is that the system's output should scale linearly with the amplitude of its input. The graph in Figure 7.1 shows that the CCR does not behave exactly in this way. At low stimulus amplitudes, EMG output rises rapidly. Then, as the amplitude exceeds approximately 2°, the rate of rise becomes much less. As will be discussed below, this nonlinear behavior is interesting because it resembles the behavior of muscle spindles (Matthews and Stein, 1969; Hasan and Houk, 1975).

According to Figure 7.1, the CCR is linear for stimuli up to 2°. It can also be said to be *approximately* linear for stimuli in excess of 15°, for which the effect of the high sensitivity region at low amplitudes will be relatively small. Peterson et al. (1985b) chose to analyze the CCR in this latter range. They also chose an input stimulus that consisted of the sum of 10 sinusoids, which demonstrates another aspect of superposition. When presented with such a complex stimulus, some nonlinear systems will exhibit intermodulation distortion, defined as output at frequencies that are sums and differences of the input frequencies. The CCR did not do this and thus passed another test of its linearity. In fact, system linearity was improved by the sum-of-sines stimulus. This was because at different times cycles of rotation at each individual frequency were superimposed upon differing amounts of neck rotation produced by the other nine frequencies. Thus the response was averaged over different parts of the nonlinear input–output curve of Figure 7.1 and gave the appearance of scaling more linearly with input. Overall, then, by using an appropriately large sum-of-sines stimulus, Peterson et al. (1985b) were able to treat the CCR as an approximately linear system and to analyze its frequency response.

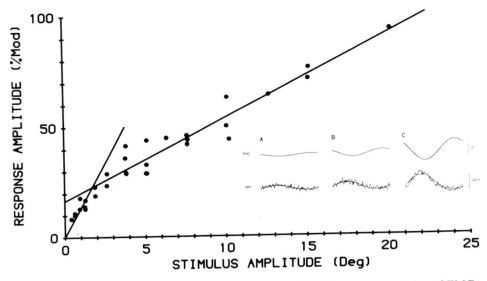

Figure 7.1.   Linearity of CCR. Traces in (A), (B), and (C) illustrate modulation of EMG of a neck muscle by small, medium, and large neck rotations with the head held fixed in space. The top traces indicate angular deviation of the platform holding the animal's body. Irregular lines in the lower traces are averaged, rectified EMG signals of muscle scaled so that deviations are proportional to percentage modulation of background EMG activity. Smooth lines are sinusoidal waves fitted to data. Notice that apparent gain (EMG modulation/platform) falls with increasing stimulus intensity. The graph plots percentage modulation of muscle EMG activity by CCR against stimulus amplitude. Stimuli were 0.5 Hz neck rotations with the head held fixed in space. Two least-squares fitted lines are superimposed on the data. The line with the lower slope was fitted to data for stimulus amplitudes above 2°. The steeper line is the best fitting line through the origin and remaining points. It indicates the high sensitivity region of the CCR. (Modified from Peterson et al., 1985b.)

FREQUENCY RESPONSE OF THE CERVICOCOLLIC REFLEX

Frequency–domain analysis is a powerful technique based upon measuring a system's response to sinusoidal inputs with a range of different frequencies. Its power derives from the principle of Fourier decomposition, which states that any time-varying signal can be represented as a sum of sinusoidal signals with appropriately chosen frequencies, amplitudes, and phase relationships. Thus, because of the superposition property, one can determine a linear system's response to any input by measuring its response to sinusoidal inputs over an appropriately wide range of frequencies.

Figure 7.2A shows the EMG response of a left complexus muscle to sinusoidal horizontal neck rotations at 10 frequencies that were presented as a sum-of-sines stimulus. Each response is fitted with a sine wave at the input frequency. These responses can be characterized by an amplitude and phase. Phase represents the timing of the peak of the response wave with respect to some portion of the input wave, the peak rightward rotation in this case. It is measured in degrees with a full cycle being 360° and phase leads specified by positive values. For the sake of generality in characterizing a linear system, response amplitude is usually expressed as a ratio of output to input amplitude. Where the input and output are in the same units (e.g., degrees, volts) this ratio is the gain. Some authors have generalized gain to refer to any output–input ratio as in Figure 7.2B, where "gain" is in EMG units per degree of neck rotation. Gains are often expressed in decibels in which $dB = 20 \log_{10} (\text{gain})$.

The variations in gain and phase as a function of frequency can be conveniently expressed using a Bode plot, as shown in Figure 7.2B. EMG responses produced by the CCR at lower frequencies characteristically have a constant gain and are in phase with the peak neck rotation in the direction that stretches the muscle. The reflex output therefore resembles the input, which is an angular position signal. In this frequency range, the CCR acts as a stretch reflex which activates muscles in response to stimuli that lengthen them.

At frequencies above 0.3 Hz, the CCR output begins to change. Phase advances until it leads the input by more than 120° and gain rises at a slope approaching 40 dB/decade change in frequency. The slope of the gain implies that output is increasing as the square of the frequency. The EMG output at high frequency thus resembles the angular *acceleration* of the neck rotation, which increases with the square of frequency and leads angular position by 180°. Similar frequency responses have been observed in a variety of dorsal neck muscles in decerebrate cats (Peterson et al., 1981a, 1985b; Ezure et al., 1983).

Once a system's frequency response has been determined, that response can be compared to those of systems containing known elements such as low or high pass filters. Such elements are usually referred to by their transfer functions written in LaPlace nomenclature (Marmerelis and Marmerelis, 1978). The simplest elements are the pure differentiator and integrator whose transfer functions are (s) and $(1/s)$, respectively, where s is the LaPlace variable. The differentiator converts a position signal input to a velocity signal output with 90° phase advance and gain slope of 20 dB/decade whereas output of the integrator has a 90° phase lag and -20 dB/decade slope. Slightly more complex are the zero (LaPlace form $s + 1$) and pole or low pass filter (LaPlace form $1/s + 1$) which act as the differentiator and integrator but in a frequency-dependent way. For instance, the zero, which is used to model the response in Figure 7.2B, leaves its input signal unchanged at low frequencies and differentiates its input at high frequencies. The "corner" frequency, f_c, where its action changes can be found from its time constant τ by the equation $f_c = 1/2\pi\tau$ where the time constant is measured in seconds.

The solid lines in Figure 7.2B plot the frequency response of a system containing two zeros with 0.06 sec time constants ($f_c = 2.7$ Hz). This system leaves the input signal unchanged at low frequencies and differentiates it twice at high frequencies, thus converting a position input to an output related to acceleration. As the solid lines show, it closely approximates the data. The correspondence is interesting and instructive, because previous investigators have shown that the

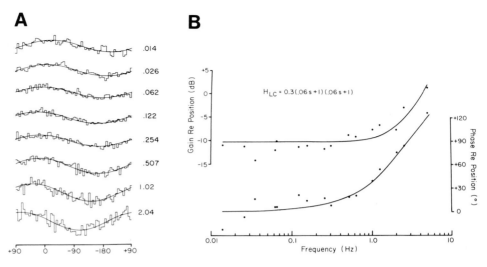

Figure 7.2.   Modulation of the left complexus muscle by CCR. Data at left show rectified EMG responses obtained from muscle during multiple frequency neck rotation. Each trace shows cycle-averaged data and best-fitting first harmonic sinusoid calculated by a least-squares fitting algorithm for muscle response at one of eight frequencies in the compound waveform. Frequencies are indicated by numbers at the right. Phases and gains of responses have been adjusted by the plotting program to reflect true phase and gain with respect to peak rightward neck deviation (i.e., peak muscle stretch). Note the gain increase and phase advance at higher frequencies. The Bode diagram at right plots gains and phases of responses shown at the left and of other responses of the same muscle against stimulus frequency. Solid lines indicate behavior of transfer function given above the plot that was fitted to the data. (Modified from Peterson et al., 1985b.)

transfer function of muscle spindle primary afferents is also well approximated by a system containing two zeros (Matthews and Stein, 1969; Poppele and Bowman, 1970). Although the zeros that best fit the responses of hindlimb muscle spindles have somewhat different time constants than those of the CCR, Peterson et al. (1985b) have argued that the time constants are similar enough to suggest that the frequency response of the CCR may be largely determined by characteristics of the afferent input it receives from neck muscle spindles. This argument is supported by the input–output curve shown in Figure 7.1, in which output increases rapidly for small stretches as does the output of muscle spindles.

    The frequency response of the CCR also provides important information concerning the role of the reflex in stabilizing the head. Typically, such stabilization occurs in conjunction with the vestibulocollic reflex, which is activated along with the CCR when the head moves on the body, producing a reflex output that sums with that of the CCR (Peterson et al., 1981b, 1985b). This issue will therefore be discussed in more detail in Chapter 12. Evidence will be presented that the high-frequency behavior of the CCR is adapted to compensate for mechanical properties of the head–neck system and its musculature in order to improve head stabilization in a critical frequency range between 0.5 and 5 Hz.

NEURAL PATHWAY MEDIATING THE CERVICOCOLLIC REFLEX

Studies of EMG responses elicited by neck rotation have also provided information about the organization of neural pathways that produce the CCR. Following up on studies of the organization of monosynaptic reflex connections between the four compartments of the splenius muscle (cf. Chapter 6), Bilotto et al. (1982b) and Ezure et al. (1983) investigated the EMG response of each of the four compartments to horizontal rotations of the neck either about the C1–C2 joint or about an axis 4 cm more posterior. As shown in Figure 7.3a, rotation about the C1–C2 axis produced the greatest modulation of EMG activity in compartment 1, and modulation decreased progressively in compartments 2–4. In contrast, rotation about the more caudal axis produced its strongest activation in compartments 3 and 4 (Figure 7.3b). In both cases, each compartment had a frequency response such as that in Figure 7.2.

The pattern of CCR activation illustrated in Figure 7.3 is consistent with the finding that monosynaptic activation of splenius motoneurons following stimulation of neck muscle afferents (presumably muscle spindle afferents) from a given compartment occurs primarily in that compartment and to a lesser extent in more anterior compartments (Brink et al., 1981b). This suggests that a significant role

Figure 7.3. Modulation of the four compartments of splenius by stimuli containing multiple sine waves. Gain and phase are expressed with respect to position; −180° phase corresponds to maximal contralateral flexion of the neck, i.e., stretch of the tested muscle. In (a) rotation was about the C1–C2 joint and maximum modulation occurred in compartment 1, the most anterior compartment. In (b) rotation was about C4–C5 and modulation was greater in the more posterior compartments (3 and 4). (Modified from Ezure et al., 1983.)

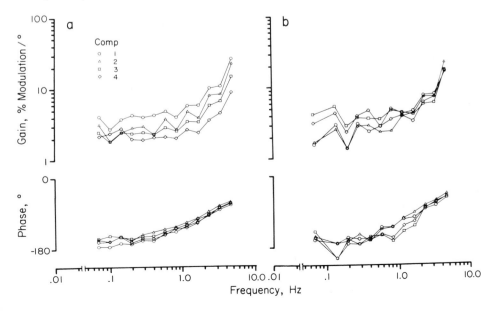

in generating the CCR may be played by monosynaptic and other relatively direct pathways that preserve the segmental specificity of the reflex in distinction to pathways such as those relaying vestibular or visual signals to the neck, which do not (Wilson et al., 1983). However, the pathways producing the CCR are not entirely homosynaptic, i.e., they do not activate a muscle only when its own receptors are stimulated. Ezure et al. (1983) showed that an isolated, splenius muscle held at constant length still responded to rotation of the neck about the C1–C2 axis with a pattern such as that illustrated in Figure 7.3a, although the response was much reduced.

In addition to monosynaptic reflex connections at the spinal level, electrophysiological studies have revealed a long-loop pathway that could link neck afferent input to neck motoneurons. This involves neck afferent input to neurons in the medial, lateral, and descending vestibular nuclei (Pompeiano and Barnes, 1971; Rubin et al., 1977; Brink et al., 1980; Boyle and Pompeiano, 1981a; Kasper and Thoden, 1981; Anastasopoulos and Mergner, 1982), some of which have been shown to project to neck motoneurons (Brink et al., 1981b). Another possible route is through reticulospinal neurons projecting to the neck (Peterson et al., 1978, 1980), since these neurons are activated by the cerebellum, which receives extensive neck afferent input (Wilson et al., 1976; Hirai et al., 1978). Nevertheless, long-loop connections are not a necessary part of the CCR because the reflex can still be observed after sectioning the spinal cord at the C1–medullary junction (Ezure et al., 1983).

THE CERVICOOCULAR REFLEX

The preceding section discussed the possibility that neck afferent projections to the vestibular nuclei might contribute to the cervicocollic reflex. Since vestibular neurons also project to structures controlling movements of the limbs and eyes, neck–vestibular projections could also play a role in neck–limb reflexes, which are the subject of Chapter 8, or in COR. Hikosaka and Maeda (1973) provided proof that neck–vestibular pathways do act upon vestibular neurons projecting to extraocular motor nuclei. They applied electrical stimuli to the vestibular nerves and recorded the resulting activation of lateral rectus motoneurons produced by excitatory disynaptic vestibuloocular connections. When stimuli were applied to neck afferent nerves just prior to the vestibular stimuli, the vestibuloocular responses were facilitated, indicating that neck inputs were exciting those vestibuloocular relay neurons which activated contralateral lateral rectus motoneurons. The effective neck stimuli were contralateral to the side on which the vestibular nerve was stimulated. Thus, the neck–lateral rectus pathway crosses twice: stimulation of *left* neck afferents, for instance, excites vestibuloocular relay neurons in the *right* vestibular nuclei, which then cross to activate *left* lateral rectus (abducens) motoneurons. If we assume that left neck afferents are excited by the stretching of left neck muscles that occurs when the head is turned to the right, the pathway described by Hikosaka and Maeda would act in a compensatory fashion: rightward head movements would cause activation of the left lateral rectus motoneurons and thus move the eye to the left.

Although electrophysiological evidence indicates that the COR acts to produce eye movements that compensate for head rotations, functional considerations raise doubts about the role of the COR in gaze stabilization. As pointed out by Fuller (1980a), the problem arises because the COR must interact with strong vestibuloocular and vestibulocollic reflexes (VOR and VCR). If we assume that the gain of the VOR is too low to produce eye movements that precisely counter rotation of the head in space, then a compensatory COR would help in achieving gaze stability when the head rotates on a stationary body (VOR and COR add). But consider the case when the animal's body is rotating. Then, as described in Chapter 12, the VCR will cause the head to rotate in a direction *opposite* to the rotation of the body. A "compensatory" COR responding to this head rotation would produce eye movements that are in precisely the wrong direction to aid the VOR. Thus no single appropriate action of the COR will aid the VOR and VCR in maintaining gaze stability under all conditions.

In line with his theoretical argument, Fuller (1980a) found in the rabbit, cat, and bush baby (a lower primate) that the COR observed at frequencies from 0.2 to 1.0 Hz was weak and could change directions during a single recording session. Correspondingly, other investigators studying the COR in various animals have reported low gains in either the compensatory (minus gains) or anticompensatory (positive gains) direction. Gains reported in the rabbit include +0.06 (Fuller, 1980a), +0.05 (Gresty, 1976) and −0.07 (Barmack et al., 1981). In cats, the gains of the COR have been reported to be +0.2 (Fuller, 1980a) and approximately 0 (Baker et al., 1982). In primates, Fuller (1980a) reported a gain of 0.02 in the bush baby and Dichgans et al. (1973) observed a gain of 0.03 in Rhesus monkeys.

The animal studies listed above studied slow-phase eye movements produced by the COR as distinct from rapid, saccadic movements produced by quick phases. Studies in humans have a longer history, going back to Barany (1906), and include both measurements of isolated slow-phase responses and measurements of total gaze shifts due to the combination of both slow and quick phases. In the 0.2–1.0 Hz range, studies emphasizing slow-phase measurements have reported gains of −0.05 (Meiry, 1971; Barnes and Forbat, 1979), whereas studies that measured total gaze shifts have reported gains of +0.02 (Barlow and Freeman, 1980), −0.19 (Barnes and Forbat, 1979), and 0.08 (Takemori and Suzuki, 1971). Thus, humans, like other species, have only modest CORs whose signs vary in the mid-frequency range of head movements.

A few of the studies discussed above measured the frequency response of the COR over a range of a decade or more. In humans, Miery (1971) observed eye movements with phases that were almost directly opposite to those of head turning with respect to the body from 0.02 to 1.5 Hz and gains that fell from −0.3 at 0.02 Hz to −0.05 at 0.2–1.5 Hz. He modeled the system as the combination of a pole and a zero with time constants of 1.7 and 0.4 sec, respectively. Baker et al. (1982) examined the cat's COR from 0.1 to 2.5 Hz and reported very small gains over the entire range.

The most complete set of frequency responses was reported by Barmack et al. (1981) who studied both horizontal and vertical (roll rotations) COR in rabbits over a range from 0.005 to 0.8 Hz. As shown in Figure 7.4, they observed typically low gains (−0.03 to −0.05) at higher frequencies, but found significantly

higher compensatory responses at very low frequencies of 0.005–0.05 Hz. At
these latter frequencies, inputs from semicircular canals decline sharply. It is
therefore possible that in this low-frequency range the COR contributes significantly to gaze stabilization. Such a contribution would be less crucial for vertical
rotations, during which vestibular otolith inputs maintain the responsiveness of
the VOR and VCR (cf. Wilson and Melvill-Jones, 1979; Chapter 9). This may
account for the lower peak gain of the vertical COR observed by Barmack et al.
(1981).

Thus it appears that the COR plays a negligible role in gaze stabilization
except under conditions in which the VOR and VCR are weak or absent. In normal animals, such conditions occur only at very low frequencies of rotation. However, when labyrinthine function is impaired by labyrinthectomy, semicircular canal
plugging, or vestibular pathology, the situation described by Fuller is altered and
a compensatory COR becomes appropriate under all conditions. In response to
this altered situation, plastic changes occur in the COR, and the reflex develops
a significant compensatory gain in the mid-frequency range in cats (Baker et al.,
1982), monkeys (Dichgans et al., 1973), and humans (Kasai and Zee, 1978; Botros, 1979). Baker et al. (1982) and Dichgans et al. (1973) observed that the
adaptive changes developed very slowly with a time constant of 2 weeks or more.
This observation is surprising since appropriate pathways are already available
(Hikosaka and Maeda, 1973) and other forms of oculomotor plasticity occur much
more rapidly (Miles and Eighmy, 1980; Optican and Robinson, 1980).

Figure 7.4.   Comparison of the phase and gain of the HCOR and VCOR. The mean gain
and phase of the HCOR (circles) and VCOR (triangles) are illustrated for 11 rabbits. The
larger of the standard deviations is indicated for each data point. (From Barmack et al.,
1981.)

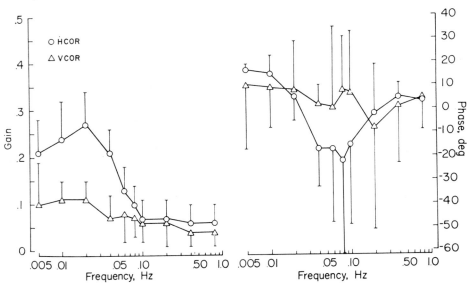

Baker et al. (1982) also suggest that CCR gain can show plastic increases after canal plugging. Here, too, the need for such changes is obvious. After plugging, the absence of the horizontal VCR causes violent horizontal head oscillations following any attempted head movement. An increased CCR gain would stiffen the neck and help to damp out such oscillations as would cocontraction of the neck muscles. The recordings of Baker et al. (1982) indicated that both CCR gain increases and cocontraction occur and allow the animals to regain head stability within a few days of the lesion.

SUMMARY

Afferent fibers from neck muscles and joints provide a sensory input that is used to control neck muscle activity by way of cervicocollic reflexes. In these reflexes, EMG activities of different neck muscles are modified in a predictable way by changes in head and neck position. The relationships between the head movement and consequent muscle activity can be determined by rotating the head according to sinusoidal patterns of controlled frequency and then studying the EMG activities of muscles using systems analysis techniques. At low frequencies of head movement, reflex output changes in a manner that reflects the position of the head. At frequencies above 0.3 Hz, the EMG patterns are influenced by the velocity and acceleration of the movement. The output of the cervicocollic reflex can be described in engineering terms by a transfer function that is similar in its form to the transfer function that described the sensory behavior of primary afferents from muscle spindles. Such a similarity might be expected if muscle spindle afferents contribute to the development of cervicocollic reflexes.

The simplest spinal circuit that might be responsible for cervicocollic reflexes is the monosynaptic pathway that links spindle afferents to motoneurons of the same muscles. However, receptors in other structures, particularly in tissues close to vertebral joints, can also affect the activities of neck muscle motoneurons. Multisynaptic pathways may also mediate cervicocollic reflexes through spinal, brainstem, or cerebellar circuits.

Cervicoocular reflexes are also initiated by changes in the activity of neck receptors and cause the eyes to rotate in a direction opposite to that in which the head is turned. Cervicoocular reflexes would seem to be useful for stabilizing the gaze during head movements. However, the reflexes are relatively weak and probably play little role in the stabilization of gaze during most types of head movement. However, such reflexes may become more important at very low velocities of movement when more powerful reflexes mediated by the vestibular system become weak or absent. Both cervicoocular and cervicocollic reflexes become more potent when the vestibular apparatus is damaged. Reflexes initiated from neck receptors therefore can provide some degree of compensation after the loss of vestibulocollic and vestibuloocular reflexes.

8

The Tonic Neck Reflex: Spinal Circuitry

V. J. WILSON

Interference with muscles and receptors in the neck can cause profound postural disturbances, as has been known since the work of Magendie and others in the first half of the nineteenth century (Longet, 1845; Bernard, 1858) and amply documented in recent years (e.g., Cohen, 1961; Abrahams and Falchetto, 1969; DeJong et al., 1977). This chapter is concerned with the role of neck receptors in normal posture, particularly with the tonic neck reflex (TNR) acting on the limbs, discovered and studied in detail by Magnus and his colleagues (see Magnus, 1924). They observed that turning the body with the head stationary in space produced a stereotyped pattern of responses in both fore- and hindlimbs.

The TNR is present in experimental preparations such as the decerebrate cat (e.g., Lindsay et al., 1976), but a pattern of muscular activity consistent with the reflex is also observed in behaving animals (Roberts, 1978). An asymmetrical posture of the limbs that corresponds to the TNR is seen in the human infant during the first few months of life (Gesell, 1938; Gesell and Ames, 1950) and there is evidence that the TNR is part of the complement of postural reflexes of adult humans (Hellebrandt et al., 1956, 1962; Fukuda, 1983).

WHAT IS THE REFLEX?

The TNR is brought about by movement of the body with respect to a stationary head, and, as its name implies, it is mainly tonic. Changes in position of the body cause changes in the position of the limbs; transient changes of muscle length may also take place during the movement itself (e.g., Lindsay et al., 1976). Once it was determined that the TNR is sufficiently linear to be studied by sinusoidal analysis, dynamics were studied with sinusoidal rotation of the head in cats that had been labyrinthectomized so that the rotation activated only neck receptors (Ezure and Wilson, 1983). As expected from the strong tonic nature of the reflex, peak modulation of forelimb extensor muscle EMG is approximately in phase with head position over a wide frequency range. Above 0.1 Hz a small phase lead may develop, and gain, which is flat up to this frequency; above it increases with a slope of about 10 dB/decade (Fig. 8.1). The increase in phase lead and gain that appear with increasing stimulus frequency indicate that the reflex has some sen-

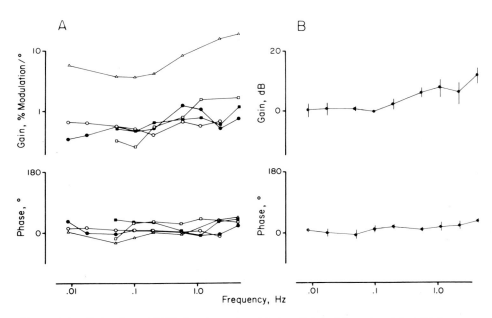

Figure 8.1.   Behavior of TNR in triceps brachii (medial and long heads). (A) Average response of one triceps muscle in each of five cats. Responses of both right and left muscles are shown, and phase is normalized so that it is 0 when the chin is rotated to the ipsilateral side. (B) Average response (±SE) of left and right triceps muscle in five cats. Note that gain in (B) is normalized. (Modified from Ezure and Wilson, 1983.)

sitivity to the velocity of the stimulus. Therefore, the reflex is not only tonic but also has a small phasic component.

The pattern of reflex action on the limbs was described by Magnus (1924), von Holst and Mittelstaedt (1950), and Roberts (1978). When the stimulus is roll rotation of the body, fore- and hindlimbs respond in the same manner: the limbs toward which the chin points extend and the contralateral limbs flex. When the stimulus is pitch, dorsiflexion of the neck causes extension of the forelimbs and flexion of the hindlimbs and ventriflexion of the neck causes the reverse. The direction of tonic vestibulospinal (tilt) reflexes acting on the limbs is opposite to that of the TNR, and Roberts and his colleagues have suggested that cancellation of the two reflex actions enables the head to rotate on a stable platform (Lindsay et al., 1976).

The reflex pattern evoked by neck rotation in roll has been confirmed in different laboratories (e.g., Ezure and Wilson, 1983; Manzoni et al., 1983a). There has been much less study of the response to pitch. Wilson et al. (1986) have recently investigated the responses of forelimb and shoulder muscles to combined vertical rotations in the roll and pitch axes over a wide range of frequencies. Stimulation was by head rotation in acutely and chronically labyrinthectomized cats, and by body rotation in animals with intact labyrinths. As earlier work had suggested that the same muscles may respond to both roll and pitch, the aim of

Table 8.1.   Response Vectors of Forelimb Muscles in the Tonic Neck Reflex[a]

Forelimb (heads of triceps brachii)	
L long	18 ± 9 (10)
R long	160 ± 8 (8)
L medial	-14 ± 7 (9)
R medial	-176 ± 8 (8)
L lateral	-11 ± 6 (5)
R lateral	-161 ± 6 (5)
Shoulder	
L infraspinatus	-24 ± 5 (8)
R infraspinatus	-150 ± 6 (7)
L supraspinatus	-38 ± 3 (12)
R supraspinatus	-148 ± 6 (11)

[a]Vector orientations for stimuli of 0.1 and 0.2 Hz, $\pm$ SE, are shown for each muscle. The number of experiments averaged is shown in parentheses. L, Left; R, right. (Modified from Wilson et al., 1986.)

these experiments was to determine whether forelimb and shoulder muscles were stimulated best by stimuli in a particular plane, i.e., had a direction of maximum sensitivity, or response vector. Similar experiments had recently demonstrated that the excitation of neck muscles by the vestibulocollic reflex was characterized by such a vector (Baker et al., 1985). In the experiments of Wilson et al. (1986) the orientation component of the vector was defined with a head-centered coordinate system, with 0° corresponding to the right ear, 90° to the nose, 180° to the left ear, and −90° to the tail, i.e., a vector of 0° indicates that maximum excitation was obtained with the head tilted right ear down (and chin to the left); similarly a vector orientation of −45° indicates that a nose up and a right ear down stimulus are equally effective (see Fig. 1 in Suzuki et al., 1985). The results, which were similar in labyrinth-intact and labyrinthectomized preparations, show that two out of three heads of triceps brachii (medial and lateral) as well as the shoulder extensors supra- and infraspinatus have vectors between nose up pitch and contralateral ear down (chin to the ipsilateral side); vectors of elbow muscles tend to be closer to roll than those of shoulder muscles (Table 8.1). The long head of triceps is excited by contralateral ear down roll and nose down pitch. With the exception of the response of the long head, the pattern observed by Wilson et al. (1986) is consistent with the results of earlier investigators. There are two additional points of interest. First, the orientation of muscle vectors is stable over a wide frequency range, showing that the receptors that give rise to the reflex themselves have directional sensitivities that are stable with frequency. Second, although muscle vectors remained stable for most of the duration of the experiment, they could differ from this central, stable period at the early and late stages of recording. Such variation shows that for any muscle the vector orientation is not fixed, which has implications for the circuitry producing the vector.

WHAT ARE THE RECEPTORS FOR THE REFLEX?

Since the work of McCouch et al. (1951) it has been accepted that the receptors for the reflex are in tissues very near the vertebral column, and from this grew the belief that they were neck joint receptors. Some time ago Wyke (1979) described Ruffini endings around the upper cervical vertebrae; these receptors are generally considered slowly adapting. Richmond and Bakker (1982) were unable to confirm these observations. On the other hand, there are great numbers of spindles in the small perivertebral muscles (Richmond and Abrahams, 1979a; Bakker and Richmond, 1982; Richmond and Bakker 1982; see Chapter 4) and these may provide an important afferent input for the TNR. Recent experiments (V. J. Wilson and Y. S. Chan, unpublished observations), in which the activity of afferents was recorded in the C2 dorsal root ganglion during head rotation, show that the dynamics of afferents identified as originating from spindle endings are quite similar to those of the reflex and of central neurons believed involved in the reflex pathway (see below).

WHAT IS THE SPINAL CIRCUITRY OF THE REFLEX?

Magnus' experiments (1914) showed that the TNR can be evoked in the spinal animal, in other words that it can be produced by a purely spinal pathway. It is also likely, a priori, that the pathway includes a supraspinal loop, because neck afferent information influences vestibulospinal and reticulospinal fibers (Brink et al., 1980; Boyle and Pompeiano, 1981a; Pompeiano et al., 1984), which in turn influence limb motoneurons directly or indirectly (see Wilson and Person, 1981). Whether the spinal circuitry can, by itself, produce a reflex with appropriate dynamics and spatial pattern in all four limbs is doubtful. Electric stimulation of neck afferents evokes a different pattern of synaptic activity in forelimb motoneurons in animals with intact and transected neuraxis (Nakajima et al., 1981) and the presence or level of activity of the brain stem modifies the response of spinal neurons to natural stimulation of neck receptors (see below). Before considering the role of descending pathways we must first describe the present knowledge of the spinal circuitry.

Intraspinal Pathways

Stimulation of neck afferents can produce synaptic potentials in forelimb and hindlimb motoneurons via fairly simple polysynaptic pathways (Kenins et al., 1978; Nakajima et al., 1981). There is no certainty that these responses are related to the TNR. However, it seems likely that they are, and that the synaptic potentials are produced by short and long propriospinal neurons, i.e., by neurons whose cell bodies are located in C3 and C4 and whose axons terminate at different segmental levels including the cervical and lumbar enlargements. Propriospinal neurons located in the lateral region of the gray matter in C3–C4 and acting monosynaptically on forelimb motoneurons have been studied in detail by Lundberg and his colleagues (e.g., Illert et al., 1977; Grant et al., 1980; Alstermark et al., 1984). We have now identified, in C4 and in L3–L4, populations of neurons, including some propriospinal neurons, whose activity is modulated by neck rotation (Wilson et al., 1984; Brink et al., 1984b, 1985; Suzuki et al., 1985). These neurons are located medially in the gray matter. Figure 8.2A shows the behavior of such a

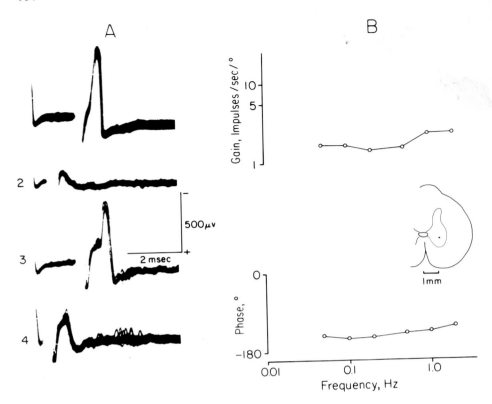

Figure 8.2.   Response of a propriospinal neuron in C4 to neck rotation. This neuron, whose location is shown in the inset, was excited by chin rotation to the contralateral side. (A) Antidromic response to stimulation in C5 (1) and C7 (3) is blocked by collision with spontaneous action potential at the start of sweep (2, 4). (B) Bode plot of response. A phase of −180 indicates peak chin rotation to the contralateral side. (From Brink et al., 1985.)

neuron, which could be activated antidromically from C5 and from C7, but not from more caudal electrode locations. Axons of cervical propriospinal neurons may terminate in the cervical enlargement, as in the case of the illustrated neuron, or project as far as the lubosacral cord; lumbar propriospinal neurons have been activated antidromically from the lumbosacral enlargement. The targets of these neurons are not known, and it remains to be determined whether their axons make synapses with motoneurons.

As illustrated in Figure 8.2B, the dynamics of cervical and lumbar neuron responses to sinusoidal neck stimulation are very similar to TNR dynamics, with the exception that the neuron phase is usually somewhat advanced with respect to that of muscle (compare with Figure 8.1). Although in the otherwise intact decerebrated cat the gains of cervical and lumbar interneurons are similar, experimental manipulations can differentially modify the gain of these populations. As shown by Table 8.2, acute labyrinthectomy causes a greater drop in gain in

Table 8.2.   Effect of Labyrinthectomy and Spinal Cord Section on Cervical and Lumbar Neurons[a]

	Gain (impulses sec^{-1} deg^{-1} of the response of spinal neurons to neck rotation)	
	C4	L3–L4
Intact labyrinth	2.5 ± 0.5 (22)[b]	2.5 ± 0.3 (44)
Labyrinthectomized	1.1 ± 0.4 (34)	0.6 ± 0.1 (44)
Rostral C1 section	1.1 ± 0.2 (23)	—

Number of modulated neurons found in C4 and in L3 in a series of three cats with the spinal cord transected rostrally in C1

C4	12/23
L3–L4	2/73

[a]Data from Brink et al. (1985), Suzuki et al. (1985), and Wilson et al. (1984).
[b]Value ± SEM. The number of the neurons is in parentheses.

lumbar than in cervical neurons; spinal transection at the rostral border of C1 has no further effect on cervical neurons, but makes it almost impossible to find modulated lumbar neurons (Wilson et al., 1984; Brink et al., 1985; Suzuki et al., 1985). Obviously the response of lumbar neurons to neck stimulation is much more dependent on the presence, or the activity level, of the brain stem.

The activity of many spinal neurons is modulated not only by neck rotation but also by vestibular stimulation (whole body tilt). As with the reflexes themselves, the directions of the two actions are always opposite, so that if the head is rotated on a stationary body, neck- and vestibular-evoked activities tend to cancel (Wilson et al., 1984; Suzuki et al., 1985). In addition, the activity of some neurons carrying neck-rotation signals, at least in the cervical cord, is influenced by input from the periphery, as shown, for example, by the effects of limb manipulation and stimulation of forelimb nerves (E. E. Brink, B. R. Park, I. Suzuki, and V. J. Wilson, unpublished observations).

Construction of the Motoneuron Vector

Each modulated neuron has a response vector, or direction of maximum sensitivity (Suzuki et al., 1985, 1986). Comparison of the vector distributions of cervical and lumbar neurons determined in labyrinthectomized cats reveals an important difference: there are many more nose-up than nose-down vectors for cervical neurons, whereas the reverse is true for lumbar neurons. The presence of many nose-up vectors in C4 neurons may be related to the fact that many of these neurons receive short-latency afferent input from the C2 dorsal root ganglion. Nose-up vectors are particularly prominent in neurons with such input (Suzuki et al., 1986). It is of some interest that the pattern of vector orientation of cervical and lumbar neurons parallels that of extensor muscle excitation by the TNR: recall that the reflex produces forelimb extension with nose-up, hindlimb extension with nose-down pitch.

Supraspinal activity influences not only the gain of the response of spinal neurons to neck rotation, but also the distribution of directional sensitivities. Table

Table 8.3. Influence of Labyrinthectomy on Distribution of Vectors
of Lumbar Neurons[a]

Response vectors	Intact cats	Labyrinthectomized cats
Roll, 0 or 180 ± 30°	28	17
Pitch, 90 or −90 ± 30°	6	16
Between roll and pitch	12	18

[a]Each column shows the number of neurons in each category. Data from Suzuki et al. (1985).

8.3 shows that the vectors of a greater fraction of lumbar neurons tend to be close to roll in cats with intact labyrinths than in labyrinthectomized cats (Suzuki et al., 1985).

The question arises, how is the motoneuron vector constructed? A likely model resembles the one proposed by Georgopoulos et al. (1983) for cortical control of movements. We have suggested (Wilson et al., 1986) that motoneuron directional sensitivity is produced by vectorial addition of the input from an array of premotor neurons, perhaps including propriospinal, reticulospinal, and vestibulospinal neurons. Modulation of the activity of the pool of premotor neurons by peripheral feedback and by central bias may change the vector of premotor neurons or determine which ones are active, and ultimately determine motoneuron vectors (Fig. 8.3). This model is consistent with the observations that muscle response vectors may change in the course of an experiment and that both gain and response vectors of populations of spinal neurons can be modified by supraspinal control.

In summary, experiments have demonstrated that medially located proprios-

Figure 8.3. Proposed model for motoneuron vector determination. A pool of premotor neurons receives input from vestibular and neck receptors. Each premotor neuron has a neck response vector, as shown, and many have vestibular response vectors that are opposite in direction. A bias of central origin, together with peripheral feedback, can determine which premotor neurons are active and perhaps change their vectors. The active premotor neurons determine the directional sensitivity of the motoneuron by vectorial addition.

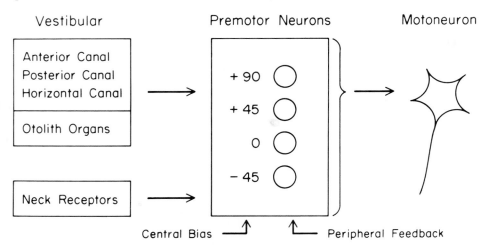

pinal neurons have properties that make them likely candidates to be part of the spinal circuit of the TNR. We can hypothesize a circuit similar to that described in 1941 by Lloyd for the bulbospinal correlation system, in which propriospinal neurons act in series and in parallel with descending pathways, particularly the vestibulospinal and reticulospinal tracts. The role of these pathways is described in detail in the next chapter.

SUMMARY

Afferent input from the neck plays a significant role in a set of stereotyped postural reflexes called tonic neck reflexes. Characteristically, in these reflexes, roll rotation of the head leads to extension of the limbs on the side to which the chin is turned, and flexion of the limbs on the opposite side. Dorsiflexion of the head leads to extension of the forelimbs and flexion of the hindlimbs, whereas ventriflexion elicits a reverse pattern. The nature of the postural responses can be described using linear systems analysis. These studies show that EMG responses in forelimb muscles follow sinusoidal changes in head position quite faithfully at low frequencies; at higher frequencies above 0.1 Hz, the patterns of response suggest that the reflex is sensitive to the velocity of the movement as well as the position of the head. The magnitude of the reflex response in an individual muscle is affected by the plane in which the head is moved. The direction of movement that evokes a maximal response has been identified for a range of forelimb muscles and varies in a predictable way for different muscles crossing the shoulder and/or elbow.

Historically, the receptors responsible for tonic neck reflexes have been considered to lie in the intervertebral joints of the neck, but the numerous spindles in intervertebral muscles may also play a significant role. The afferent information from this receptor system can affect the activities of forelimb and hindlimb motoneurons through intraspinal pathways. Certain types of interneurons that are interposed in such pathways respond with firing patterns that reflect the dynamic properties of tonic neck reflexes. However, a number of brain stem pathways are also involved in the development of tonic neck reflexes. Of particular significance in the ultimate expression of tonic neck reflexes is the contribution made by the vestibular system, because head movement will elicit vestibular reflexes that are opposite in sign to tonic neck reflexes. Thus, vestibular and tonic neck reflexes tend to modify or cancel each other during head movements in the normal animal.

9

The Tonic Neck Reflex: Supraspinal Control

O. POMPEIANO

Descriptions of tonic neck reflexes presented in the previous chapter have highlighted propriospinal mechanisms that may underlie the characteristic changes of posture evoked by head movement. However, any discussion of tonic neck reflexes would be incomplete without exploring the potentially significant roles of medullary structures that may also influence the postural activity of spinal motoneurons. Of particular interest are two pathways that project onto α and static γ motoneurons supplying extensor muscles. The first is the vestibulospinal (VS) pathway that originates from the lateral vestibular nucleus of Deiters (LVN) and projects to all segments of the spinal cord (Pompeiano and Brodal, 1957). This pathway exerts an excitatory influence by way of monosynaptic or polysynaptic connections onto motoneurons innervating extensor muscles (cf. Pompeiano, 1975; Chapter 11). The second pathway, the inhibitory reticulospinal (RS) pathway, originates from the medial aspect of the medullary reticular formation (RF) (Magoun and Rhines, 1946) and produces postsynaptic inhibition in extensor motoneurons (cf. Pompeiano, 1975; Chapter 11).

It has been well established that many neurons in the vestibular nuclei (Fredrickson et al., 1966; Hikosaka and Maeda, 1973; Mori and Mikami, 1973; Rubin et al., 1975, 1977, 1978; Schwarz et al., 1975; Thoden et al., 1975; Thoden and Wirbitzky, 1976; Brink et al., 1980, 1981a) and in the medullary RF (Thoden et al., 1975; Thoden and Wirbitzky, 1976; Coulter et al., 1977) receive an input from neck afferents. The following section describes the responses observed in excitatory VS neurons and *presumably* inhibitory RS neurons during sinusoidal rotation of the body in a manner that excites neck receptors. The contributions of these pathways to postural adjustments of the neck and limbs are then discussed.

RESPONSES OF VESTIBULOSPINAL NEURONS TO NECK ROTATION

When the head moves, the firing patterns of brain stem neurons involved in tonic neck reflexes might be expected to change in a fashion appropriate for producing the changes in extensor muscle tone. In tonic neck reflexes, axial rotation (around an animal's longitudinal axis) with the head held stationary or axial rotation of the head in the labyrinthectomized animal predictably increases the activity of forelimb extensors on the side to which the chin points and excites the dorsal neck extensors on the opposite side (see Chapter 8 for review). Hindlimb extensors are less influenced by the reflex; in decerebrate cats, they either fail to respond or show a pattern of modulation similar to that of forelimb extensors but with a much smaller amplitude (Manzoni et al., 1984).

To explore the role of descending vestibulospinal pathways in neck reflexes, Boyle and Pompeiano (1980b) recorded the responses of 120 LVN neurons as the body was rotated slowly (at 0.026 Hz, $\pm$ 5–10°) around the longitudinal axis with the head held fixed. The proportion of responsive neurons was higher in the rostroventral LVN (rvLVN, 74%) than in the dorsocaudal LVN (dcLVN, 49%). The rvLVN projects mainly, although not exclusively, to the cervical spinal cord, whereas the dcLVN projects primarily to lumbosacral segments (Pompeiano and Brodal, 1957). The difference between rvLVN and dcLVN neurons may be related to the fact that tonic neck reflexes have more effective actions on neck and forelimb extensors than hindlimb extensors. The responses of LVN neurons were primarily related to neck position, as shown by an average phase lead of 19° with respect to the extreme neck displacements. In addition, LVN neurons are known to respond to sinusoidal lateral bending of the cervical axis (Kasper and Thoden, 1981).

In order to relate the response patterns of LVN neurons with postural adjustments, Marchand et al. (1987) studied the effects of slow neck rotations on 109 LVN neurons activated antidromically by electrical stimulation of the spinal cord between T12 and L1, and thus identified to project into lumbosacral segments of the spinal cord (lVS neurons). The response characteristics of these neurons are shown in Table 9.1(A). The lVS neurons showed an average phase lead of 52° with respect to the extreme neck displacements, which was higher than that previously obtained from unidentified LVN neurons. This difference can be understood if we consider that the majority of recorded lVS neurons (86/109, i.e., 79%) were located in the dcLVN, which is particularly under the direct inhibitory control of the cerebellar vermis (Ito, 1972; Fanardjian and Sarkissian, 1980; Akaike, 1983a).

Most of the responsive lVS neurons (79%) were maximally excited during *side-up* neck displacement; only 11% showed the opposite response pattern (Fig. 9.1A). Thus, the responses of neurons projecting to lumbosacral levels resemble the response of limb motoneurons to neck rotation. In contrast to the strong preponderance of neurons excited by side-up displacement in the lVS population, the more inclusive population of LVN neurons studied by Boyle and Pompeiano (1980b), whose projections were not identified, had approximately equal numbers of neurons responding to side-up (54%) and to side-down (44%) rotations. This suggests that the latter population contains an admixture of cells with the limb extensorlike response pattern of lVS neurons and cells with the opposite response which could contribute to the side-down activation pattern observed in ipsilateral neck extensors.

RESPONSES OF MEDULLARY RETICULOSPINAL NEURONS TO NECK ROTATION

Srivastava et al. (1984) studied the effects of slow neck rotation on the activity of neurons in the ventrocaudal and medial aspects of the medullary RF, corre-

Table 9.1. Responses of Lateral Vestibulospinal Neurons[a] and Medullary Reticulospinal Neurons[b] to Neck Rotation at Standard Parameters of Stimulation (0.026 Hz, ±10°)

	(A) LVN neurons[c]			(B) Medullary reticular neurons[c]		
	Antidromic IVS	Nonantidromic LVN	Total LVN	Antidromic IRS	Nonantidromic RF	Total RF
Number of units	109	13	122	85	47	132
Responsive (R) units	75 (68.8)	7 (53.8)	82 (67.2)	66 (77.6)	31 (66.0)	97 (73.5)
Unresponsive units	34 (31.2)	6 (46.2)	40 (32.8)	19 (22.4)	16 (34.0)	35 (26.5)
Conduction velocity of R units	89.8 ± 21.0	—	—	66.3 ± 27.7	—	—
Base discharge frequency of R units (mean ± SD)	21.6 ± 17.6	17.6 ± 20.3	21.3 ± 17.7	10.4 ± 8.2	13.1 ± 11.1	11.3 ± 9.2
Gain of R units (mean ± SD)	0.49 ± 0.40	0.48 ± 0.56	0.49 ± 0.42	0.52 ± 0.45	0.32 ± 0.27	0.45 ± 0.41
Sensitivity of R units (mean ±SD)	3.30 ± 3.42 (n = 63)	3.08 ± 2.97 (n = 5)	3.28 ± 3.37 (n = 68)	5.70 ± 4.73 (n = 61)	3.35 ± 3.42 (n = 30)	4.90 ± 4.47 (n = 91)
Phase angle of R units						
From +90° to −15° (LVN)	8 (10.7)	3 (42.9)	11 (13.4)			
From +90° to −30° (RF)				47 (71.2)	23 (74.2)	70 (72.2)
From +165° to −90° (LVN)	59 (78.6)	4 (57.1)	63 (76.8)			
From +150° to −90° (RF)				13 (19.7)	6 (19.35)	19 (19.6)
From +90° to +150° and from −30° to −90° (LVN)	8 (10.7)	0	8 (9.8)	6 (9.1)	2 (6.45)	8 (8.2)

[a]Marchand et al. (1987).
[b]Srivastava et al. (1984).
[c]Abbreviations: antidromic IVS and IRS, vestibulospinal and reticulospinal neurons activated antidromically by spinal cord stimulation at T12–L1; nonantidromic LVN and RF, lateral vestibular nucleus and reticular formation neurons not antidromically activated by stimulation of the spinal cord at T12–L1. Conduction velocity of axons is in meters per second; base discharge frequency, mean firing rate in impulses per second evaluated during standard parameters of neck rotation; gain of first harmonic, change of the mean firing rate per degree of displacement (impulses per second per degree); sensitivity o the first harmonic, percentage change of the mean firing rate per degree (%/degree); phase angle of the first harmonic, in degrees of phase lead (positive values) or phase lag (negative values) with respect to the side-down neck displacement. Numbers of units without parentheses are slightly lower than the corresponding numbers of R units due to silent or slowly discharging neurons showing a cut-off of their response, so that their sensitivity could not be evaluated. Numbers in parentheses are percentages.

sponding to the inhibitory area of Magoun and Rhines (1946). The majority of these neurons (85/132) were activated antidromically by electrical stimulation of the spinal cord between T12 and L1 and thus projected to the lumbosacral segments of the spinal cord (lRS neurons). Table 9.1(B) illustrates the response characteristics of these identified neurons. Most neurons (71%) increased their firing rate during *side-down* neck rotation, but 20% showed an increase during *side-up* neck rotation (Fig. 9.1B). The responses of the two main populations of lRS neurons to neck rotation showed an average phase lead of 40° with respect to the extreme neck displacements, which did not greatly differ from that of lVS neurons.

It is not yet possible to establish conclusively that the recorded lRS neurons belong to the medullary inhibitory system, but several lines of evidence support this position (cf. Srivastava et al., 1984). In particular, the lRS neurons were found to increase their firing rates during episodes of postural atonia associated with postsynaptic inhibition of extensor motoneurons that occured after intravenous injection of an anticholinesterase in decerebrate cats (Srivastava et al., 1982; cf. Pompeiano, 1980). The fact that these presumably inhibitory lRS neurons responded in a pattern exactly opposite to that of excitatory lVS neurons suggests that the two effects might be complementary at the level of extensor motoneurons. During neck rotation, hindlimb motoneurons on the side to which the chin is turned would not only be excited by an increased discharge of excitatory lVS neurons, but also disinhibited by a reduced discharge of presumably inhibitory RS neurons.

ROLE OF MEDULLARY RETICULOSPINAL NEURONS IN THE GAIN REGULATION OF THE NECK REFLEX

Recent evidence suggests that the activity of the lRS system may have an important influence upon the gain of neck reflexes in limb motoneurons. In the decerebrate animal, in which the activity of lRS neurons is low (Srivastava et al., 1984), reflex gain is also quite low (Boyle and Pompeiano, 1984; Manzoni et al., 1983a, 1984; d'Ascanio et al., 1985a; Pompeiano et al., 1985b, c). Following systematic administration of small doses of eserine sulfate, an anticholinesterase, the resting discharge of lRS neurons increased and the activity of limb extensor muscles decreased as expected given the presumed inhibitory action of lRS neurons (Pompeiano, 1980; Srivastava et al., 1982). In addition, the drug caused a large increase in neck-reflex modulation of extensor muscles in the forelimbs (Pompeiano et al., 1983a) and the hindlimbs (Manzoni et al., 1984). However, no change in the phase angle of the electromyographic responses was observed. It is reasonable to assume that increased modulation of lRS inhibitory action on the limb extensors played a significant role in this enhancement of reflex gain.

The cholinergic neurons responsible for the increase in lRS neuron activity have been shown to be located in the dorsal pontine RF, which is the origin for a tegmentoreticular tract ending in the medullary inhibitory area (Sakai et al., 1979; cf. Sakai, 1980) (Fig. 9.2A). An electrolytic lesion limited to this pontine tegmental structure not only decreases the response gain of the triceps brachii to

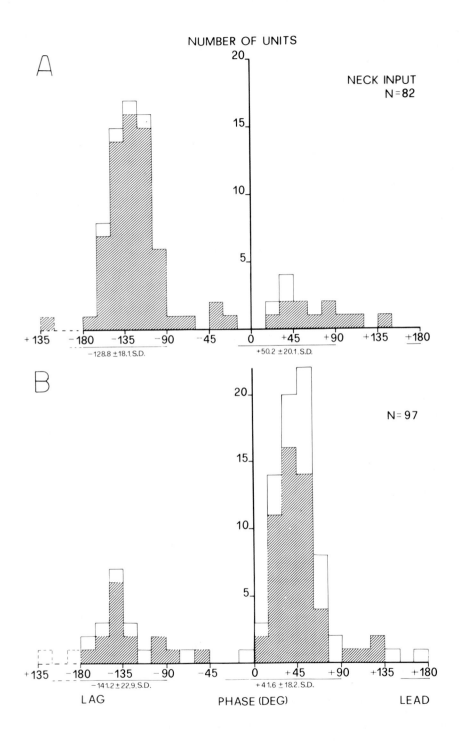

neck rotation in decerebrate cats, but also suppresses the increase in gain following injection of anticholinesterase (d'Ascanio et al., 1985b; cf. Pompeiano, 1985). In contrast, increased activity of dorsal pontine reticular neurons produced by local injections of cholinomimetic substances such as carbachol or bethanechol greatly enhances the response gain of the triceps brachii to neck rotation (Barnes et al., 1985).

It is of interest that the cholinergic pontine tegmental neurons described above are, in turn, inhibited by neurons in the noradrenergic locus coeruleus (LC) (cf. Pompeiano, 1980; Sakai, 1980) (Fig. 9.2A). Thus destruction of the LC increases the resting discharge of both the cholinergic pontine tegmental structure and the related inhibitory RS neurons of the medulla and also increases the gain of responses in limb extensors to neck rotation (d'Ascanio et al., 1985a). Similar results were also obtained after functional inactivation of the noradrenergic LC neurons either by injecting clonidine (an α_2-agonist) into the LC (Fig. 9.2B and C) or injecting prazosin (an α_1-antagonist) into the dorsal pontine RF (Pompeiano et al., 1985a).

In conclusion, the available data indicate that inhibitory RS neurons are tonically excited by cholinergic pontine tegmental neurons, which in turn are inhibited by noradrenergic LC neurons. An increased discharge of these inhibitory RS neurons following either activation of the cholinergic pontine tegmental structure or inactivation of the noradrenergic LC neurons would lead to a greater disinhibition of limb extensor motoneurons during side-up neck rotation. These motoneurons would then respond more efficiently to the same excitatory VS volleys elicited by given parameters of neck stimulation, thus increasing the response gain of the corresponding muscles to neck rotation. The system described above may thus operate as a "variable gain regulator" modulating motoneuronal activation during the neck reflex. The shifting levels of reticulospinal inhibition produced by the pontine tegmentum may also influence neck reflex gain by altering transmission of signals by spinal interneurons such as Renshaw cells (cf. Pompeiano et al., 1985b, c).

Pompeiano et al. (1985b, c) postulated that in decerebrate preparations the excitatory VS volleys driven during side-up neck rotation activate not only ipsilateral hindlimb extensor motoneurons, but also the Renshaw cells which mediate

---

Figure 9.1.   Distribution of the phase angle of the first harmonic of responses of LVN neurons (A) and medullary reticular neurons (B) to neck rotation at 0.026 Hz, ± 10°. Among these responsive neurons, 75 out of 82 LVN neurons and 66 out of 97 medullary reticular units were antidromically activated by stimulation of the spinal cord at T12–L1 (IRS neurons: hatched columns), whereas the remaining units were not identified antidromically (RF neurons: open columns). The phase angle of responses was evaluated with respect to the extreme side-down position of the neck, indicated by 0°. The positive and negative numbers on the abscissa indicate the phase lead and lag of responses, respectively. Mean value and standard deviation of the phase angles corresponding to populations of neurons excited by side-down or side-up displacement of the neck are given below each histogram. (From Marchand et al., 1987, and Srivastava et al., 1984).

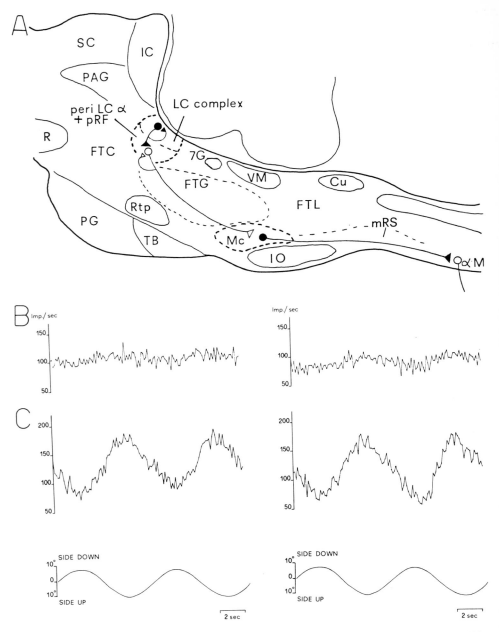

Figure 9.2.   Structures involved in the gain regulation of the neck-to-forelimb reflex. (A) Schematic sagittal section of the brain stem, showing anatomical connections between the noradrenergic locus coeruleus (LC) neurons and the cholinergic neurons located in the dorsal aspect of the pontine reticular formation (pRF); this structure projects to the magnocellular part of the medullary RF (Mc), from which the inhibitory reticulospinal system (mRS) ending on extensor α-motoneurons (M) originates. Both LC and pRF neurons give rise to self-inhibitory and self-excitatory recurrent collaterals, respectively; inhibitory or excitatory neurons are actually indicated by filled or empty symbols. SC, superior colliculus; IC, inferior colliculus; PAG, periaqueductal grey; R, red nucleus; PG, pontine grey;

recurrent inhibition; these Renshaw interneurons would then fire in phase with the VS neurons, thus contributing to the low response gain of the corresponding muscle to neck rotation. However, after cholinergic activation of the inhibitory RS neurons, the Renshaw cells would be decoupled from their input motoneurons to undergo the most efficient excitatory control of the RS pathway. In this instance these Renshaw cells would fire in phase with the RS neurons, thus decreasing their firing rate during side-up neck rotation. The resulting disinhibition of limb extensor motoneurons would then be responsible for the increased gain of response of the corresponding muscles to neck stimulation (cf. Pompeiano, 1984b).

COMMON RESPONSE FEATURES OF VESTIBULOSPINAL AND MEDULLARY RETICULOSPINAL NEURONS

Both the lVS (Marchand et al., 1987) and the medullary lRS neurons (Srivastava et al., 1984) that showed the predominant response pattern to neck rotation had on the average higher gains than those neurons displaying the opposite response pattern (Table 9.2). This finding indicates that afferent pathways originating from different populations of neck receptors that respond to side-up or side-down neck rotation are not homogeneously distributed among the lVS and the lRS neurons. However, independent of the response pattern, both the resting discharge as well as the dynamic characteristics of responses of lVS and lRS neurons to neck rotation were in part at least related to the cell size (Pompeiano et al., 1983b, 1987).

The responses of LVN (Boyle and Pompeiano, 1980b) and medullary RF neurons (Srivastava et al., 1984) to increasing frequencies of neck rotation were also investigated. In both populations, both the gain and phase angle of responses remained relatively stable as the frequency of neck rotation was gradually changed from 0.008 to 0.05 Hz. Their gain and phase lead then increased as frequencies were raised further from 0.05 to 0.3 Hz (see Fig. 9.3 for responses of medullary reticular neurons). These data suggest that responses are strongly influenced by neck position, but at higher frequencies of rotation they may also be influenced

---

Rtp, tegmental reticular nucleus (pericentral division); TB, trapezoid body; IO, inferior olive; 7G, genu of the facial nerve; FTG, gigantocellular tegmental field; FTL, lateral tegmental field; Cu, cuneate nucleus; VM, dorsal motor nucleus of vagus. (B and C) Decerebrate cat. Sequential pulse density histograms showing averaged multiunit EMG responses of the right triceps brachii to neck rotation at 0.15 Hz, $\pm$ 10°; the lower traces monitor the neck displacement. (B) illustrates control records with an average base frequency of 96.6 impulses/sec, a response gain of the first harmonic of 0.68 impulses/sec/deg, and a phase lag of $-165.6°$ with respect to the ipsilateral side-down neck rotation. (C) illustrates responses to the same parameters of neck rotation obtained 52 and 54 min after local injection in the ipsilateral LC of 0.25 μl of the α_2-adrenergic agonist clonidine at a concentration of 0.015 μg/μl. In this instance the average base frequency corresponded to 123.0 impulses/sec, the response gain was 4.31 impulses/sec/deg, and the phase angle corresponded to a lag of $-178.8°$. (From Pompeiano and coworkers, unpublished.)

Table 9.2. Comparison of the Responses of Lateral Vestibulospinal Neurons[a] and Medullary Reticulospinal Neurons[b] Displaying Different Response Patterns to Neck Rotation at Standard Parameters of Stimulation (0.026 Hz, ±10°)

Phase angle of neck responses[c]	Responsive (R) units	Nonresponsive units	Conduction velocity of R units (mean ± SD)	Base discharge frequency of R units (mean ± SD)	Gain of R units (mean ± SD)	Sensitivity of R units (mean ± SD)	Phase angle of R units (mean ± SD)
(A) Vestibulospinal neurons[c]							
From +90° to −15°	8		89.4 ± 11.2	22.9 ± 17.8	0.34 ± 0.32	1.57 ± 1.54 (n = 6)	+55.9 ± 21.0°
From +165° to −90°	59		91.7 ± 20.9	20.8 ± 17.6	0.53 ± 0.43	3.66 ± 3.54 (n = 49)	−128.5 ± 18.1°
From +90° to +165° and from −15° to −90°	8		93.5 ± 18.7	25.9 ± 18.2	0.26 ± 0.14	2.36 ± 3.43 (n = 8)	
Total population (n = 109)	75 (68.8)	34 (31.2)	91.6 ± 19.7	21.6 ± 17.6	0.49 ± 0.40	3.30 ± 3.42 (n = 63)	
(B) Reticulospinal neurons[c]							
From +90° to −30°	47		76.5 ± 26.5	10.9 ± 7.9 (n = 43)	0.63 ± 0.46	6.84 ± 4.87 (n = 43)	+39.0 ± 14.8°
From +150° to −90°	13		56.3 ± 18.0	10.8 ± 10.5 (n = 12)	0.25 ± 0.21	3.72 ± 3.72 (n = 12)	−137.7 ± 19.7°
From +90° to +150° and from −30° to −90°	6		53.2 ± 15.2	7.1 ± 4.6 (n = 6)	0.11 ± 0.09	1.61 ± 0.98 (n = 6)	
Total population (n = 110)	66 (60.0)	44 (40.0)	70.4 ± 25.8	10.5 ± 8.2 (n = 61)	0.52 ± 0.45	5.70 ± 4.73 (n = 61)	

[a]Pompeiano et al. (1987).
[b]Pompeiano et al. (1983b).
[c]Abbreviations as in Table 9.1. Vestibulospinal and reticulospinal neurons are activated antidromically by spinal cord stimulation at T12–L1.

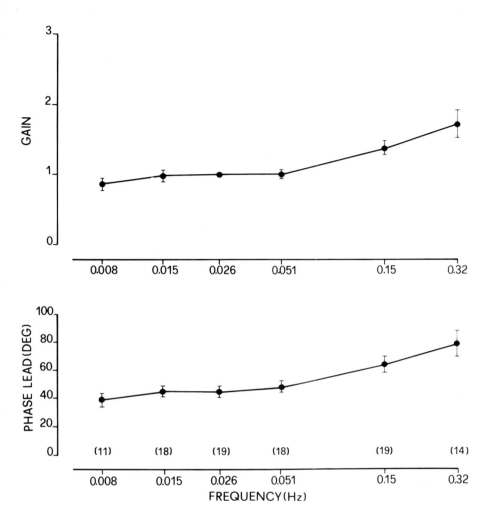

Figure 9.3. Effects of changing frequency of sinusoidal neck rotation on the gain and phase angle of responses of medullary reticular neurons. The upper diagram shows the average gain of responses of 19 medullary reticular neurons, 18 of which were antidromically identified as IRS neurons, to increasing frequencies of sinusoidal neck rotation at the peak amplitude of 10°. Among these units, 16 were excited by side-down neck rotation and depressed during side-up neck rotation, whereas 3 showed the opposite response pattern. The gains of unit responses were normalized at 0.026 Hz. The lower diagram shows the average phase angle of corresponding responses for the extreme side-down or side-up position; the phase angles of units excited by side-up neck rotation were reversed by 180° before averaging. Note the moderate increase in gain of responses from 0.86 impulses/sec/deg at 0.008 Hz to 1.73 impulses/sec/deg at 0.32 Hz. The phase angle of responses increased from an average lead of +38.7° at 0.008 Hz to a lead of +70.9° at 0.32 Hz. Both mean values (closed circles) and standard errors (bars) of responses have been plotted; the numbers of units tested for each parameter of stimulation are in parentheses. (From Srivastava et al., 1984.)

by the angular velocity of neck rotation. These findings are consistent with the results of recent experiments in which the dynamics of the neck reflexes acting on limb and neck extensors had been investigated (Peterson et al., 1981b; Ezure and Wilson, 1983).

The afferent signals responsible for eliciting responses in both LVN and medullary RF neurons probably originate from deep neck receptors innervated from C1 and C2 as discussed in Chapter 8. The nuchal input could be transmitted to the LVN and medullary RF by way of one or more of the transcerebellar pathways that are relayed through group x of the medulla (Mergner et al., 1982), the external cuneate nucleus (Murakami and Kato, 1983), or the central cervical nucleus (Hirai et al., 1984b). Information related to neck position could also be carried out by the uncrossed cervical spinoreticular pathway, which may not only activate neurons of the medullary inhibitory RS system, but also inhibit neurons of the excitatory VS system, by utilizing the precerebellar lateral reticular nucleus (LRN) and the corresponding cerebellar loop (cf. Pompeiano, 1979). Recent experiments have, in fact, shown that side-down neck rotation excites most precerebellar LRN neurons (Kubin et al., 1981a; cf. Pompeiano, 1981) and Purkinje cells located in the ipsilateral vermal cortex of the cerebellar anterior lobe, including those which project to the LVN (Denoth et al., 1979a, 1980). In turn, the Purkinje cell discharge inhibits the corresponding fastigial neurons (Stanojević, 1981) as well as the dcLVN neurons projecting to the lumbosacral segments of the spinal cord (Marchand et al., 1987). Therefore it appears that during side-down neck rotation the proprioceptive excitatory input, which acts on neurons in the medial RF, is transformed through the cerebellum into an inhibitory input acting on the dcLVN neurons. The role that the cerebellum exerts on the dynamic characteristics of responses of LVN neurons to neck rotation has been evaluated by comparing the results obtained in normal decerebrate animals with those obtained after cerebellectomy (Boyle and Pompeiano, 1980b, 1981b,c; Marchand et al., 1987; Pompeiano et al., 1987).

Nuchal afferent input is not the only sensory system to influence the activity of LVN and presumably inhibitory RF neurons. Both LVN (Boyle and Pompeiano, 1980a; Schor and Miller, 1982; Marchand et al., 1987; Pompeiano et al., 1987) and RF neurons (Manzoni et al., 1983b) also respond to stimulation of labyrinthine receptors that are excited selectively by rotating the whole animal around its longitudinal axis, but the responses elicited by this stimulation are opposite to those elicited by rotating the neck in the same direction (cf. Pompeiano, 1984a). This finding is consistent with the observation that the postural adjustments involving limb and neck extensors during animal rotation (Schor and Miller, 1981) are opposite in sign to those elicited during neck rotation (Ezure and Wilson, 1983), for the same direction of animal and neck orientations. Reciprocal patterns of convergence of both labyrinth and neck inputs were also obtained at the level of precerebellar LRN neurons (Kubin et al., 1980, 1981a,b; cf. Pompeiano, 1981), Purkinje cells projecting the LVN (Denoth et al., 1979a, 1980) and fastigial neurons (Stanojević, 1981). When neck and labyrinthine inputs are elicited concurrently, their effects can be predicted by summing the response vectors corresponding to each input (Denoth et al., 1979a; Boyle and Pompeiano, 1981a; Kubin et al., 1981b; Stanojević, 1981; Pompeiano et al., 1984; Stampacchia et al., 1987; cf. Pompeiano, 1981, 1984a). The cancellation of the two inputs would tend to keep the posture stable as the head is in motion (Lindsay et al., 1976; Manzoni et al., 1983a; Ezure and Wilson, 1984; cf. von Holst and Mittelstaedt, 1950).

SUMMARY

Some of the pathways implicated in the development of tonic neck reflexes relay in medullary structures. Of particular interest are two pathways, an excitatory pathway that originates from the lateral vestibular nucleus and an inhibitory pathway from the medial part of the medullary reticular formation. Both pathways are influenced by sensory signals from the neck. When the body is rotated with respect to the head, neurons of the excitatory vestibulospinal system increase their rate of firing on the side to which the chin is pointed, whereas neurons presumed to contribute to the inhibitory reticulospinal system show a reduced rate of firing. Both systems project onto spinal motoneurons in which their effects are complementary. For example, hindlimb motoneurons on the side to which the chin is pointed are excited by the augmented input of the vestibulospinal system and disinhibited by the reduced input from the inhibitory reticulospinal system. Both systems also receive input from receptors in the vestibular apparatus. This input modulates the firing of medullary neurons in a pattern reciprocal to that elicited by neck receptors. Thus, in a situation in which the head moves on the body, vestibular and neck inputs would tend to cancel one another so that posture remains stable.

The role played by the inhibitory pathway originating from the medullary reticular formation has recently come under much study. This work suggests that inhibitory reticulospinal neurons may act to regulate the degree to which motoneurons can be activated by tonic neck reflexes. Reticulospinal neurons are excited tonically by cholinergic neurons in the pontine tegmentum, and these cholinergic neurons can be inhibited in turn by noradrenergic neurons in the locus coeruleus. Thus, changes in the activity of neurons in either the pontine tegmentum or the locus coeruleus can modify the degree to which reticulospinal neurons inhibit limb extensor motoneurons during body-on-head movements. Experimental evidence also suggests that the inhibitory reticulospinal pathway could influence the magnitude of reflex responses during head movements by altering the transmission of information through spinal interneurons such as Renshaw cells.

10

Chronic Recording of Neck Sensory Input to Vestibular Neurons

J. H. FULLER

Afferent input from the muscles and/or joints of the neck plays an important role in a number of reflexes including local cervicocollic reflexes and more generalized postural reflexes. To understand the motor effects of these reflexes, much attention has been focused on the influence of neck sensory afferents on the activity of neurons in the brain stem and spinal cord. Most of these studies, summarized in the previous three chapters, have been carried out in anesthetized or reduced preparations in which neck receptors are stimulated by passive deviations of the neck with and without concomitant labyrinthine stimulation. Because the effects of nuchal input interact with those of the labyrinth during most natural head movements, many previous studies have examined the relative weighting between convergent vestibular and neck inputs. The present chapter explores the way in which stimulation of receptors in the neck or the vestibular apparatus influences the activity of single brain stem neurons in conscious cats that are executing active, voluntary head movements.

In active movements neuronal activity can be influenced not only by primary sensory responses, which result directly from the stimulus, but also by the centrally derived, or internally generated, efferent components, and by secondary sensory responses or reafference, which result from motor commands. An example of this motor–sensory delineation can be seen when recording central activity related to a putative spindle input. A primary sensory response would result directly from perturbation of the spindle. There are two other possibilities: first, the recorded neural activity could be premotor and related to α or γ motor output; second, the neuron could reflect sensory activity secondarily, not from the stimulus itself, but from reafference due to γ drive or unloading in the case of α activation. Recordings from vestibular neurons with neck sensory inputs (Fuller, 1978) have revealed a class of neurons in which this problem is exemplified. Before describing these data, the general problem of distinguishing motor–sensory phenomena in chronic recordings will be examined.

Three areas of the brain have been the subjects of experiments in which complex interactions of sensory and motor signals have been related to movements and/or receptor activation. These examples will show that "higher level" (e.g., higher than the γ effect of spindles) centrally generated signals alter single neuron responses to constant stimuli, and that the motivational state of the animal plays a critical role in relatively direct, short latency sensory responses to carefully controlled stimuli.

The experiments of Goldberg and Wurtz (1972) on monkey superior colliculus provided one of the earliest demonstrations that an internally generated signal could influence sensory input. They observed that the response to a visual stimulus was enhanced when the animal was prepared to make an eye movement to a point in visual space corresponding to the receptive field of the recorded neuron. They termed this the enhancement effect, and showed that the effect was specific to a predetermined motivational state of the monkey. Later work revealed similar effects in other regions of the brain, including the parietal cortex, about which more will be said below.

The work of Evarts and Tanji (1974) on limb sensory inputs to the monkey cortex provides a second example of motivational (internally generated) effects upon sensory input to central neurons. The experiments were initially based on Hammond's (1956) observation that the amplitude of the stretch reflex of the arm was altered depending on the subject's predetermined intention to resist or assist perturbation of limb position, with the resist state producing the larger reflex amplitude. Recording in monkey motor cortex, Evarts and Tanji found that some motor cortical neurons increased their activity in response to instructions that an ensuing trial was about to begin, which they termed the "set." They also found that the sensory response to the perturbation was magnified if the "set" were similar to Hammond's "resist" state. Thus, the neurons in the motor cortex showed an enhanced response to proprioceptive sensory inflow in a manner related to the subject's internally generated activity.

A final example comes from studies of the posterior parietal cortex, in which differences in semantics and interpretation have led to serious questions about what constitutes a sensory, sensory-enhanced, or motor-related response in single neurons recorded in this cortical association area. In an initial set of experiments Yin and Mountcastle (1978) examined sensory and motor-related activity of Areas 5 and 7, in part motivated by the observation that humans suffering unilateral damage to this area had clinical deficiencies related to their immediate extrapersonal space, typically on the side opposite the lesion. They found neurons in monkey Area 7 which increased their firing rate when movement of an extremity and/or the eyes was made to a point in space within narrowly defined boundaries. They proposed that such neurons were part of an ensemble that identified the point in space and that initiated movement toward that point in response to a stimulus or target. However, a different interpretation was suggested by Robinson and Goldberg (1978)—that the heightened activity was the result of an enhanced sensory response and was prerequisite to, not the cause of, the initiation of movement.

In each of the above examples, sensory-related activity recorded in single neurons was altered as a result of an internally generated signal. Consideration of such effects is a concern mainly when recording from awake animals—although "biasing" of reflexes may also be seen in acute preparations (see Wilson, Chapter 8). Studies of vestibular neurons have revealed that the animal's behavior (or, i.e., "set") may also affect the response to a controlled stimulus. Before

discussing these neurons, it is necessary to describe methods for the initial characterization of the source of afferent input; in the case of motor cortex and superior
colliculus, an initial advantage is gained because the topographic disposition of
neurons is correlated with the type of afferent input that they receive. No such
topography related to receptor origin appears to be present in the vestibular nucleus; thus standard tests to identify putative vestibular semicircular canal and
neck proprioceptive inputs are reviewed.

Fuller (1978) recorded the activity of brain stem neurons in cats trained to
make ballistic head movements between visual targets. Neurons were found that
were related to eye or head movement. Characteristics of neurons associated with
eye movements are covered elsewhere (Fuller et al., 1983; Shimazu, 1983); only
those neurons related to head movement are described here. Four categories of
neurons were identified according to the input that they received from semicircular
canal and neck receptors and to the relation of their firing rates to head motor
output. Neurons in Categories 1 and 2 were distributed throughout the medial
vestibular nucleus and nucleus prepositus hypoglossi, and received input from
both canal and neck receptors. However, Category 1 neurons were responsive
almost exclusively to canal input, whereas those in Category 2 were influenced
either equally by sensory input from the neck and the canal, or more strongly by
neck sensory input. Category 3 neurons were found in the descending vestibular
nucleus; their activities were modulated by active and passive neck perturbations.
These neurons had sensory responses that were very sensitive to vibration and
thus were presumably from a Paciniform-like receptor input. Category 4 neurons
showed no consistent modulation when canal or neck receptors were activated.
However, they showed intense activity during active head turns. Category 4 neurons were located in the medial reticular formation beneath Category 1 and 2
neurons, and are included to illustrate activity related to internally generated signals.

The above classification of four categories of neurons is based in part on
passive tests shown in Figure 10.1 and in part on active tests shown in Figure
10.2. Two standard passive tests consisted of (1) whole body rotation (WBR, Fig.
10.1A) with the head fixed on the trunk, thus passively stimulating the canals;
and (2) rotation of the trunk beneath an earth-fixed head, or head fixed in space
(HFS, Fig. 10.1B), thus passively stimulating neck afferents. Neurons in Categories 1, 2, and 3 clearly modulate their firing rate in response to WBR, whereas
those in Categories 2 and 3 show a response to HFS rotation. As expected, Category 4 neurons showed no consistent modulation during either test.

In the testing procedure proposed above, there may be some question concerning the origin of sensory-related signals. Thus, a more definitive test for vestibular input was developed. Electrical stimulation of the vestibular nerve has been
previously used to provide an unequivocal demonstration of vestibular input.
However, although this type of stimulation may be effective in provoking neuron
discharge, it does not solve the problem of proving that the activity seen during
natural stimulation is from the same source. For example, a neuron with no sensitivity to whole body rotation may have a short latency response to eighth nerve
stimulation; this may be due to activity evoked simultaneously in many thick afferent fibers near the stimulating electrode, which have low electrical thresholds
but do not necessarily originate from the canal of importance. Another neuron

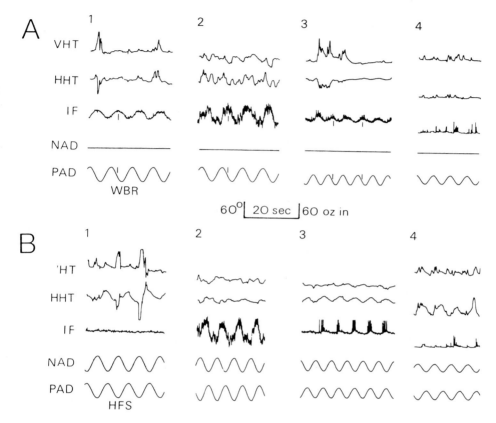

Figure 10.1. Four categories of neurons. Characterization based on relative sensitivity to passive vestibular afferent (A) and neck afferent (B) stimulation. (A) Whole body rotation (WBR) for each of four neurons (Categories 1, 2, 3, and 4, in respective columns). Traces are of single, unaveraged trials. Instantaneous frequency peak-to-peak modulation in each of the columns is (1) 40–80 spikes/sec, (2) 5–30, (3) 30–60, and (4) 0–100. Vertical tics in WBR of columns 1, 2, and 3 indicate peak PAD velocity. In column 3 a second tic is added to show phase variation; note also the first cycle differs from the others, due to attempted head movements (VHT and HHT). Time and amplitude calibration below the middle columns applies to all panels. (B) Head fixed in space (HFS) rotation. The procedures and conventions are the same as in (A). Rightward and upward signals are represented by positive deflections in all traces. Abbreviations: VHT, vertical head torque; HHT, horizontal head torque; IF, instantaneous frequency; NAD, neck angular deviation or head movement on trunk; PAD, platform angular deviation.

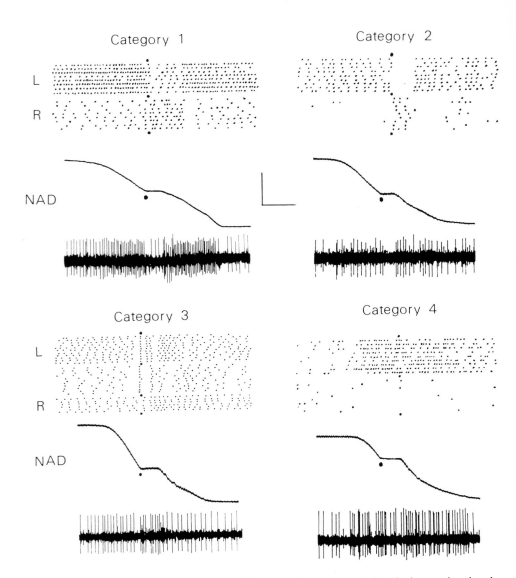

Figure 10.2. Active head movements. Rasters of neuron activity during active head movements with interruption of the movement by an electronic brake. Categories 1–4 are same neurons shown in Figure 10.1. The large dot above, in the middle, and below each set of rasters marks the onset of the brake. Each raster is 500 msec in duration, except in Category 3, in which the expanded time base of the lower one-half of L is 250 msec in duration. Below each group of rasters are analog traces of single head movements representing one line of the raster above. The dot below the neck angular deviation (NAD), or head movement, trace corresponds to the large dots in the rasters above designating brake onset. The head was braked a second time at the end of the trace in Category 1 neuron. Calibration bar is 150 msec (abscissa) and 20° for all four analog traces. Rasters show left (L) and right (R) head movements separately.

with WBR sensitivity, due to multiple asynchronous inputs with optimal summation, may show no response to nerve stimulation. Thus a second test using a more extreme form of natural stimulation was incorporated to characterize further the input from the horizontal semicircular canals, and is illustrated in Figure 10.2.

Voluntary (active) ballistic head movements were interrupted by an electronic brake (Fig. 10.2). A vestibular response to the arrest of movement (Categories 1 and 2) should occur at a short latency and have a clear leading and trailing edge of altered activity. The activity should be symmetrical during on- and off-directional head movements, with an even reduction of firing when the on-movement is interrupted and elevation of firing when the off-movement is interrupted. Neurons in Categories 1 and 2 satisfy these criteria and thus were considered conclusively to have an input from the vestibular canals. Note that these two neurons discharge more strongly during the braked interval in the off-direction (rightward) than in the on-direction (leftward). Although this is unexpected (one would assume equal rates), it represents a consistent finding in neurons with canal inputs.

Neurons in Category 3 show a time-locked response to the brake (Fig. 10.2), but the response (neither symmetrical nor even) comprised a series of bursts. This category of neurons will be discussed further below. Category 4 neurons show a symmetrically altered discharge, beginning before the head movement, but show no alteration of activity during the braked interval. As suggested by the data in Figure 10.1, these reticular neurons are related to the motor aspects of head movement, and have no canal or neck sensory inputs.

The above cursory description shows that in three groups of neurons a vestibular and neck sensory input can be characterized (Categories 1 and 2) and segregated from activity related to internally generated motor commands (Category 4). However, Category 3 neurons deserve special consideration, because the data present many of the motor–sensory and primary–secondary sensory distinctions discussed earlier in this chapter. Data presented in detail below will illustrate this dilemma, which is common in the analysis of recordings from alert animals.

The expanded raster time base and analog trace in Figure 10.2 (Category 3 neuron) show a relatively reliable single spike response that is almost synchronous with the brake application and precedes the arrest of head movement by 4 msec; it is followed by a burst of two to three spikes some 10 msec later, and by a more variable burst of three to four spikes in the next 30 msec. The earliest spike suggests that the response is due to the activation of the brake itself, not the stoppage of head movement. Indeed, application of the brake while the head is stationary elicits the same short latency response, although less reliably. Simply tapping the head holder lightly with a pencil also produces the same short latency response. Other forms of perturbation were applied. Square wave pulses of whole body rotation also produced short latency responses of three to five spikes. Although the platform had moved only 0.4° when these spikes appeared, examination of torque sensors with high amplification revealed minute oscillations of the platform prior to its movement, and in some cases the three- to five-spike train had a frequency (20–50 Hz) similar to that of the vibration. The same square wave was applied with HFS rotation (eliminating the 0.4° vestibular stimulus) and similar results were obtained. Finally, a small solenoid-activated probe was placed against the neck to deliver rapid and repeatable mechanical perturbations to the neck.

Probing at different neck sites proved effective in producing qualitatively different responses, but no focal location of a receptor site was found. This is not surprising, since given their extreme sensitivity, any disturbance should excite these receptors. All of these observations suggest that a Paciniform receptor is responsible for some of the response; such receptors have been described in the neck (Richmond and Bakker, 1982).

An additional complexity arose from the observation that during the tests performed to identify sensory responses of Category 3 neurons, there were frequently rapid changes in head torque closely following all forms of perturbations, regardless of whether the stimuli were delivered by the servo motor of the platform, by engagement of the brake, or by the muscle probe. The amplitude of these head torque inflections varied by an order of magnitude in response to sequential, identical stimuli. Latency of the torque responses was less variable (5–10 msec), although each form of stimulus provoked responses at different latencies, varying between 25 and 50 msec. The variability in amplitude and the 10 msec jitter in latency show that these torque changes were due to a response of the cat, rather than direct activation of the strain gauges due to mechanical perturbations. The rapidity of the responses (25–50 msec) was initially surprising. However, short neck and limb reaction times have been described previously in cats following the application of stimuli to the vibrissae or the limb (Ghez and Vicario, 1978).

The remarkably quick responses of the cat to the test stimuli used in classifying Category 3 neurons raise the previously stated question: are the responses of these neurons entirely of sensory origin, or are they at least partially associated with premotor activity? For example, the initial burst of activity beginning less than 5 msec after brake activation is clearly a primary sensory response; however, the burst beginning 15 msec after the onset of the brake could be either a primary sensory response or a premotor output, which will subsequently be relayed by the spinal cord to neck muscles, thus producing the head torque peaks seen 15–25 msec later. This latency for a motor response is not unreasonable, considering the conduction time, a few synaptic delays, and, most important, the excitation–contraction coupling of the muscle. Although the separation of activity related to sensory or motor activity may seem arbitrary, the issue of whether these neurons play a role in the initiation of movement (premotor) or whether they relay sensory information is similar to the questions concerning the posterior parietal cortex, summarized earlier.

Setting aside the issue of cause, a second important consideration is the extreme sensitivity of Category 3 neurons, which would predispose these neurons to respond to almost any active perturbation of the neck; in this case, certain forms of muscle activity related to the stimuli could produce a secondary sensory response. For example, small neck muscle contractions are induced by vestibulocollic reflexes during WBR (Vidal et al., 1982); these may be too weak to be seen in the head torque signal, yet these contractions could cause sensitive neck receptors to discharge in a fashion that could be mistaken for a vestibular effect. In fact, some Category 3 neurons showed presumptive "vestibular" modulation for several cycles that alternated with no modulation; this pattern is suggestive of the waxing and waning vestibulocollic reflex seen in animals with a free head

(Fuller, 1981). Another form of stimulus-related muscle contraction has been attributed to the animal's voluntary response to WBR, termed the "slow velocity component" (Fuller, 1981). Sensitive neck receptors could be systematically activated by neck muscle contractions due to this nonreflex behavior. Thus WBR modulation in Category 3 neurons may not necessarily represent a primary vestibular response, but rather the influence of other receptors that are secondarily activated, and are more or less effective depending on the "set" of the animal. In a similar vein, the responses to head movement interruption, which are unlike the archetypal responses of Category 1 and 2 neurons, may represent a mixed input from vestibular and neck receptors, or a single input from neck receptors, or, incorporating the arguments in the preceding paragraph, a mixed sensory–motor response.

Neurons with a purely motor association (e.g., the present Category 4 neurons) can also have false associations with certain stimuli; they can systematically modulate their firing rate during "passive" head movements if the animal actively anticipates the stimulus with systematic neck muscle contraction. Indeed, Category 4 neurons occasionally show stimulus-related modulation when the animal's head is forcably moved (by the experimenter) or during WBR. In the former case the patterns of neuronal activity are opposite to those seen during voluntary movements, because the animal is resisting movement, whereas in the latter case WBR generates the voluntary "slow velocity component" mentioned above. In both circumstances recordings of head torque indicate that the activity is related to a motor response rather than to the stimulus.

One objective in recording the activity of single neurons is to identify the sensory inputs to different subsets of neurons. Analysis of vestibular inputs is relatively easy because macular (e.g., Boyle and Pompeiano, 1981a) or canal inputs (e.g., Rubin et al., 1977; Kasper and Thoden, 1981; Anastasopoulos and Mergner, 1982) can be specifically identified. The isolation and identification of neck sensory inputs are more difficult. However, the elegant experiments of Ezure et al. (1983), in which neck muscle responses to specific stimuli were isolated, represent a significant first step. A second more comprehensive objective of neuronal recording in alert animals is to map the neuronal pathways that produce specific behaviors. Detailed analysis of neuronal activity related to eye movements has led to much progress in defining specific neuronal networks responsible for oculomotor activity (see Shimazu, 1983). The present experiments do not lend themselves to such specificity, but rather represent the earliest stage in describing the detailed characteristics of sensory inputs and their interactions with motor outputs in the more complicated context of active movement. With such descriptions, one hopes to be able to compare and contrast data for vestibular and neck sensory inputs to specific, reliably identified, brain stem neurons: ultimately the ensemble of neural activity that regulates head movement will be identified from such information.

SUMMARY

In the past, the reflex effects of sensory input from the neck have usually been studied in anesthetized, decerebrate, or spinalized animals. However, such effects can also be examined by recording patterns of neuronal firing in conscious cats that have been trained to make head movements. In the brain stem can be found at least four categories of neurons that differ in their patterns of input from neck and vestibular receptors and in their relationship to active head movements.

Two categories of responses are characteristic of cells in the medial vestibular nucleus and nucleus prepositus hypoglossi. Cells in both categories respond to vestibular or neck sensory inputs. However, one type of cell receives its dominant input from the semicircular canals, whereas the other type is affected more strongly by sensory input from the neck. A third category of response is recorded from cells in the descending vestibular nuclei. These responses are modulated by active and passive head movements and are particularly sensitive to vibration. The fourth category of neuron is found in the medial reticular formation. The responses of these neurons are not influenced consistently by vestibular neck input but show intense activity during active head turns.

The responses of the latter two categories of neurons are not simple to understand. In the conscious, behaving animal, responses can be influenced not only by a direct sensory input, but also by centrally generated motor signals and by sensory signals that result from the movement itself. These problems complicate the analysis of inputs to neurons in the normal animal, but underscore the fact that neuronal processing may not be as simple as is sometimes concluded from analyses in unconscious animals whose heads are moved passively.

11

Vestibular and Reticular Projections to the Neck

V. J. WILSON and B. W. PETERSON

Afferents from the three semicircular canals and two maculae terminate in different, partly overlapping regions in the four vestibular nuclei: the lateral (Deiters'), medial, descending, and superior nuclei (for review, see Wilson and Melvill Jones, 1979). Except for the superior, all nuclei project to the spinal cord via the lateral and medial vestibulospinal tracts (LVST and MVST). Of the two tracts, the MVST is the one closely related to the neck, although the upper cervical segments also receive a projection from the LVST. This dual innervation of the neck has been studied extensively by neuroanatomical and electroanatomical methods, which have also been used to study a parallel projection of reticulospinal fibers. In this chapter we review this literature only briefly, with emphasis on recent developments.

THE VESTIBULOCOLLIC PROJECTION

Origin of Axons Projecting to the Neck

Petras (1967) observed degeneration in C1–C4 after lesions in Deiters' nucleus, as did Nyberg-Hansen (1964) after lesions in the medial nucleus. It was originally believed that Deiters' nucleus was the origin of the LVST and the medial nucleus was the origin of the MVST, but antidromic stimulation experiments subsequently showed that the origin of the MVST is more widespread and includes the medial, Deiters', and descending nuclei (Akaike, 1973; Akaike et al., 1973a; Rapoport et al., 1977a; Akaike, 1983b). In addition, some LVST fibers come from the descending nucleus (Rapoport et al., 1977a). The MVST is bilateral whereas the LVST is mainly ipsilateral with only some crossed fibers.

Terminations in Neck Segments

Lesions of Deiters' nucleus cause widespread ipsilateral degeneration in the ventral horn of C1–C4 (Petras, 1967), whereas those of the medial nucleus cause bilateral degeneration, mainly medially in Laminae 7 and 8 (Nyberg-Hansen, 1964). Recent experiments with intraaxonal injection of horseradish peroxidase (HRP) show that MVST axons (to the contralateral side) give off collaterals 1–2 mm apart that terminate in the ventromedial nucleus (containing dorsal neck motoneurons) and in the spinal accessory nucleus (containing trapezius motoneurons) (Fleming and Rose, 1983).

Action of Vestibulocollic Axons on Motoneurons

The literature dealing with synaptic actions of vestibulospinal axons on neck motoneurons has already been reviewed in detail (Wilson and Melvill Jones, 1979; Wilson and Peterson, 1981). In brief, evidence drawn from experiments utilizing techniques ranging from electrical stimulation of the vestibular nuclei (Wilson and Yoshida, 1969a,b) to spike-triggered averaging from single vestibular neurons (Rapoport et al., 1977b) has shown that LVST and MVST neurons make synapses with dorsal and ventral neck motoneurons and that there are both excitatory and inhibitory connections (Fig. 11.1). The prevalence of monosynaptic connections is similar to the situation with other axial motoneurons (Wilson et al., 1970) and is in contrast to what has been seen so far in limb motoneurons. Some monosynaptic connections to hindlimb motoneurons were described as far back as 1968 by Lund and Pompeiano, but none to forelimb motoneurons has been identified as yet in physiological experiments (Wilson and Yoshida, 1969a; Maeda et al., 1975). The situation in the cervical enlargement may need to be reexamined in light of recent observations based on intraaxonal HRP injections, which show that some LVST axons branch profusely among forelimb motor nuclei and seem to terminate on motoneurons (Shinoda et al., 1986).

The organization of the vestibulocollic projection is summarized in Figure 11.1. Axons linking neurons in the vestibular nuclei and neck motoneurons are mainly, but not only, in the MVST. Experiments with electrical stimulation have demonstrated that several types of vestibular nucleus neurons project in the MVST: (1) those monosynaptically excited by stimulation of the horizontal and posterior semicircular canals and making synapses with ipsilateral or contralateral dorsal neck motoneurons, and (2) those excited by anterior canal stimulation and making synapses with contralateral dorsal neck motoneurons. In contrast, neurons excited from the anterior canal and acting on ipsilateral dorsal neck motoneurons project in the LVST (Wilson and Maeda, 1974). Projections to ventral neck (sternocleidomastoid) motoneurons, on the other hand, seem to be entirely via the MVST (Fukushima et al., 1979). The LVST and MVST may both relay otolith information, but the MVST is apparently responsible for all contralateral connections (Akaike et al., 1973a; Wilson et al., 1978a).

Recent work demonstrates that monosynaptic connections of vestibulocollic axons are not restricted to neck motoneurons. The C3 and C4 segments contain short and long propriospinal neurons, whose axons terminate in the cervical enlargement and thoracolumbar cord, respectively. The activity of some of the propriospinal neurons is modulated by natural vestibular stimulation (Chapter 8) and this modulation may, at least in part, be due to monosynaptic projections from the vestibular nuclei (Sasaki et al., 1983).

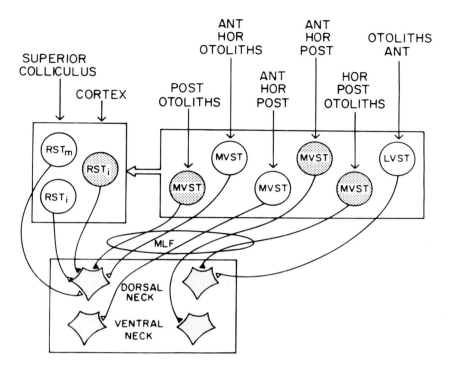

Figure 11.1.   Diagrammatic representation of vestibular and reticular projections to neck motoneurons. Circular profiles indicate different groups of VST and RST neurons (for definitions, see text) with inhibitory neurons and terminals indicated by shading. Neurons are located in the right vestibular nuclei (large box) and left medullary-pontine reticular formation (small box). Their projections to motoneurons controlling dorsal and ventral muscles of the left and right neck are shown. Ant, Hor, and Post are afferents from anterior, horizontal, and posterior canals, respectively. Information on connections of canal afferents is much more complete than that on connections of otolith afferents.

Stimulation of individual canal nerve branches in the labyrinth has shown that the MVST and, to a lesser extent, the LVST transmit a pattern of activity to dorsal and ventral neck motoneurons appropriate to produce the head movements normally elicited by electrical stimulation of the same canals (Suzuki and Cohen, 1964; Wilson and Maeda, 1974; Fukushima et al., 1979). For example, stimulation of nerves from the horizontal canal evokes contralateral head turning in alert cats and the appropriate ipsilateral inhibitory postsynaptic potentials (IPSPs) and contralateral excitatory postsynaptic potentials (EPSPs) in splenius and other dorsal neck motoneurons. Studies exploring the physiological signals carried by vestibulospinal neurons will be described in Chapter 13.

Branching of Vestibulocollic Axons

Abzug et al. (1974) showed that LVST axons may branch to widely separated spinal levels: many fibers with collaterals ending in the cervical enlargement extend to the lumbar cord. Vestibulocollic axons also branch widely, but, in contrast to LVST axons to the cervical enlargement, few reach the lumbar cord. However, many (62%) extend to the cervical enlargement, and some as far as the upper thoracic cord (Rapoport et al., 1977a).

Vestibulocollic axons may also be branches of axons projecting to the extraocular nuclei. This possibility was first suggested by the observation that vestibulocollic and vestibuloocular neurons were both located in the same area of the medial nucleus (Rapoport et al., 1977a; Nakao et al., 1982). McCrea et al., (1980), using intraaxonal injection of HRP, identified second-order vestibular neurons

Figure 11.2.   Branching of the same neurons to the oculomotor nuclei and upper cervical cord. (A) Although some anterior canal neurons in the vestibular nuclei project only to the oculomotor nucleus, others bifurcate. Abbreviations: ACN, anterior canal nerve; C1–C3 DR, upper cervical dorsal rami; D, descending nucleus; IO, inferior oblique muscle; M, medial nucleus; MLF, medial longitudinal fasciculus; S, superior nucleus; SR, superior rectus muscle; Vestibular N, vestibular nuclei; III, oculomotor nuclei. (B) Branching and spinal action of a bifurcating neuron. (1) Orthodromic response of the neuron to stimulation of ACN, and antidromic spike evoked by weak stimuli to electrodes in the contralateral C1 DR and inferior oblique motoneuron pools. Negative up. (2) Spike-triggered averaged unitary EPSP evoked in a C1 DR motoneuron (652 sweeps averaged). Upper trace intracellular and lower trace juxtacellular recording. Positive up. (Modified from Uchino and Hirai, 1984.)

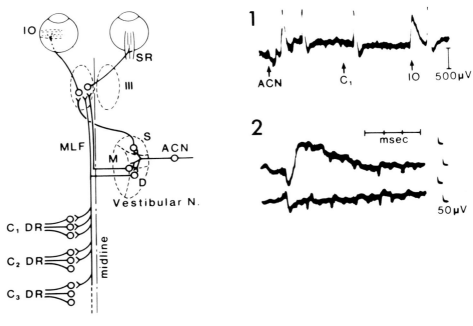

projecting to the abducens nucleus; some of these neurons had collaterals that could be activated antidromically from C2. It was postulated that such "vestibuloocular" neurons contributed to vestibulocollic reflexes. Bifurcation of axons of vestibular neurons to extraocular nuclei and spinal cord has now been studied in detail for the horizontal and anterior canal systems. For the former, Isu and Yokota (1983) studied a population of medial nucleus neurons activated by ipsilateral horizontal rotation (Type I neurons) and projecting to the contralateral abducens nucleus. Some neurons projected to the abducens nucleus only; others projected only to the spinal cord. Over 40% of neurons projecting to the abducens nucleus had a spinal collateral extending as far as C1. Fewer collaterals reached C2 and C3, and none extended to the cervical enlargement. Collaterals terminating in the upper cervical segments branched within the motor nuclei, and it is safe to assume that they made synapses with neck motoneurons. Very similar observations were made for the anterior canal system by Uchino and Hirai (1984) who found neurons projecting to both the inferior oblique nucleus and upper cervical cord in the descending, medial, and Deiters' nuclei (Fig. 11.2). Once again, the cervical projections were predominantly to C1, although a substantial fraction of axons originating in the descending nucleus reached C4 and even the cervical enlargement. Uchino and Hirai (1984) obtained direct evidence that the spinal collaterals excited neck motoneurons monosynaptically (Fig. 11.2).

Thus there is abundant evidence that vestibulocollic axons (1) may project to the cord only, (2) often branch to the cervical enlargement, and (3) may themselves be a branch of a neuron projecting to the extraocular nuclei. As yet there is insufficient evidence to determine to what extent these different neuron types carry different signals. It is tempting to speculate that branching, which ensures that the same signal is sent to widely separate destinations and perhaps to more than one effector system, may underlie coordinated responses of, e.g., eyes and head. This remains no more than speculation because the function of the short-latency connections made by vestibular nucleus neurons with neck motoneurons is not yet known (see below).

Summary

The anatomical and physiological data described above identify two major vestibulospinal projections to the neck. The properties of these projections may be summarized as follows.

1. The LVST originates from neurons in the lateral vestibular (Deiters') nucleus. These neurons receive input from anterior semicircular canal and otolith receptors in the labyrinth and project to and excite ipsilateral dorsal neck motoneurons.
2. The MVST contains multiple components shown in Figure 11.1. MVST neurons receiving horizontal semicircular canal input excite contralateral neck motoneurons and inhibit ipsilateral neck motoneurons.
3. MVST neurons receiving anterior canal input excite contralateral dorsal and ventral neck motoneurons and inhibit ipsilateral ventral neck motoneurons.

4. MVST neurons receiving posterior canal inputs excite contralateral ventral neck motoneurons and inhibit ipsilateral dorsal and ventral neck motoneurons and contralateral dorsal neck motoneurons.
5. MVST neurons also mediate inhibition of ipsilateral neck motoneurons and excitation and inhibition of contralateral neck motoneurons by the otolith organs.
6. LVST and MVST neurons that project to the neck may also send axon branches to other levels of the spinal cord or to brain stem nuclei including the oculomotor nuclei.

THE RETICULOCOLLIC PROJECTION

Origin of Reticulospinal Projections to the Neck

A large number of cell groups within the region classically called the brain stem reticular formation project to the spinal cord where they may impinge on neurons in a number of motor pools. These reticulospinal pathways have now been characterized extensively by neuroanatomical techniques involving retrograde (Torvick and Brodal, 1957; Coulter et al., 1979; Peterson, 1977; Martin et al., 1979a,b, 1981; Tohyama, 1979a,b) and anterograde (Nyberg-Hansen, 1965; Petras, 1967; Basbaum et al., 1978; Basbaum and Fields, 1979; Holstege et al., 1979; Martin et al., 1979a,b, 1981) tracing of connections. Retrograde labeling following injection of tracers into the neck segments has been described both in regions that project primarily to the neck, including nucleus reticularis (n.r.) parvocellularis, n.r. lateralis, n.r. dorsalis, and nucleus supraspinalis, and in regions that also project to lower spinal levels, including n.r. pontis oralis, n.r. pontis caudalis, n.r. gigantocellularis, n.r. ventralis, nucleus cuneiformis, nucleus parabrachialis, and the ventral nucleus of the lateral lemniscus (Peterson, 1977; Coulter et al., 1979; Martin et al., 1981). Anterograde studies indicate that reticulospinal projections terminate in Rexed's (1954) Laminae I and II of the dorsal horn and throughout the ventral horn including the motoneuron pools in Lamina IX (Petras, 1967; Basbaum et al., 1978; Basbaum and Fields, 1979; Holstege et al., 1979; Martin et al., 1979a,b, 1981). They are thus likely to be involved both in regulation of neck sensory input and in generation of neck motor activity.

Although it is possible that a number of reticulospinal pathways influence the activity of neck motoneurons, detailed neurophysiological information is available concerning only the rapidly conducting reticulospinal projections originating within the medial pontomedullary reticular formation (MPRF) consisting of nuclei reticularis pontis oralis, pontis caudalis, gigantocellularis, and ventralis (Brodal, 1957). These projections will be the focus of the present discussion. As indicated above, neurons in n.r. pontis oralis, pontis caudalis, and dorsorostral gigantocellularis project in the ventromedial funiculus and are therefore termed RSTm (RST, reticulospinal tract) neurons (Ito et al., 1970; Peterson et al., 1975a). Neurons in n.r. gigantocellularis and ventralis project in the ventrolateral funiculus of the ipsilateral and ipsilateral and contralateral side and are therefore termed RSTi and RSTc neurons. These three projections terminate throughout the ventral horn of the upper cervical segments and therefore potentially influence neck motoneurons. Their fibers conduct relatively rapidly so that impulses in them reach the neck within 0.4–1.6 msec following activation of the cell soma (Ito et al., 1970; Peterson et al., 1975b).

Only a fraction of the reticulospinal terminals observed in the upper cervical segments are likely to arise from axons targeted solely for the neck. Figure 11.3A–C shows the results of a study in which electrodes were implanted at multiple levels of the spinal cord to determine the approximate level of descent of RSTm and RSTi neurons (Peterson et al., 1975b). The data reveal one reticulospinal projection that appears to be targeted specifically for the neck. This consists of

Figure 11.3.   (A–C) Locations of reticulospinal neurons. Locations of reticulospinal neurons projecting in RSTc, RSTm, and RSTi are shown on three drawings of a schematic parasagittal section through the pons (right) and medulla (left). Asterisks indicate neurons projecting to the neck; diamonds, squares, and circles indicate neurons projecting to cervical, thoracic, and lumbosacral levels, respectively. Diagonal dashed lines indicate the border between two reticular regions labeled Zone 1 and 2 in (A). (D–F) Reticular regions from which monosynaptic excitation or inhibition of neck motoneurons could be evoked. Stimuli of 100 μA applied at points located 1 to 2 from the midline within darkly shaded areas evoked monosynaptic excitation (D) or inhibition (E) in >50% of motoneurons tested. Stimulation in lightly shaded regions excited or inhibited 10–49% of motoneurons. (F) Five reticulospinal projection zones described in the text. Abbreviations: IO, inferior olivary nucleus; NRTP, nucleus reticularis tegmenti pontis; PH, prepositus hypoglossi nucleus; TB, trapezoid body; VI, abducens nucleus; VII, genu of facial nerve; XII, hypoglossal nucleus. (From Peterson, et al., 1975b; and Peterson and Fukushima, 1982.)

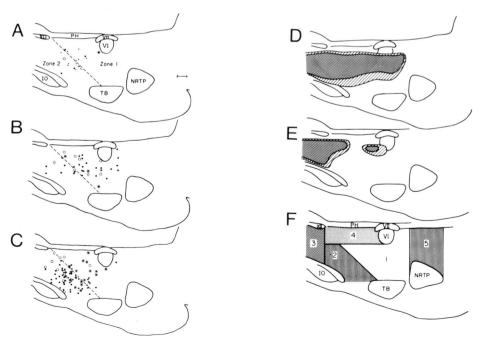

RSTi neurons that are found in the vicinity of the abducens nucleus, anterior to the long-projecting neurons of this tract. These neurons may account for direct inhibition of neck motoneurons that is evoked from the region behind the abducens nucleus (see below). In most other regions of the MPRF, the great majority of the neurons continue to lumbosacral levels, which suggests that many terminals in the neck are branches of reticulospinal axons that also project to lower levels, as in the case of branching vestibulospinal axons. The same study also demonstrated extensive branching of lumbar-projecting reticulospinal neurons within the cervical enlargement, supporting the idea that the reticulospinal system is a highly branched network. Branches of reticulospinal axons are not restricted to the spinal cord: data presented in Chapter 18 will show extensive arborization of reticulospinal axons to brain stem nuclei, including abducens and facial nuclei and the vestibular complex (Grantyn et al., 1980). The anatomical data thus suggest that the reticulospinal system should be viewed as a system that activates neck motoneurons as part of broad synergies involving activation of muscle groups throughout the body.

Action on Neck Motoneurons

As indicated above, reticulospinal projections from the MPRF have three components. The RSTm projection was initially identified as the source of direct excitatory input to hindlimb motoneurons (Grillner and Lund, 1968; Wilson and Yoshida, 1969; Grillner et al., 1971). Subsequently, Peterson et al. (1978) showed that stimulation of regions containing RSTm neurons (Zone 1 of Fig. 11.1) produced monosynaptic excitation in the majority of dorsal neck motoneurons on the ipsilateral side. The same region also directly excites forelimb and back motoneurons (Wilson and Yoshida, 1969a,b; Peterson et al., 1978), suggesting that this region activates the neck as part of a generalized orienting response.

RSTi and RSTc neurons have a more posterior origin (Zones 2 and 3 of Fig. 11.3) than RSTm neurons. Stimulation of this more caudal region excites dorsal neck motoneurons via pathways that descend lateral to the RSTm projection (Peterson et al., 1978). The same stimuli also activate back but not limb motoneurons, suggesting that RSTi and RSTc pathways may produce axial muscle activation such as occurs during righting reflexes.

The RSTi population also contains inhibitory neurons (Ito et al., 1970), which have been shown to directly inhibit dorsal neck motoneurons but not motoneurons at lower levels (Peterson et al., 1978). The effective region includes Zones 2, 3, and 4 of Fig. 11.3, which led Peterson et al. (1978) to speculate that the neck receives two inhibitory reticulospinal projections. The first of these originates from Zone 4, is related to eye–head coordination, and involves the specific reticulo–neck projection discussed above. The second originates more posteriorly in the classic inhibitory area of Magoun and Rhines (1946), which corrsponds to Zones 2 and 3, and may be related to generalized inhibitory control of the neck, including neck muscle atonia seen during rapid-eye-movement (REM) sleep.

It should be emphasized again that the projections described above are only a subset of the reticulocollic system. There are other areas, such as n.r. supraspinalis, whose roles in neck motor control require investigation. It is also important to recognize that reticulocollic projections may act upon other neuronal populations in the neck such as C3–C4 propriospinal neurons described above. These neurons have been shown to receive both reticulospinal excitation (probably from both RSTm and RSTi neurons) and reticulospinal inhibition from regions corresponding to Zones 2 and 3 (Alstermark et al., 1983a,b).

Sources of Afferent Input to Reticulospinal Neurons

While vestibulospinal pathways received particularly strong input from the vestibular labyrinth, reticulospinal pathways are more polymodal, receiving input from many premotor structures. Strong direct excitatory inputs reach reticulospinal neurons throughout the MPRF from the sensorimotor region of the cortex, the superior colliculus, and the cerebellum (Magni and Willis, 1964; Peterson et al., 1974; Eccles et al., 1975; Grantyn and Grantyn, 1982). Studies by Anderson et al. (1971) and Alstermark et al. (1983a,b) suggest that reticulospinal neurons are the major relay from the superior colliculus and motor cortex to neck motoneurons (cf. Chapter 18). Thus, these neurons form the site of convergence of motor commands related to visually triggered orienting and voluntary movement of the neck.

As illustrated in Figure 11.4, activation of semicircular canals with electrical polarization modulates the activity of the same RSTm neurons that serve as relays of superior colliculus activity to the neck (Peterson et al., 1980; Peterson and Fukushima, 1982). This pattern of convergent input is consistent with the idea that RSTm neurons are involved in whole body orienting movements requiring movement of many parts of the body. Polarization of the canals produced relatively weak modulation of neurons in Zone 2, but these neurons did respond vigorously to electrical stimulation of the entire vestibular nerve. Therefore, they may be activated by otolith inputs, which would be expected if they played a role in righting reflexes as suggested above. Zones 2 and 3 also receive much somatosensory input (Magni and Willis, 1964; Peterson, 1975a), which appears to play an important role in spinal–bulbospinal reflexes, a kind of startle response (Shimamura and Livingston, 1963; Shimamura and Kogure, 1979).

Summary

The anatomical and physiological data described above suggest that there are four projections from the MPRF that directly control dorsal neck motoneurons via monosynaptic connections.

1. An inhibitory RSTi projection to neck only, originating in Zone 4 of Figure 11.3. This may be involved in coordinated eye–head movements during gaze shifts.
2. An excitatory RSTm projection to neck, back, and limb motoneurons originating in Zone 1. This may be involved in whole body movements associated with orienting responses.
3. An excitatory RSTi projection to neck and back motoneurons originating in Zones 2 and 3. This may be involved in righting reflexes and startle resonses.

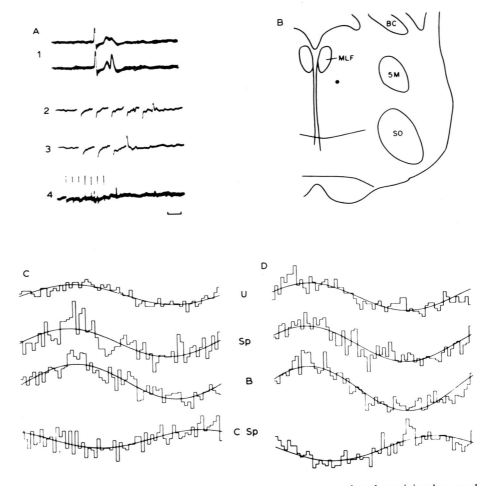

Figure 11.4. Reticulospinal neuron receiving convergent tectal and semicircular canal input. The neuron, located at site shown in (B), was identified as an RSTm neuron by its antidromic response to stimulation of the ventromedial funiculus at C2 (Al, lower trace). In the upper trace, the neuron fails to respond to slightly weaker spinal stimulus. (A2) and (A3) show responses to trains of stimuli applied to anterior and posterior portions of the contralateral superior colliculus, respectively. (A4) shows response to trains of stimuli applied to an electrode implanted close to the contralateral horizontal semicircular canal ampulla. The time base for A1 is 1 msec, for A2 and A3 2 msec, and for A4 5 msec. (C) and (D) show the responses of the neuron and neck muscles to sinusoidal polarization of contralateral horizontal semicircular canal afferents at 0.2 Hz (C) and 3.0 Hz (D). Modulation of unit activity (U) is in phase with activity of right splenius (Sp). Abbreviations in B: BC, brachium conjuctivum; MLF, medial longitudinal fasciculus; SO superior olive; 5M, trigeminal motor nucleus. (From Peterson and Fukushima, 1982.)

4. An inhibitory RSTi projection to neck motoneurons and probably to spinal interneurons at other levels. This may be related to changes in muscle tone such as those occurring in sleep.

These projections are summarized in Figure 11.1, in which the two inhibitory RSTi projections have been combined. Only connections with motoneurons controlling ipsilateral dorsal neck muscles are shown. Direct actions on contralateral dorsal neck muscles were much weaker and could have been due in part to coactivation of VST fibers by the brain stem stimuli. No data are available on reticulospinal actions on ventral neck muscles.

FUNCTIONAL ROLE OF VESTIBULOCOLLIC AND RETICULOCOLLIC PROJECTIONS

The role of VSTs in defined neck motor behaviors is still not fully understood; work on this problem is now underway in several laboratories and will be described more fully in Chapters 12, 13, and 14. One approach has been to make lesions that interrupt specific descending tracts and then evaluate their effect upon neck motor output. Ezure et al. (1978) initiated a series of studies to evaluate the effect of transecting the descending medial longitudinal fasciculus (MLF) upon the vestibulocollic reflex (VCR). As indicated in Figure 11.1, this lesion interrupts all VST fibers except for the LVST projection to the ipsilateral neck. Since the latter carries anterior canal and otolith signals, the lesion will eliminate all VST participation in the horizontal VCR. When Ezure et al. (1978) found that this lesion did not modify the low-frequency dynamics of horizontal vestibulocollic reflexes it immediately became clear that the reflex did not depend on this direct pathway. Extension of these experiments further showed that this statement was also true for responses to high-frequency stimulation (Wilson et al., 1979; Bilotto et al., 1982a). Lesion experiments are difficult to interpret because the fact that a behavior survives transection of a tract tells us little about the role of this tract in normal function. Nevertheless, because many reticulospinal neurons have dynamics similar to those of the VCR (Peterson et al., 1980) and because gain of the VCR is not reduced unless spinal lesions impinge on the area of the reticulospinal tracts (Bilotto et al. 1982a), it seems reasonable to assume that the latter are an important component of the pathways producing the VCR.

Another line of experimentation involves searching for VST or RST neurons that carry specific signals that have been observed during EMG recordings from neck motoneurons. As described in Chapter 17, Vidal et al. (1982) observed that neck EMG signals are modulated by eye position; for example, right neck muscle activity increases when the eyes are deviated toward the right. This activity might be produced in part by branching VST neurons that project to both abducens nucleus and neck because these neurons carry an eye position signal. In addition, however, Grantyn and Berthoz (1980) have found a specific group of RSTm neurons that carry eye position signals and project to abducens, facial, vestibular, and neck motor nuclei (see Chapter 18).

A similar analysis was applied to the VCR, resulting in the hypothesis that branching VST neurons and RSTm neurons might contribute the low-frequency phase-lagging portion of the reflex modulation of neck motoneurons, while the high-frequency phase-advanced portion could be carried by VST neurons that project only to the neck (cf. Chapter 10). However, the lesion studies described above showed this hypothesis to be incomplete: both low- and high-frequency signals must be carried by non-VST pathways. This finding indicates that caution is required in interpreting experiments correlating neural activity with motor output: until appropriate lesion studies are performed, it cannot be concluded that pathways identified are necessary for (or even involved in) the behavior under study.

SUMMARY

This chapter is divided into sections describing the role of vestibulospinal and reticulospinal pathways in transmitting signals from the vestibular labyrinth to neck motoneurons. The reader will find summaries of these projections following each section.

12

Reflex Stabilization of the Head

R. H. SCHOR, R. E. KEARNEY, and N. DIERINGER

Head stabilization in the face of perturbations introduced by the environment or by movements of the body is a complex process involving the interaction of reflexes elicited by vestibular, visual, and proprioceptive signals. This chapter examines this process from a number of viewpoints. The first section focuses on the cornerstone of the stabilization process, the vestibulocollic reflex (VCR). It explores the dynamic properties and neuronal substrates of head-stabilization reflexes that originate from sensors of gravity (otolith organs) and of angular acceleration (semicircular canals) within the vestibular labyrinth. The second section takes a systems analysis approach to explain how the VCR interacts with head–neck mechanical properties, voluntary movements, and other reflex systems (cervicocollic and optocollic) to determine head position. The last section examines head stabilization in submammalian species, in which differences related to phylogeny and to differing behavioral strategies shed light on the general problem of how stabilization is maintained.

THE VESTIBULOCOLLIC REFLEX

The vestibulocollic reflex (VCR) is the name given to a set of reflexes acting on muscles of the neck that arise from stimulation of vestibular receptors in the labyrinth. The reflexes activate neck muscles in such a manner as to counteract any head movement sensed by the vestibular apparatus; this activation helps to maintain head stability in space. Its task is similar to that of the better studied vestibuloocular reflex (VOR) which stabilizes the eye position in space when the head moves. To describe these reflexes, it is useful to start by examining their properties as control systems. Simple block diagrams of these two reflexes are presented in Figure 12.1. For simplicity and consistency, the input and output of these reflexes will be called "position," meaning position as a function of time; by taking appropriate time derivatives, velocity and acceleration control loops result.

The VCR operates as a closed-loop negative feedback system: its output, compensatory (−) head position, opposes (and partly cancels) the input driving signal. The output of the VOR, compensatory eye position, has no direct influence

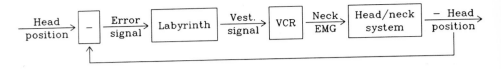

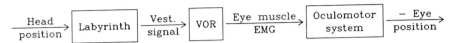

Figure 12.1.   Block diagrams of the vestibulocollic reflex (top) and vestibuloocular reflex (bottom). The diagrams have been drawn to emphasize the similarities between the two reflex systems. Head position in this figure is assumed to be a function of time: note in particular that whereas the otolith organs are modulated directly by head position, the semicircular canals respond to changes in position.

on the input head position signal: the VOR operates as an "open-loop" system. For ideal operation, an open-loop reflex such as the VOR should have a gain of 1; this causes the output (eye movement) to exactly compensate for the input (head movement), so that the eye is fixed in space. For closed-loop systems such as the VCR, it becomes slightly more difficult to compute the gain of the reflex. Although the reflex gain is still the ratio of the output to the input signal, the closed nature of the loop implies that the signal that gets transformed by the system is the difference between the input and output, an "error" signal that shows how far the reflex is from its desired goal (keeping the head fixed in space). The "loop gain" of the reflex is the product of the gains of each of three processing steps: transduction of head movements by the labyrinth, central processing to produce neck EMG, and the muscle mechanics that provide the actual movement. The gain of each subsystem is not large, since each step must accommodate a wide range of inputs without saturating its output. Thus the loop gain is probably fairly small (perhaps 2–10), although it is difficult to measure directly. Most studies of the VCR have measured the reflex with the head immobilized; this opens the feedback loop and allows neck EMG to be recorded as a measure of "open-loop" gain.

What are the implications of a closed-loop reflex system? The reflex gain, defined as the ratio of the output response to the input signal, can be expressed in terms of the loop gain. If the loop gain is symbolized by A, then the reflex gain G is simply

$$G = A/(1 + A) = 1/(1 + 1/A) = 1 - 1/A + 1/A^2 - \cdots$$

Most closed loop systems operate with large loop gains (A much larger than 1), in which case the above formula simplifies to $G = 1$. Such a "servo" mode forces the output to follow the input, independent of loop gain (or the gain of any of the components comprising the feedback loop). This feature of closed-loop systems, that the system gain G does not vary strongly with the gain of any internal component, means that questions of "adaptive gain plasticity" necessary to set the (open-loop) gain of the VOR may not be as important for the VCR system.

The above formula treats loop and reflex gains as constants. When they are expressed as functions of frequency (by specifying their amplitude and phase as functions of frequency), the reflex gain G is usually called the system transfer function. For a stable system, which does not oscillate, certain restrictions must be placed on the frequency properties of the loop gain. In particular, no large phase shifts may be introduced in the loop without a severe reduction in gain. One way to accomplish this is by having the VCR produce a neck EMG signal that compensates for the load introduced by the head–neck mechanical system, giving a loop gain that is constant with frequency. The head–neck system presents a load made up of the inertial mass of the head plus the viscoelastic properties of the neck musculature, and can be modeled as a simple second-order system (involving first and second derivatives with respect to time, namely velocity and acceleration). It differs from the second-order system model of the mechanical load of the eye presented to the VOR by being an "underdamped," rather than an "overdamped," system. The signals necessary to compensate for the head–neck and eye load are plotted in Figure 12.2, using data drawn from work on the monkey.

The VCR is not only frequency dependent, but also direction specific. Suzuki and Cohen (1964) demonstrated that electrical stimulation of a single semicircular canal caused the head to move in the plane of the canal, and in the direction opposite that which normally activates the canal (thereby canceling the imposed "movement" stimulus). Studies in the cat have utilized electrical and natural stimulation to activate various combinations of vestibular afferents in order to characterize the spatial and temporal properties of the reflex. Earlier studies focused on describing the VCR with respect to the cat axes of symmetry, which allowed simple stimulus paradigms to be employed (see Table 12.1). More recently, attempts have been made to look along more than one spatial dimension, to understand the head–neck system as it behaves in the freely moving animal.

VCR Due to Horizontal Canal (Yaw Stimulus)

The early systematic investigations of VCR dynamics were performed on decerebrate cats by using whole body rotations about a vertical (yaw) axis, with the head prevented from turning on the neck (Ezure and Sasaki, 1978; Bilotto et al., 1982a). These studies showed that at high frequencies, gain of the neck EMG signal increased whereas phase advanced with respect to position. These properties would "match" the inertial load of the head. In addition, the EMG signal developed a phase lead at the lowest frequencies (Fig. 12.3). The simplest models that could mimic this response require two first-order lead terms (in which output depends on the input position and velocity—see Chapter 7) for the high-frequency response, and two high-pass filter terms that produce the phase lead observed at the lowest frequencies. Part of the high-pass filtering and perhaps one lead term are due to transduction in the horizontal semicircular canals (Fernandez and Goldberg, 1971; Tomko et al., 1981b); similar canal-like dynamics have been observed in the vestibular nuclei during yaw (Shinoda and Yoshida, 1974). An additional

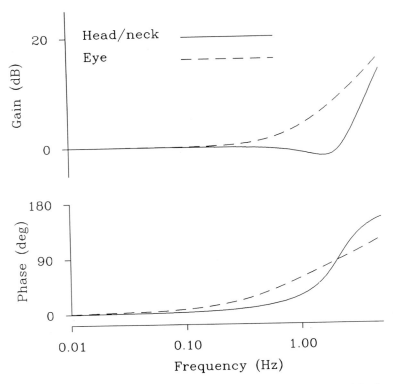

Figure 12.2.   Signals necessary to compensate for the mechanical load of the head–neck (solid curves) and oculomotor (dashed curves) systems. Head and eye mechanics were modeled as a simple second-order mass-dashpot-spring system. Estimates of the relative system parameters (inertia, viscosity, and spring constants) are from Robinson (1981) and Bizzi et al. (1978).

lead term is needed to produce the high-frequency acceleratory neck muscle EMG signal appropriate for driving the inertial mass of the head; it is probably produced somewhere in the pathway from the vestibular nuclei to neck muscles.

In parallel experiments, the horizontal VCR was evoked by applying sinusoidal polarizing currents directly to the horizontal canal on one side; the response of vestibulospinal and reticulospinal neurons were simultaneously recorded (Wilson et al., 1979; Peterson et al., 1980). This stimulus effectively bypasses the dynamics introduced by canal mechanics and allows a wide frequency range to be tested conveniently. At lower frequencies the response of second-order vestibulospinal neurons, which receive monosynaptic labyrinthine input, shows a variable phase lead compared to neck muscles. This suggests that some form of neural integration (perhaps after additional neural filtering) takes place to remove the phase lead. Other vestibulospinal neurons, mainly located in the lateral vestibular nucleus (and projecting in the lateral vestibulospinal tract), have response dynamics similar to the reflex (see Fig. 12.3); a population of reticulospinal neurons

Table 12.1. Paradigms for Natural Stimulation of the VCR[a]

Stimulus	Movement	Activated Receptor
Yaw	Rotation, vertical axis	Horizontal canal
Roll	Rotation, longitudinal axis	Vertical canals, utricle
Pitch	Rotation, transverse axis	Vertical canals, utricle
Horizontal	Linear, fore–aft, left–right	Utricle
Vertical	Linear, up–down	Saccule

[a]This table illustrates movements used to study the VCR, and the primary vestibular receptor activated by such movements (assuming a cat that is lying down in a normal prone position, the rotation axes pass through the labyrinth, and that roll and pitch rotations are of small amplitude).

Figure 12.3. Frequency response of neck EMG to yaw rotations. These data, from the complexus muscle of decerebrate cats, are taken from Bilotto et al. (1982) and are plotted with respect to head position (0° phase being perfect compensation). These points can be adequately fit by a model having two lead terms and two high-pass filter terms. One lead and filter term arises from the transfer properties of the horizontal canals. The extra lead term, producing additional high-frequency gain increase and phase lead, helps to overcome the inertial load of the head (compare with Fig. 12.2).

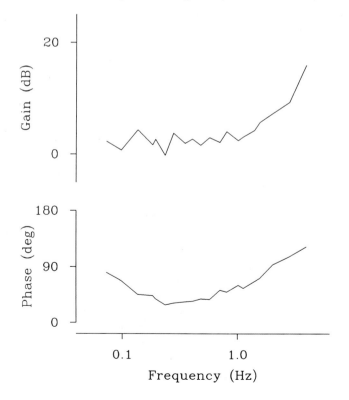

also has reflex-like dynamics, although reticular neurons are usually not modulated at higher frequencies. The roles of these vestibular and reticular neurons in the production of the reflex are as yet not fully known; remarkably, interrupting the direct vestibulospinal pathways from the horizontal canals to the neck by severing the medial vestibulospinal (Ezure et al., 1978; Wilson et al., 1979; Bilotto et al., 1982a) or the lateral vestibulospinal (Peterson et al., 1980) tracts produces little change in reflex dynamics, and only modest decreases in gain.

Responses Due to Vertical Canals (Roll and Pitch)

In response to roll tilt, which activates both canals and otolith organs, the VCR produces increased electromyographic (EMG) activity of dorsal neck muscles on the elevated side (Berthoz and Anderson, 1971; Schor and Miller, 1981; Miller et al., 1982). The dynamics of the reflex at frequencies above 0.1 Hz are similar to those of the horizontal VCR, suggesting that the vertical semicircular canals provide the dominant vestibular input at these frequencies. At lower frequencies, however, the additional position signal from utricular afferents keeps the response nearly in phase with position (Fig. 12.4, solid curves; compare with Fig. 12.3).

When the stimulus is pitch, the dorsal neck muscles are activated during nose-down tilt. Response dynamics observed using such a pitch stimulus are similar to those for roll (Anderson and Pappas, 1978; J. H. Anderson, unpublished observations; Dutia and Hunter, 1985). The responses to yaw, roll, and pitch, particularly at higher frequencies, have all been modeled by two terms consisting of a lead plus high-pass filter, one set reflecting the transformed head-rotation signal from the semicircular canals, and one due to neural processing in the VCR. The actual time constants used in these models differ slightly; it is difficult to know, at present, if this represents slight differences in the preparation or reflects inherent differences between the yaw, roll, and pitch responses.

The vertical VCR was also examined using electrical polarization of the anterior semicircular canal nerve (Wilson et al., 1979; Peterson et al., 1980). There were no obvious differences from responses obtained with horizontal canal stimulation. As was true for the horizontal component of the VCR, lesioning the medial longitudinal fasciculus (MLF) (medial vestibulospinal tract, MVST) or lateral vestibulospinal tract (LVST) appeared to cause only minor modifications of response dynamics to electrical (Wilson et al., 1979; Peterson et al., 1980) or roll (Miller et al., 1982) stimuli.

Studies of the dynamics of vestibular neurons possibly involved in the transmission of the vertical VCR are complicated by the dual activation of canal and otolith receptors. Boyle and Pompeiano (1980b) have described neurons with an increasing gain with respect to position as the frequency increased to 0.325 Hz. This could suggest a dual canal–otolith input, but similar response dynamics can also occur in the otolith neurons of canal-plugged cats (Schor, 1974; Schor and Miller, 1982). More recent studies (discussed below, and in Chapter 13) have specifically examined how canal and otolith signals interacting within the vestibular nuclei produce a variety of spatial and temporal response characteristics.

Responses to rotations in vertical planes (including roll and pitch) have also been observed in spinal interneurons at the C3–C4 levels (Schor et al., 1986).

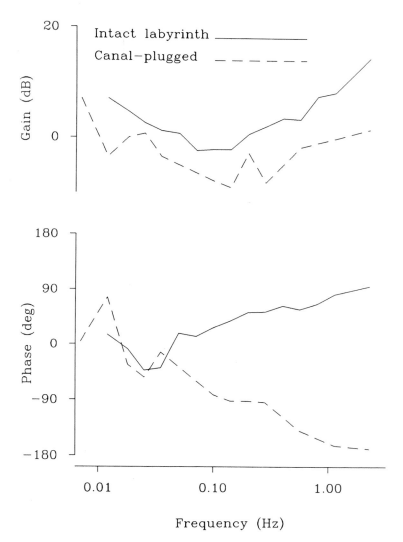

Figure 12.4. EMG response of biventer cervicis muscle to roll tilt. Responses from de-cerebrate cats with intact labyrinths (solid curves) and from decerebrate canal-plugged cats (dashed curves) are taken from the work of Schor and Miller (presented in Schor, 1981). Data are plotted with respect to position; 0° phase implies perfect compensation (the side-up biventer, which would help right the head, is activated). Note that in the absence of the semicircular canals, the reflex produced by the otolith organs develops a large phase lag as frequency is increased.

for producing sufficient acceleration to activate the reflex) to 0.25 Hz, the muscle exhibits two peaks in the EMG response, coinciding with maximal upward and maximal downward velocity. As the stimulus frequency increases to 1 Hz, the two peaks coalesce to a single peak that slightly lags peak upward movement (or peak downward acceleration). Since the action of splenius is to raise the head, it may seem that the reflex is anticompensatory (since splenius activity is greatest during the highest head position). At these frequencies, however, the role of the reflex is probably to accelerate the mass of the head, leading to the observed activation during downward head acceleration. The double activation at lower frequencies is at present a mystery—perhaps it represents a different head-stabilization strategy involving co-contraction of dorsal and ventral neck muscles to stiffen the neck during periods of peak velocity, regardless of the direction.

Neck Muscles Respond Best to Particular Spatial Orientation of Stimulus

Thus far, the VCR has been presented in terms of a simplified, animal-centered coordinate system. More recent studies have examined more carefully the encoding of spatial information within the reflex. For example, if a neck muscle responds to both roll and pitch, might there be some intermediate angle that provides the "best" stimulus, and is there a simple rule for describing the response to an arbitrary angle?

Vestibular afferents can be characterized by a polarization vector that describes the stimulus producing the maximal response. For example, horizontal canal afferents have vertical angular rotation vectors, whereas a utricular afferent may have a linear acceleration vector that points out the ipsilateral ear. These afferents all obey a "cosine rule": their response to an arbitrarily directed stimulus is proportional to the cosine of the angle between the stimulus and the polarization vector. If the VCR response arises from a linear combination of three angular acceleration vectors from the semicircular canals (Estes et al., 1975) and linear polarization vectors from otolith organs arranged roughly in horizontal and sagittal vertical planes (Fernandez and Goldberg, 1976a; Tomko et al., 1981a), a VCR response vector whose orientation and dynamics are simply given by the convergence "coefficients" of afferent polarization vectors should result.

Baker, Peterson, and their colleagues have, in fact, demonstrated that neck muscles in the cat can be characterized by such a stimulus orientation, which produces the maximal VCR at a given frequency (Baker et al., 1985). Changing the direction of the stimulus changed the amplitude and phase of the response according to the "cosine rule" observed in vestibular afferents and within the vestibular nuclei. These directional coding properties remained stable for frequencies above about 0.5 Hz, but for lower stimulus frequencies (at which perhaps input from the semicircular canal contribution did not overwhelm that from the otolith organs), the orientation of the most effective stimulus was either poorly defined (different orientations giving equal responses, but with the phase of the response varying with orientation) or was shifted to a markedly different direction. These results are consistent with a convergence of inputs from canal and otolith systems which have different spatial orientations and different temporal properties. For example, a "roll position" signal from the otolith organs combined with a "pitch velocity" signal (such as from both anterior canals) would produce a response vector aligned with roll at low frequencies, but as the canal response begins to dominate, the direction of the most effective stimulus will shift from roll to pitch.

Such convergence between semicircular canals, and between canals and otolith organs, is partly organized within the vestibular nuclei; both multiple canal convergence (Curthoys and Markham, 1971; Baker et al., 1984a) and the interaction of spatial and temporal coding that probably arises from canal and otolith convergence (Baker et al., 1984b) have been observed in cats. Convergence may also play a role in shaping the spatial properties of signals arising from the otolith organs, narrowing the range of polarization vectors from the relatively uniform distribution observed in utricular afferents (Tomko et al., 1981a) to the greater concentration of vectors near roll seen in the region of the lateral vestibular nucleus (Schor et al., 1984, but see also Chan et al., 1985) and in spinal interneurons (Schor et al., 1986). Since the otolith response vector orientations within the lateral vestibular nucleus of canal-plugged cats does not vary with frequency (Schor et al., 1985), whatever convergence is present must involve otolith signals with dynamics or spatial orientations similar to each other.

Response Dynamics Are Modified by "Closing the Loop"

In the behaving animal, the VCR rarely occurs by itself. A head movement will provide a vestibular signal that gives rise to a VCR acting to slow, or stop, the movement. In addition, rotation of the head on the neck will activate the cervicocollic reflex, which acts as a stretch reflex (Chapter 7), as well as optocollic reflexes (Wilson et al., 1983), to oppose the applied disturbance. Visual and vestibular stimuli caused by the head movement can also activate ocular-stabilizing reflexes; since signals related to eye position have been recorded in neck muscles (Vidal et al., 1982), an explicit optocollic or vestibulooptocollic reflex may play a role in head stabilization. Furthermore, the head–neck system rides on the body: neck rotation produces both a tonic neck and a vestibular reflex on limbs, and any body movement that also moves the head–neck system can, in turn, provide additional vestibular stimulation.

Goldberg and Peterson (1986) measured head movements produced by whole body rotation in alert and deeply anesthetized cats. The responses resembled a second-order underdamped high-pass system. In the anesthetized animal, the resonant frequency was 1–2 hz, and the gain at low frequencies fell at 40 dB/decade. In contrast, in the alert animal the resonant frequency was about 4 Hz, presumably because of the higher viscoelasticity of the active neck musculature. Furthermore, the low-frequency gain stabilized at 0.5; this value was attributed to an interaction of a VCR and cervicocollic reflex with similar gain and dynamics.

The interaction of the VCR with other reflexes to control the position of the head has been examined most extensively in experiments performed on primates, including humans. The next section examines the interactions of visual, vestibular, and proprioceptive systems in the overall head control strategy.

CONTROL OF HEAD POSITION

The control of head position is a complex process that integrates information from a variety of sources to generate functionally appropriate motor commands. Figure 12.5 presents a block diagram description of the system's operational structure; it includes the VCR diagram of Figure 12.1 in a modified form. Inputs to the head control system enter the block diagram from the left and include central commands to the motoneuron pool, movements of the body in space, movements of the visual environment with respect to the head, and external torques applied to the head. These inputs are not controlled directly by the head system and therefore can be manipulated experimentally without interfering with its operation.

There are two main subsystems in the forward pathway from central motor commands to head position: the muscle activation dynamics (M), which transform neural activation into active muscle force, and the head plant mechanics (P), which generate a movement in response to the net torque applied to the head. The muscle and plant dynamics may interact; M can change with head position and P will vary with the level of torque generated by M. These interactions must be recognized, although it may be possible to ignore them for small perturbations about an operating point.

Three feedback subsystems relay information about head position by means of different sensory modalities. The cervicocollic reflex (CCR) subsystem uses somatosensory information to monitor the position of the head with respect to the body; the vestibulocollic reflex (VCR) and optocollic reflex (OCR) subsystems signal movement of the head in space, using vestibular and visual signals. These feedback systems undoubtedly connect centrally as well as peripherally and may therefore contribute to the formulation of central "voluntary" commands as well as "reflex" responses. Distinguishing between "reflex" and "voluntary" responses is not always easy, particularly at latencies longer than those required to subserve purely spinal pathways. It may be useful to consider the feedback pathways as representing all responses that occur automatically for a given mental set. Sensory contributions toward the formulation of less automatic, voluntary commands should be considered as part of the strategy that generates the central command input.

Because the head control system contains a number of feedback loops, the behavior of individual subsystems can be examined directly only by opening the feedback pathways. In some cases this can be done readily (e.g., visual inputs can be masked); in other cases feedback pathways are difficult to eliminate without interfering with the operation of the system (e.g., somatosensory inputs can be reduced by fixing the head with respect to the body, but this obviously changes the normal operation of the system).

Either head position in space or neck position (the position of the head with respect to the body) can be employed as the functional output of the system. The neural command to the neck muscles and the net torque applied to the head are two other variables that may be regarded as outputs under some conditions. The neural command to the neck muscles cannot be measured directly, although an indirect measure is available in terms of the EMGs of the neck muscles. The net torque applied to the head can be measured only by preventing movement of the head. It may be estimated from an analysis of head movements provided that a

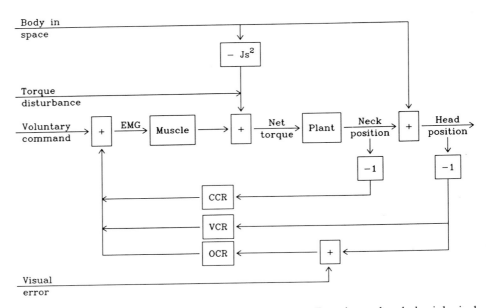

Figure 12.5.   Block diagram of the head control system. Experimental and physiological inputs are on the left, the outputs of head and neck position on the right. The feedback loops include the cervicocollic reflex (CCR), the vestibulocollic reflex (VCR), and an optocollic reflex (OCR). The moment of inertia of the head, J, produces a torque on the neck during head angular accelerations (s^2).

good model of the plant mechanics is available. Finally, by embedding the head control system in a larger system, other outputs, such as gaze, can be developed.

In a normal behavioral situation, many of the inputs to the head control system will change at the same time. It is advantageous to manipulate experimental conditions so that only one input changes at any time. Individual input–output relations can be derived for each experimental case and are presented in Table 12.2. These relations clearly indicate that M (the muscle dynamics) and P (plant mechanics) terms play important roles in determining the behavior of the system.

The foregoing discussion suggests that a full understanding of the head control system requires (1) the characterization of the system's response to each of the input modalities, applied either separately or together; and (2) the determination of the dynamics and relative gains of each subsystem. As we shall see, investigations to date have provided some insight into each of these aspects, but much remains unknown.

The open loop mechanics of the monkey head (P) during vertical axis (yaw) rotations have been modeled as a second-order mechanical system having inertia, viscosity, and elasticity (Bizzi et al., 1978). The elasticity and viscosity have two components: an active component, which varies with the level of neural activation, and a passive, unvarying, component. Inertia of the head was estimated from the dynamics of a severed, perfused head, whereas elastic and viscous parameters were obtained from responses to step torque perturbations in animals in which

Table 12.2. Input–Output Relations for the Head Control Diagram of Figure 12.5[a]

Input	Output	Transfer Function
Voluntary command	Neck, head	$$\dfrac{MP}{1 + (CCR + VCR + OCR)MP}$$
Visual error	Neck, head	$$\dfrac{OCR\ MP}{1 + (CCR + VCR + OCR)MP}$$
Torque disturbance	Neck, head	$$\dfrac{P}{1 + (CCR + VCR + OCR)MP}$$
Body movement	Neck	$$\dfrac{-Js^2P - (VCR + OCR)P}{1 + (CCR + VCR + OCR)MP}$$
Body movement	Head	$$\dfrac{1 - Js^2P + CCR\ MP}{1 + (CCR + VCR + OCR)MP}$$

[a]The effect of each input, taken alone, on the two output systems, head and neck position, is presented. Note that for the first three inputs, voluntary command, visual error, and a torque disturbance of the head–neck system, the response of both head and neck (which carries the head) are the same. Head and neck react differently, however, to imposed body movements. M, Muscle activation dynamics; P, head plant mechanics; CCR, VCR, OCR, reflex contributions due to cervicocollic, vestibulocollic, and optocollic systems; J, moment of inertia of the head; s^2, Laplace frequency variable, signifying that angular acceleration is the relevant movement parameter.

sensory feedback had been eliminated by vestibulectomy and dorsal rhizotomy. Head mechanics, plotted in Figure 12.2, were found to have a natural frequency of about 2 Hz and to be quite underdamped (damping factor of about 0.4). Although amplitude-dependent nonlinearities were noted in these experiments, they were ignored in subsequent analysis. Trajectories of orienting head movements were then recorded under normal conditions and with unexpected load disturbances. Normal and loaded trajectories were always significantly different, indicating that the monkeys were not able to compensate fully for unexpected loads, as might be expected if the cervicocollic reflex acted as a powerful servo mechanism. Furthermore, most of the incremental torque developed in the loaded movements could be predicted from the open-loop model of head mechanics. This suggested that the gain of the cervicocollic reflex was normally low; models describing plant mechanics could largely ignore somatosensory feedback. The gain of the CCR may also be reduced prior to the onset of a voluntary movement, as has been reported for stretch reflexes in limb muscles (e.g., Gottlieb and Agarwal, 1980).

For the human head in the sagittal (pitch) plane, the transfer function relating head position to applied force shows two resonances at about 3 and 6 Hz (Viviani and Berthoz, 1975). In this study, sensory feedback was not eliminated, leading to closed-loop behavior corresponding to that described by the third equation of Table 12.2. The double resonance was interpreted as resulting from the kinematics of head movement in the sagittal plane, which is thought to occur about two distinct centers of rotation. A two-degree-of-freedom model, with each degree of freedom having distinct elastic and viscous components, provided a good fit to the experimental data at low frequencies; at higher frequencies, at which the elastic and viscous properties varied with frequency, the fit was poor. This nonlinear behavior could arise from interactions between the two degrees of freedom in the system. Alternatively, the poor fit at high frequencies could arise because the analytic model used was too simple to describe the behavior of the system with intact sensory feedback. Although visual feedback was shown to be unimportant, vestibular and somatosensory effects remained and could contribute to the observed dynamics. Fitting a second-order model to data from the resulting higher order system would cause parameter estimates to vary with frequency. Another possibility is that the observed dependence of elasticity and viscosity on frequency resulted from the use of force inputs. The amplitude of the displacements evoked by a torque of constant amplitude will decrease with increasing frequency because of inertial effects. This could cause an apparent change in head mechanics with frequency, since the stiffness of joints and muscles is known to decrease with an increasing amplitude of displacement (Rack and Westbury, 1974; Kearney and Hunter, 1982).

A more complex, sixth-order nonlinear model to describe combined open-loop muscle and head dynamics was developed to investigate voluntary control of rapid head movement in humans (Zangemeister et al., 1981c). As a major innovation, the model incorporated the activation dynamics of agonist and antagonist muscles, and its parameters were adjusted to reproduce the trajectories observed in voluntary head movements. This model then was used to investigate the pattern of "motor commands" required to produce various head trajectories. However, it was not possible to verify independently many of the parameters of the model, including those describing muscle dynamics.

The relative contributions of visual, vestibular, and voluntary mechanisms during head stabilization in humans have recently been reported in normal subjects and in patients with bilateral loss of vestibular function (Guitton et al., 1986). Responses in both the time and frequency domain to whole-body rotations about a vertical axis were examined using different behavioral tasks. In the "Gunsight" task, the subject was instructed to hold the head fixed in space under normal visual conditions: visual, vestibular, and voluntary (Vi + Ve + Vo) systems could all be employed. The "Imaginary Gunsight" task also required that the head be held fixed, but visual cues were removed (Ve + Vo). In the "Mental Arithmetic" task, designed to activate the vestibular control system (Ve) in isolation, vision was obscured and subjects were given a mental arithmetic task to distract them. For the final task, "Visual Tracking," the chair was fixed and a moving target was displayed to generate a visual input to be followed by the head, giving rise to a primarily visual and voluntary (Vi + Vo) input signal.

Figure 12.6A shows typical gain curves relating head position (with respect to the target) to the stimulus input for all four cases. When all three systems were

$\longrightarrow$

Figure 12.6.   Frequency responses of a normal human experimental subject. Typical gain curves (from Guitton et al., 1986) are illustrated in (A) for four behavioral paradigms, designed to selectively stimulate visual (Vi), vestibular (Ve), and voluntary (Vo) systems in various combinations. The responses in (B) were derived from a simple model of head control after adjusting the static gains corresponding to the VCR and OCR loops.

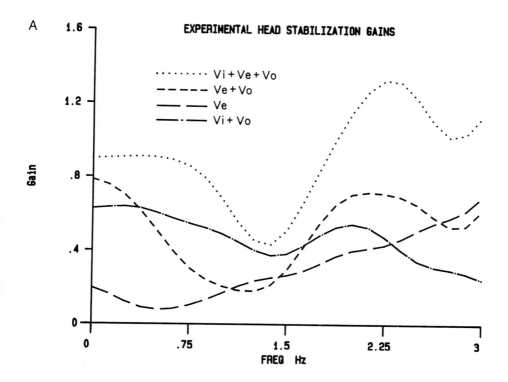

A

EXPERIMENTAL HEAD STABILIZATION GAINS

Gain

$\cdots\cdots\cdots$ Vi + Ve + Vo
$-----$ Ve + Vo
$-$ $-$ $-$ Ve
$-\cdot-\cdot-$ Vi + Vo

FREQ Hz

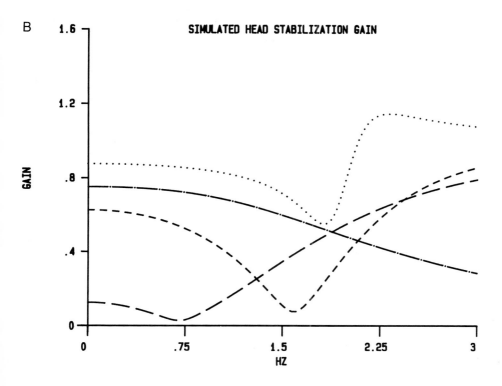

B

SIMULATED HEAD STABILIZATION GAIN

GAIN

HZ

155

employed ("Gunsight," or Vi + Ve + Vo), the gain at low frequencies was close to one. The low-frequency gains during the other "active" tracking tasks ("Imaginary Gunsight," Ve + Vo and "Visual Tracking," Vi + Vo) were substantial, although lower; when mental arithmetic was used in the vestibular paradigm (Ve), however, the gain was close to zero. At high frequencies, the response gains for the three tasks involving chair rotation (Vi + Ve + Vo, Ve + Vo, and Ve) increased, presumably because head inertia began to dominate the response and aided in holding the head fixed in space. In contrast, in the visual tracking task (Vi), in which the head must be actively moved, causing inertia to work against the task, the gain decreased with increasing frequency. At lower frequencies (below 1 Hz), at which inertial effects are less important, the gain should be determined by the relative importance of the different feedback systems and the elastic properties of the head (Table 12.3). The major findings for both normal and vestibular-loss subjects were as follows:

1. The gain during the mental arithmetic task (Ve) was very low for both normal and vestibular-loss subjects, indicating that the vestibulocollic gain was low.
2. The gain during active tracking in the dark (Ve + Vo) was quite high in normal subjects, whereas for the vestibular patients it was very low. Thus, subjects can stabilize the head in space quite effectively at low frequency without vision, but require vestibular function to do so.
3. When all three systems were available (Vi + Ve + Vo), the gain for normal subjects was somewhat higher than when one system was absent (Ve + Vo or Vi + Vo), indicating that visual and vestibular mechanisms together generate better head stabilization than either alone. In vestibular patients (whose Ve response is presumably diminished), the gain under Vi + Ve + Vo conditions was similar to that during visual tracking (Vi + Vo), and hence lower than that of normal subjects.

These findings can be plugged into the model of the head control system presented in Figure 12.5, and estimates can be made for various components of the model. Plant mechanics were modeled as a second-order low-pass system having a natural frequency of about 1 Hz and slightly less than critical damping (comparable to earlier models of human and monkey head–neck mechanics). Muscle activation and the feedback pathways associated with the vestibulocollic, cervicocollic, and optocollic reflex systems were modeled as simple constants, ignoring their dynamic, time-varying properties. Figure 12.6B shows gain curves obtained from this highly simplified model when the VCR and OCR gains were adjusted to give low-frequency responses corresponding to those observed experimentally. The similarity of the model gain curves in Figure 12.6B with the corresponding experimentally observed gains in Figure 12.6A suggests that the model, although simplified, may be a useful representation of the system.

While gain measurements in the frequency domain provide information about the relative importance of the different feedback modalities, measurements in the time domain provide insight into the latencies at which the different mechanisms act. Figure 12.7A shows step responses (computed from responses to a suitable set of random stimuli) from a typical normal subject for the four conditions de-

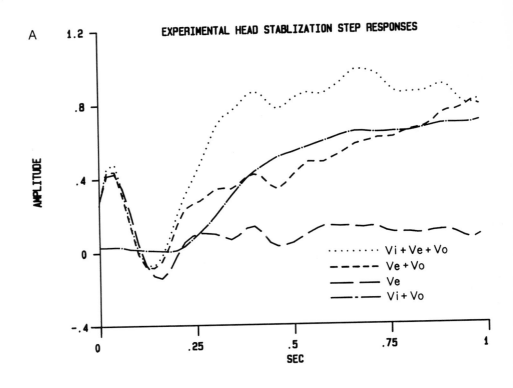

A EXPERIMENTAL HEAD STABLIZATION STEP RESPONSES

.... Vi + Ve + Vo
- - - - Ve + Vo
— — Ve
—·— Vi + Vo

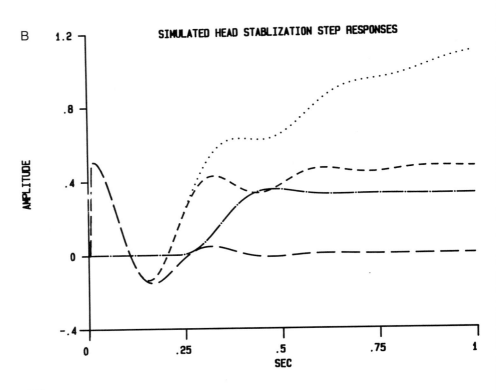

B SIMULATED HEAD STABLIZATION STEP RESPONSES

158

Table 12.3. Head Stabilization Gain of Normal Subjects and Patients with Vestibular Deficits in a Variety of Behavior Paradigms[a]

Stimulus	Task Name	Normal Subjects	Vestibular Patients
Vi + Ve + Vo	Gunsight	0.81 (0.05)	0.54 (0.23)
Ve + Vo	Imaginary gunsight	0.61 (0.15)	0.08 (0.01)
Ve	Mental arithmetic	0.12 (0.10)	0.09 (0.07)
Vi + Vo	Visual tracking	0.68 (0.06)	0.50 (0.03)

[a]The various tasks are designed to test combinations of visual (Vi), vestibular (Ve), and voluntary (Vo) contributions. The numbers represent the mean gain of the transfer function over a 0 to 1 Hz bandwidth; the standard deviation of the population of 10 normal subjects and 3 patients are indicated in parentheses. From Guitton et al. (1986).

scribed above. The responses for Vi + Ve + Vo, Ve + Vo, and Ve conditions were nearly identical for the first 120–140 msec, suggesting that the passive mechanical properties and short latency reflex mechanisms were similar in these three conditions. After about 140 msec the curves diverged: the "active" curves, Vi + Ve + Vo and Ve + Vo, rose toward unity gain, while the mental arithmetic curve, Ve, returned to zero. This divergence may be due to a relatively long-latency contribution from vestibular feedback. Step responses from vestibular patients support this interpretation, since the rise toward unity gain was delayed in Vi + Ve + Vo conditions and absent in Ve + Vo. The step response during visual tracking, Vi + Vo, did not begin to rise until about 200 msec, corresponding to the time at which the Vi + Ve + Vo and Ve + Vo curves began to diverge, suggesting that visual information can be utilized only after a delay of about 200 msec. Incorporating these delays into the simple head control model described above, the step response from the model (Fig. 12.7B) exhibits the essential characteristics of the experimental observations.

Properties of the head control system observed in the studies described above range from the relatively stereotyped servo-like action of the VCR and CCR in the cat (Goldberg and Peterson, 1986) to a more voluntary stabilization system in humans (Guitton et al., 1986). These differences may in part be related to differences in experimental paradigm, which have either used measurements during primarily voluntary head movements (Bizzi et al., 1978; Zangemeister et al., 1981b) or during responses to externally applied perturbations (Viviani and Berthoz, 1975; Goldberg and Peterson, 1986; Guitton et al., 1986). Stimulus intensities also varied between studies, a factor that may be important since the VCR has been shown to have a head velocity threshold in cats (Peterson et al., 1985b). It is also possible that species differences may play an important role, with voluntary control superseding reflex control as the phylogenetic scale is ascended.

HEAD STABILIZATION IN SUBMAMMALIAN VERTEBRATES

The cranium, the most rostral addition and perhaps the most decisive acquisition in the phylogeny of chordates (Gans and Northcutt, 1983), is equipped with a concentration of paired, specialized sense organs that made it excellent for locating predators and prey. In aquatic forms, the degree of mobility of the head on the trunk is limited by hydrodynamic and biomechanical demands. These ecological constraints were overcome in evolving quadrupeds as they became independent of an aquatic life style. In conjunction with the many modifications of the skeleton, a cervical region with increasing numbers of vertebrae (1 in amphibia, 14–15 in most birds) and greater flexibility became prominent, allowing the axis of head rotation to shift from a thoracic to a cervical level. Mechanical factors resulting from this increasing length and flexibility of the neck may have favored a change in the orientation of the cervical column from horizontal to vertical (Vidal et al., 1986).

Together with the ability to explore the environment with active head movements came the necessity to stabilize the head reflexively against passive displacements resulting from trunk movements during locomotion. Since the main function of these collicular reflexes is to assist locomotion by stabilizing posture and gaze, their properties can be expected to be adjusted to the particular requirements resulting from the locomotor repertoire of a given species.

Vestibulocollic and optocollic reflexes are particularly prominent in lower vertebrates, forming the basis for a number of early investigations. Lesion experiments, particularly those involving selective destruction of individual labyrinthine receptor organs (e.g., Tait and McNally, 1934; Ewald, 1892) revealed that resting activity from the periphery, in particular from the utricle, is important for maintaining normal posture. The OCR was used for a very extensive study of the frog's visual acuity, the development of the OCR, its response asymmetries under monocular viewing conditions, and the fatigue of these responses over time (Birukow, 1937; Birukow, 1952). Quantitative measurements of the OCR and VCR in the sagittal, pitch plane of the frog (Birukow, 1952; Butz-Kuenzer, 1958) demonstrated an increase in the gain of the VCR with frequency and a decrease in OCR gain. In the pigeon, OCR and VCR responses sum during rotation; at the end of rotation, the OCR can cancel the vestibular after-responses (Mowrer, 1935; Huizinga and Van der Meulen, 1951).

Optokinetic Reflexes

The optokinetic system is a stabilizing subsystem that converts visual image motion into eye and head movements. When activated by a movement of the visual surround relative to the retina, the system causes both eye and head to follow the stimulus, thereby reducing the velocity of the images slipping across the retina sufficiently to allow clear vision (Fig. 12.8). This system is particularly well tuned to low velocities such as those occurring during a drift of the position of the eye or head in the dark. In species with few or no spontaneous eye movements such

Figure 12.7. Step response of the head control system. As in the previous figure, (A) illustrates the response of a typical normal human subject, whereas (B) gives the response of the head model, characterized by second-order passive mechanics, static vestibular feedback with a delay of 140 msec, and a static visual feedback with a delay of 200 msec.

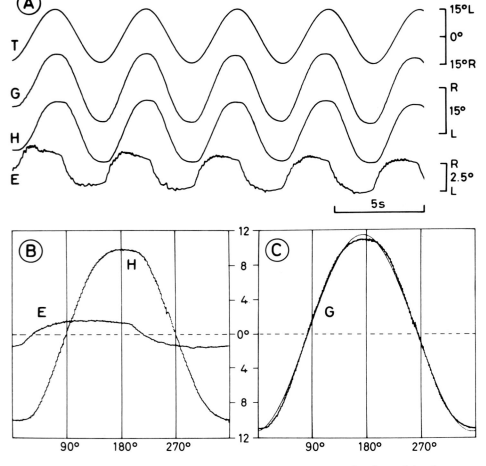

Figure 12.8. Compensatory gaze, head, and eye movements of a frog. Stimulus consisted of whole body oscillation, 0.2 Hz, 15° (T) in the horizontal plane, in front of a stationary patterned background. Simultaneous position records of gaze (G), head (H), and eye (E) as shown in (A) were averaged and plotted in (B) and (C). The averaged gaze movement in (C) was fit by a sine wave.

as crab, frog, or rabbit, it is possible to record optokinetic responses evoked by pattern movements as slow as the apparent movement of the sun (15°/hr) or even slower (Ter Braak, 1936; Horridge, 1966; Dieringer and Daunicht, 1986). This incredibly high sensitivity of the optokinetic system prevents image fading even in the absence of spontaneous saccades. Thus, it allows an effective camouflage strategy that is not jeopardized by conspicuous eye movements. At present it is not known whether this high sensitivity is a common feature among vertebrates or whether it is a specialization found only in some species. At higher pattern velocities, nystagmus, consisting of compensatory following movements ("slow phases") and rapid, repositioning movements ("fast phases"), results. During this sequence of nystagmus, fast phases of the head and eye are typically coupled (Fig. 12.9) and head movements compensate for up to 80% of the stimulus velocity in frog (Birukow, 1952; Lazar and Kolta, 1979; Dieringer and Precht, 1982a), salamander (Kopp and Manteuffel, 1984), and turtle (Dieringer et al., 1983). Head movements also exceed eye movements in other reptiles and birds (Dunlap and Mowrer, 1931; Tauber and Atkin, 1968, Flanders, 1985; Gioanni, 1986). However, these compensatory head movements still need to be complemented by adequate eye movements, particularly following head quick phases or changes in stimulus velocity or direction (Fig. 12.8 and 12.9). Compensatory eye movements can complement head movements during these periods because eye movements have much shorter reaction times at the onset of an optokinetic or a vestibular stimulus, and because ocular quick phases start earlier and have a shorter duration than head quick phases (Dieringer and Precht, 1985; Dieringer, 1987).

Saturation of the optokinetic system occurs at velocities that differ between species. In amphibia, such as frogs or salamanders, this already occurs at a few degrees per second (Dieringer and Precht, 1982a; Kopp and Manteuffel, 1984), a value 5–10 times slower than in the turtle or gecko (Dieringer et al., 1983; N. Dieringer, unpublished observations). The pigeon optokinetic system saturates at

Figure 12.9. Compensatory gaze, head, and eye movements of a turtle. Stimulus consisted of a constant velocity body rotation in the horizontal plane (T), in front of a stationary pattern projected on a cylindrical wall. The vertical dashed line indicates the time at which the projector was turned off. Note the long lasting afternystagmus of gaze (G), head (H), and eye (E), the tight coupling of eye–head fast phases, and the low gaze velocity (G) during the first few fast phases, when head slow phase velocity was low. (From Dieringer, 1986.)

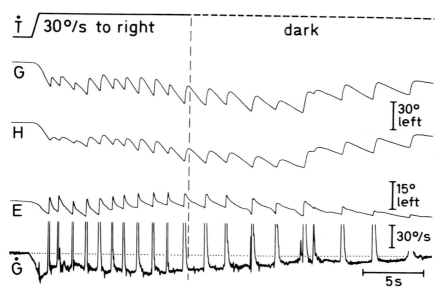

velocities similar to those in the turtle (Gioanni, 1986), as would be expected from the relation between the frequency of head nystagmus and stimulus velocity (Huizinga and Van der Meulen, 1951; Fite et al., 1979). The rather low following capacity in frogs and salamanders is likely to be representative for other amphibia as well, and might reflect the limited capacity of a rather direct, short latency brain stem pathway (Cochran et al., 1984) that is not supplemented by the action of a velocity storage network (Dieringer et al., 1983). The latter network acts as a storage capacitor that is charged up by continued image slip in one direction, expressing itself at the end of an optokinetic stimulus as an afternystagmus (in the dark) of head and eye as shown in Figure 12.9 for the turtle. As with the behavioral data, single unit data from the central vestibular nuclei contain evidence for a functioning velocity storage network in turtles, but not in frogs (Dieringer et al., 1983), and corroborate the idea, originating from lesion experiments (Cohen et al., 1973), that central vestibular neurons represent an essential link in the velocity storage system.

To maintain eccentric eye and head position, these velocity-related motor signals have to be supplemented by appropriate position commands. These position signals are thought to result from the action of a network that acts as a leaky integrator to convert velocity into position signals. Compared to mammals, the frog's velocity integrator has a particularly long time constant, on the order of 90 sec; it exhibits remarkably little "leakiness" (Dieringer and Precht, 1986). From behavioral observations it may be assumed that other amphibians and geckos (Meyer et al., 1979) have similar gaze-holding capabilities, which in turn might be correlated with their rather similar ambush strategy for prey catching.

In analogy to the organization proposed for the extraocular motor system (Dieringer and Precht, 1986), the velocity and position-related portions of the optocollic reflex appear to act on different types of the frog's neck motor units. Neck motoneurons innervating large twitch muscle fibers, which are not active at rest, can be expected to exhibit pure velocity signals. The EMG activity in neck muscles of unrestrained frogs is, in fact, present only during evoked head movements, but not when the head is at rest, regardless of whether the head is in or out of center position (for vestibular signals, see Fig. 12.10 and below). Those motoneurons, on the other hand, that innervate nonspiking, skeletal slow-tonic muscle fibers might mediate pure position signals. A remaining third group might mediate a mixed velocity plus position signal to the small twitch muscle fibers as in the case of the frog's extraocular motor system (Dieringer and Precht, 1986). Such an arrangement might be the most economical compromise between organizational demands for walking and for lurking.

Vestibular Reflexes

Vestibulocollic and vestibuloocular reflexes can supplement concomitant optokinetic reflexes in the light, because of their shorter reaction times and their higher gains at higher frequencies. In the frog, the reaction times of horizontal vestibular reflexes decrease exponentially with increasingly higher accelerations to about 35 (VOR) and 75 msec (VCR) at $1000°/sec^2$ (Dieringer and Precht, 1985). The gain of the VCR, but not of the VOR, exhibits a frequency-dependent threshold above which it increases to reach a plateau. The level of this plateau increases with

Some neurons had predominant velocity responses at high frequencies, whereas others remained nearer to position; these neurons could be carrying signals appropriate for either the high- or low-frequency portion of the vertical VCR. Although the projection of these neurons has not been examined, they could, in principle, terminate on neck motoneurons and contribute to the VCR responses.

Utricular Component of the VCR (Roll, Pitch, and Horizontal Movements)

The component of the VCR due to stimulation of the utricle has been investigated using sinusoidal roll tilt in cats with plugged, nonfunctioning semicircular canals (Schor and Miller, 1981). In such a canal-plugged preparation, the roll VCR at frequencies below 0.1 Hz shows a relatively constant gain and remains nearly in phase with position. However, at higher frequencies, the utricular component of the roll VCR develops both a progressive gain increase and phase lag (Fig. 12.4, dashed curves). This phase lag in canal-plugged cats contrasts sharply with the VCR phase lead (due in part to the phase-leading velocity signal coming from the vertical canals) observed in animals with intact labyrinths (Figs. 12.3 and 12.4).

Within the vestibular nuclei of canal-plugged cats, about one-third of the neurons exhibit dynamics characteristic of the otolith component of the VCR (Schor and Miller, 1982; Schor et al., 1985). Most of the remaining modulated neurons have relatively flat response gains, with phase near position, similar to responses recorded from otolith afferents (Fernandez and Goldberg, 1976b; Anderson et al., 1978; R. H. Schor and B. R. Park, unpublished observations). Of the neurons with muscle-like dynamics, almost all were inhibited during side-down tilt, a response that might be expected of neurons that provide an excitatory input to ipsilateral dorsal neck extensors during the VCR. Since muscle-like dynamics can be observed in such second-order vestibular neurons, yet are not present in the incoming afferent signal, some form of neural processing must be occurring, possibly involving an inhibitory side path that dominates the high-frequency response (Schor et al., 1985).

A number of laboratories are beginning to examine responses to pure linear movements in the horizontal plane. Although the data are sparse at present, both the rat (Lannou et al., 1980) and monkey (Perachio, 1981) have vestibular neurons that show progressive phase lags similar to those in the canal-plugged cat (although in the monkey, the gain of the neuron response decreases, rather than increases, with frequency).

Saccular Component of the VCR (Vertical Movements)

Because it is difficult to provide controlled vertical accelerations to selectively activate the sacculus, the vertical linear acceleration component of the VCR has only recently been studied (Lacour et al., 1987). The response in splenius, a dorsal neck extensor, shows one of two patterns: at frequencies from 0.05 Hz (threshold

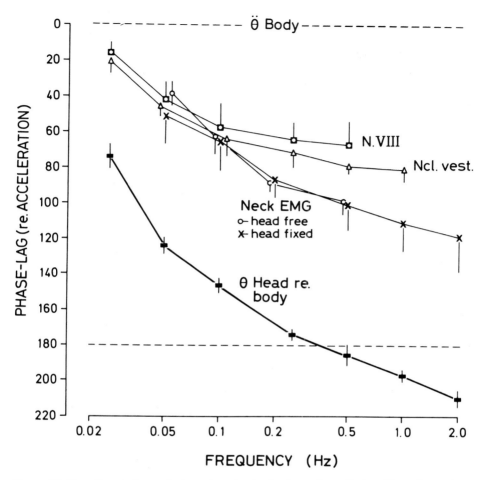

Figure 12.10.   Comparison of phase lags in the horizontal vestibulocollic reflex of the frog. Mean values are for vestibular afferents (N.VIII from Blanks and Precht, 1976) and for central vestibular neurons (Ncl. vest.) from paralyzed frogs. Neck EMG was recorded from Mm. intertransversarii capitis in head restrained and in unrestrained animals. Data for head movements are in part from Dieringer and Precht (1982a).

frequency, i.e., maximal gain is 0.04 at 0.025 Hz but 0.75 at 0.5 Hz (Dieringer and Precht, 1982a). The phase lag (with respect to angular acceleration) increases monotonically over this frequency range and exceeds 180° at frequencies above 0.5 Hz (Fig. 12.10).

The time constants of the frog's VOR and VCR, measured in the frequency and in the time domain, are about 3 sec. Similar values were measured or extrapolated from responses of central (Dieringer et al., 1983) and peripheral afferent vestibular neurons (Precht et al., 1971; Blanks and Precht, 1976) and from electromyographic records of neck muscles. These data, summarized for the frequency domain in Figure 12.10, are consistent with the interpretation that a velocity storage network is not functioning in this species and that part of the neck muscle fibers (i.e., spontaneously inactive, large twitch fibers) receives a direct head velocity signal. This velocity signal must be complemented by more indirect, position-related signals, most likely in small twitch and slow-tonic skeletal muscle fibers (see above), in order to explain the large phase difference between neck EMG and head movement at lower frequencies in Figure 12.10. At higher frequencies, no secondary phase lead develops in the frog's neck EMG signal (Fig. 12.10) nor in its extraocular motor output (Dieringer and Precht, 1982b). Thus, the increasingly larger mechanically induced phase lag is not compensated, as in the cat, and effective gaze stabilization is limited in frogs to frequencies below 1 Hz.

In species with a functioning velocity storage mechanism, such as turtle, gecko (Dieringer et al., 1983; Dieringer and Precht, 1986), or pigeon (Huizinga and Van der Meulen, 1951), the time constants of perrotatory and postrotatory head nystagmus are about two to three times longer than those of vestibular afferents and about as long as that of optokinetic head afternystagmus. Cancellation of a postrotatory nystagmus by an ongoing optokinetic afternystagmus is correspondingly good (Huizinga and Van der Meulen, 1951; Dieringer et al., 1983).

Coordination of Fast Eye–Head Movements

Quick phases of eye and head are rather tightly coupled as long as the position of the head is eccentric (Fig. 12.9). With the head around center position, however, only a suppression of the slow phase head movements occurs during ocular quick phases (Dieringer et al., 1982; Dieringer, 1987). In such a situation, the frequency of ocular quick phases can become high enough to prevent compensatory head movements in an unrestrained frog. The gain of these compensatory eye movements, however, is small (about 0.2) and does not exceed similarly low values measured in a head fixed situation (Dieringer et al., 1983). Therefore in lower tetrapods, increasingly faster stimuli require increasingly larger compensatory head movements for gaze stabilization. Because of the much larger amplitude range of head with respect to eye movements and because of the tight coupling of eye–head quick phases, the frequency of quick phases, and consequently the momentary loss of gaze stabilization, is relatively low in unrestrained animals.

Ocular quick phases of the frog start about 50 msec before head quick phases, overshoot center position by up to 100%, and reach center position by a secondary, passive movement component (Dieringer and Precht, 1982a, 1986). During these quick phases, peak head acceleration reaches up to $3000°/sec^2$ in frogs (Dieringer and Precht, 1985). The VOR must be suppressed during this period to avoid its saturation and to enable a repositioning of both eye and head simultaneously. In fact, frogs with missing vestibular reflexes in the horizontal plane (after a section of both horizontal canal nerves) exhibit parameters of optokinetically evoked head and ocular quick phases that are very similar to those of controls (Dieringer and Precht, 1985). These results demonstrate a rather efficient suppression of vestibular reflexes during quick phases in controls. After each head quick phase the faster reaction time of the eyes allows compensatory eye movements to bridge the time until head velocity has more slowly built up again (see Fig. 12.8 and 12.9).

Comparison Between Mammals and Lower Vertebrates

Reflex stabilization of the head is the result of a complex interaction of the signals from vestibular, optokinetic, and proprioceptive reflexes in both lower and higher vertebrates. For almost all vertebrates, the semicircular canals are oriented in three roughly orthogonal planes, signals from the two labyrinths combine in a reciprocal, push–pull manner, the principal VOR and VCR connections are similar, and a separate visual subsystem, the accessory optic system, is present for the mediation of optokinetic signals. These and many other structural and functional similarities may reflect similar selective pressures and a rather conservative common plan among vertebrates.

Differences, particularly major ones, are probably even more revealing. The working ranges of the frog's anatomically rather direct optokinetic and vestibular reflex systems, good for only a few degrees per second for frequencies up to about 1.0 Hz, would not allow a cat, for example, to maintain unblurred vision for faster head movements and higher speeds of locomotion. Obviously, the properties of stabilizing reflexes have to be adjusted to the animal's normal movement repertoire. This difference in the effective working range of these reflexes apparently does not result from a greater efficacy in the basic, anatomically rather direct reflex circuits. Instead, reflex properties are extended by the addition of functionally new parallel networks such as the velocity storage mechanism, the smooth pursuit system, and circuitry producing the phase lead of the VCR at higher frequencies. Contemporary amphibian and mammalian species offer model systems with differing degrees of complexity, suitable for studying particular problems more conveniently and for recognizing ecological constraints and evolutionary novelties.

SUMMARY

The three sections of this chapter examine how reflexes elicited by vestibular, visual and proprioceptive signals combine to stabilize the head.

The first section focuses upon the vestibulocollic reflexes (VCR) in which signals from otolith organs (the utriculus and sacculus) and semicircular canals generate neck muscle activity to compensate for perturbations that cause the head to move in space. Theoretical requirements for a closed-loop stabilizing system such as the VCR are compared with experimental measurements of dynamic and spatial properties of otolith–neck and canal–neck reflexes. The neural mechanisms that produce these dynamic properties and their relation to the mechanical load imposed by the head–neck system are discussed.

The second section employs systems analysis techniques to explain how vestibulocollic reflexes interact with head–neck mechanical properties, voluntary movements, and other reflexes to determine head position. Recordings from humans and other primates suggest that short latency reflexes are relatively unimportant compared to voluntary reactions that have latencies on the order of 150–300 msec. The latter are most efficient in stabilizing the head when a combination of vestibular, visual, and proprioceptive cues is present.

The third section examines phylogenetic differences in head-stabilizing strategies in a number of submammalian species. Vestibulocollic and optocollic reflexes are shown to be particularly important in stabilizing gaze in lower vertebrates. The latter is optimized to respond to very low movement velocities whereas the VCR responds to more rapid movement. These species lack the more sophisticated velocity storage and visual pursuit systems found in mammals.

13

Kinematic Properties of the Vestibulocollic Reflex

J. BAKER and C. WICKLAND

The vestibulocollic reflex (VCR) must accomplish its task of stabilizing the head (Schor, 1974; Baker et al., 1982) by producing a motor output that has both appropriate timing (dynamics) to accommodate the load presented by the head and appropriate spatial organization (kinematics) so that many neck muscles have the correct synergies to oppose a disturbance in head position. In this chapter we will consider the problems of VCR kinematics. We will begin by describing methods by which vestibular reflexes can be measured in three-dimensional rotational space. We will then give a quantitative description of measurements of the VCR motor output to several of the major neck muscles in the cat. Such a description provides useful information about the combination of semicircular canal inputs that produces excitation of each muscle during the VCR. However, it would be far more valuable to know the rule or rules by which the nervous system has arrived at a particular kinematic organization. Toward this end, the following chapter describes a tensorial model that provides an explicit set of assumptions about the neural mechanisms of the VCR. There is close agreement between the model predictions and the measured excitation of neck muscles during the VCR, suggesting that the tensorial model incorporates essential features of the brain circuitry that organizes the VCR.

ROTATIONS IN THREE DIMENSIONS

Studies of vestibular reflexes and neural responses have traditionally concentrated on the dynamics of responses to rotation about a single axis, most commonly the vertical axis of horizontal plane rotations. The spatial character of a vestibular response is explored with rotations about a number of different axes. The minimal requirement is successive measurements of responses to rotation about three different axes that do not lie in a plane. These could be the orthogonal axes defined as the pitch, roll, and yaw axes in Figure 13.1A (Baker et al., 1985), similar to the X, Y, and Z axes defined by Fernandez and Goldberg (1976a,b,c). Given the strengths of responses to rotations about the three axes, and some additional as-

A

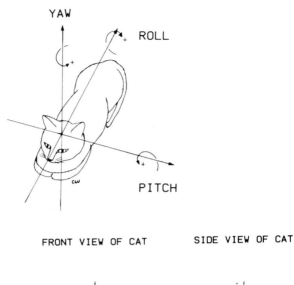

YAW

ROLL

PITCH

B

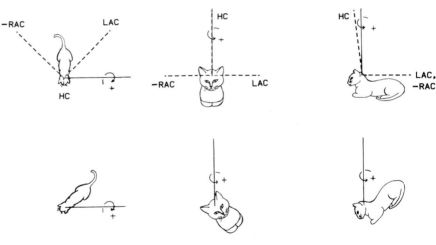

TOP VIEW OF CAT   FRONT VIEW OF CAT   SIDE VIEW OF CAT

-RAC   LAC   HC   HC

HC   -RAC   LAC   LAC, -RAC

45 deg. YAWED PITCH   45 deg. ROLLED YAW   45 deg. PITCHED YAW

Figure 13.1. (A) A rotational coordinate system. (B) Orientation of a cat and the axis about which it is rotated in yawed pitch (left), rolled yaw (center), and pitched yaw (right) sets of axes. Forty-five degree orientations are shown at the bottom. Dashed lines on the top figures show orientations of the semicircular canal pair axes. Abbreviations: LAC, left anterior minus right posterior canal pair; −RAC, left posterior minus right anterior canal pair; HC, left horizontal minus right horizontal canal pair. (Reprinted from Baker et al., 1985.)

sumptions and information, the relative strengths of neural connections that converge from the different semicircular canals to produce the response mechanism can be determined.

What are the assumptions and information we need? We must assume that the measured responses behave linearly (see Chapters 7 and 12), we must assume that only semicircular canals contribute to the responses, and we must follow the widely accepted assumption that the six semicircular canals operate as three pairs (Shimazu and Precht, 1966). In addition, we must know the relative strengths of excitation of the three canal pairs in each of the three response measurement planes. If the response strengths measured for the vestibular mechanism under study are P, R, and Y, then we can find the canal pair neural input strengths A, B, and C by solving the three equations in three variables

$$P = HCP \times A + V1P \times B + V2P \times C$$
$$R = HCR \times A + V1R \times B + V2R \times C$$
$$Y = HCY \times A + V1Y \times B + V2Y \times C$$

where HCP represents the horizontal canal pair excitation during pitch rotations, $V1P$ and $V2P$ represent the excitation of the two vertical canal pairs during pitch, and so on for roll and yaw.

Thus, the first step toward describing the spatial organization of vestibular responses is determination of the kinematics of semicircular canal responses. Canal excitations have been determined from anatomical measurements in several species (Blanks et al., 1972, 1975a, 1985; Curthoys et al., 1975, 1977) and from physiological recordings in some cases (Blanks et al., 1975b; Abend, 1977, 1978; Miles and Braitman, 1980; Baker et al., 1982, 1984a; Bohmer et al., 1985). Only the earliest physiological studies simply measured pitch, roll, and yaw responses (Lowenstein and Sand, 1940); instead responses were recorded to rotations about several axes for *null point determination* or *best-fitting sinusoids*. These techniques are based on the observations that a canal (or otolith organ) does not respond to rotations (or tilts) about axes that are orthogonal to the maximally excitatory axis (Ross, 1936; Fernandez and Goldberg, 1976b), and that the strength of the sensory response varies as a cosine function of the angle between the axis of rotation and the best excitatory axis (Loe et al., 1973; Blanks et al., 1975b).

Null point determination is done by testing several axes of rotation to find two distinct axes about which rotation produces no response. This is sufficient for calculation of the axis of best response, which is the axis perpendicular to the two null axes. An excellent example of the use of null points is the characterization of vestibular afferents by Estes et al. (1975), who found four null axes for each neuron and averaged the two axes of best response to obtain a more accurate estimate.

It has been known for many years that the strength of the gravitational stimulus to the otolith organs and the strength of their sensory responses both vary as a sinusoidal function of the orientation of the organ with respect to the earth when an animal is rotated through increasing angles about a given axis (Lowenstein and Roberts, 1950). Loe et al. (1973) successfully extended this idea to predict otolith responses to rotations about arbitrary axes in three-dimensional space (Werner et al., 1969; Loe et al., 1973), and Blanks et al. (1975b) applied it to semicircular canal responses to rotations about several axes. The typical procedure (Baker et al., 1985) is to make successive recordings of responses to rotations about several axes, all of which lie in one plane. The strength of the measured response should be a sinusoidal function of the angle of the rotation axis with respect to some reference in the plane containing the axes. Figure 13.1B shows examples from three such sets of axes lying in a yaw horizontal, roll vertical, and pitch vertical plane. The reference axes for the three sets are pitch, yaw, and yaw axes, respectively. Baker et al. (1985) have named such sets of axes according to their plane and reference axis; the sets in Figure 13.1B are yawed pitch, rolled yaw, and pitched yaw, respectively. Rotation about the pitch axis is called a 0° axis yawed pitch rotation. In our apparatus, the animal may be moved into different positions before applying rotations about one of two fixed servo-driven axes. If the animal is positioned in the rotation apparatus by turning it from the 0° orientation through a 90° angle about the yaw axis then locking the animal in place, oscillations about the horizontal axis are roll axis rotations, also called 90° yawed pitch rotations. Figure 13.1B shows the rotation axis at the 45° yawed pitch orientation.

Figure 13.2 (top) shows the sinusoidal variation in response strength of a secondary vestibular neuron stimulated by rotations about 14 of the yawed pitch axes (top left) and 12 of the rolled yaw axes (top right). The rotation stimulus in each case was sinusoidal oscillation about the axis at 0.5 Hz, and the phases of the response peaks relative to peak rotational positions are shown in the second row of graphs from the top of Figure 13.2. [The sinusoidal variation of the response strength for different axes is not related to the sinusoidal nature of the oscillatory stimulus; Blanks et al. (1975) used a constant acceleration stimulus of short duration to obtain their sinusoidal response functions of stimulus axis.] The solid lines passing through the data points are sinusoidal curves that follow the least-squares error criterion. The kinematics of the secondary neuron's responses are well described by the fitted functions. Can these methods of analyzing vestibular responses in three-dimensional rotational space be usefully applied to the VCR?

VCR RESPONSES TO HIGH-FREQUENCY ROTATIONS:
THE DIRECTION OF BEST EXCITATION

Studies of the VCR have focused on the dynamics of neck muscle electromyographic (EMG) responses to horizontal rotations (Berthoz and Anderson, 1971; Ezure and Sasaki, 1978; Bilotto et al., 1982a), although roll vertical rotations have been tested (Berthoz and Anderson, 1971), particularly in relation to responses produced by the otolith organs (Schor and Miller, 1981). Only recently have VCR EMGs been recorded during rotations about many different axes in three dimensions (Baker et al., 1985), and the resulting data have revealed several features of the kinematics and dynamics of the motor output to the VCR.

The third row of graphs in Figure 13.2 shows the gains of responses of a left biventer cervicis muscle during yawed pitch rotations at 0.4, 0.8, and 1.6 Hz, and the bottom row of Figure 13.2 shows the corresponding response phases.

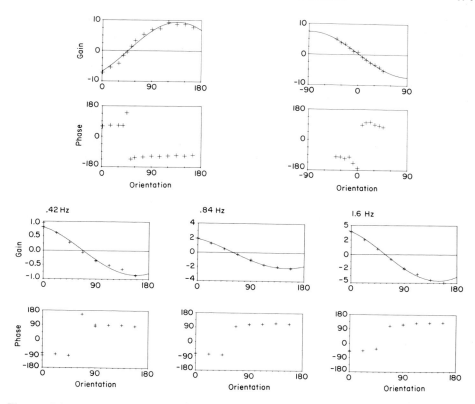

Figure 13.2. Top and second row: Gains (top row) and phases (second row) of a second-order vestibular neuron's responses to yawed pitch (left) and rolled yaw (right) rotations. Responses in the 0° yawed pitch position are to rotations about a pitch axis, 90° responses are to roll rotations. Solid curves are best fit sinusoids. Third and fourth rows: vestibulocollic reflex electromyographic responses of a left biventer cervicis neck muscle to yawed pitch axis rotations at 0.4, 0.8, and 1.6 Hz. Gains and phases are based on percentage modulation of rectified, filtered activity.

Clearly, the best fit sinusoids (solid lines) provide a good description of the spatial character of these neural responses, and the results do not vary appreciably across this range of oscillation frequencies. Other biventer cervicis muscles gave very similar data, and the spatial behavior of six other neck muscles we tested also was well described by sinusoidal functions, each muscle having a different characteristic peak response angle. Responses to rotations about vertical axes are similarly well behaved, except when the decerebrated preparation must be oriented in an extreme position (e.g., on its nose or upside down) in order to rotate about a desired axis.

Because the sinusoidal fits provided an accurate representation of the VCR EMGs, it was possible to give a shorthand description of a muscle's kinematics by using the values of the fitted functions at the standard yaw, pitch, and roll position. The best axis of rotation in three-dimensional space is specified by these values and can be displayed by a unit vector along that axis. Figure 13.3 shows how the best response axis is found for the biventer cervicis illustrated in Figure 13.2.

VCR RESPONSES TO LOWER FREQUENCY ROTATIONS: ORIENTATION DEPENDENT DYNAMICS

Neck muscle VCR EMGs at high frequencies of rotation consistently followed the behavior described above. At frequencies below about 0.4 Hz, however, response strength often did not vary as a sinusoidal function of the orientation of the rotation axis. Figure 13.4 (center) shows an example of the kind of responses often observed when 0.1 to 0.4 Hz rotation frequencies were used to measure response strength. These data were obtained from a complexus neck muscle, a muscle that often showed this type of nonsinusoidal spatial responsiveness. This behavior is not a purely kinematic phenomenon, because as can be seen from the graph of phase behavior (center, right), response dynamics vary depending on the orientation of the rotation axis. Orientation-dependent dynamics are not peculiar to the VCR of decerebrated cats (Baker et al., 1984b); Figure 13.4 (top) shows the responses of a secondary vestibular neuron recorded from the brain stem of an alert cat, and Figure 13.4 (bottom) shows EMG responses recorded from splenius in an alert cat trained to make sinusoidal head movements about the yawed pitch axes.

What is the source of orientation-dependent dynamics, and why does the VCR neural circuitry produce them? A clue to the origin of this odd behavior is its absence when rotation axes were vertical with respect to the earth. Vertical axis stimuli do not modulate the gravitational stimulus to the otolith organs. Furthermore, the change in horizontal axis rotation response phases as rotation frequency is lowered can be described as the appearance of responses that peak at peak rotational displacement, and such position phase responses are characteristic of many otolith afferents (Fernandez and Goldberg, 1976c; Schor and Miller, 1982). It appears likely that orientation-dependent dynamics are the result of an otolith contribution to the VCR at lower frequencies. A clue to the possible function of this behavior is the occurrence of position phase responses to roll rotations significantly more often than to pitch rotations. This could reflect a difference in the load presented by the head about the roll axis as compared to the pitch axis. The inertial component of the head load about the roll axis can be expected from physical considerations to be less than about the pitch axis, and the VCR may accommodate by introducing greater response phase lead for pitch than for roll.

VCR EXCITATION BEST DIRECTIONS FOR NECK MUSCLES

High-frequency rotation VCR EMG responses not only reliably showed the sinusoidal behavior outlined above, they also produced very similar best axes for the same muscle from cat to cat. This consistency of the VCR made it possible to average the best axes determined for a muscle in several experiments to produce

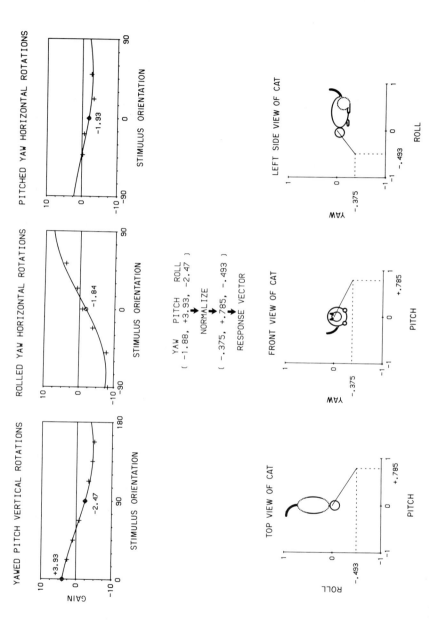

Figure 13.3. Calculation of a response axis unit vector based on responses to yawed pitch, rolled yaw, and pitched yaw rotations. Pitch and roll values (top left, circled) are taken from the sinusoidal function fitted to yawed pitch data. The yaw value is the average of values obtained from rolled yaw and pitched yaw fits (top center and right, circled). The axis vector is normalized and displayed at the bottom of the figure. (Reprinted from Baker et al., 1985.)

173

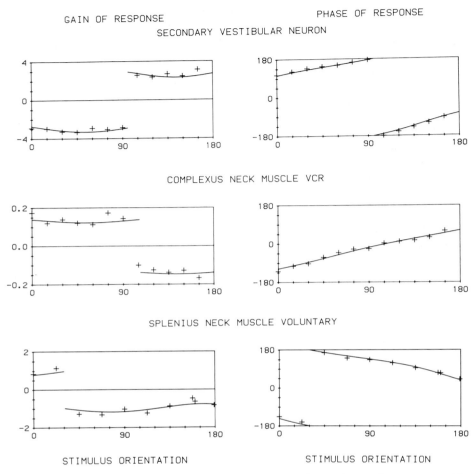

Figure 13.4.   Response gains (left) and phases (right) of complexus electromyographic vestibulocollic activity (center), secondary vestibular neuron activity (top, from Baker et al., 1984b), and splenius activity during sinusoidal voluntary movement (bottom). Responses are to rotations about yawed pitch axes. 0 = pitch, 90 = roll.

a single average best axis. The average best excitation axes for seven of the major neck muscles are shown, for the right side muscles, from three views in Figure 13.5 (top row). The muscles are biventer cervicis, complexus, longus capitis, obliquus capitis inferior, occipitoscapularis, rectus capitis major, and splenius.

The pitch, roll, and yaw values corresponding to each axis were used to estimate the relative contributions of the three pairs of semicircular canals to each muscle's VCR responses, according to the procedure outlined earlier in this chapter. The relative strengths of neural connections from the canal pairs to each muscle are shown in Table 13.1. The computations were based on data gathered with the animal at or near the normal upright position, and are based on high-frequency rotations to minimize a possible otolith influence. Table 13.1 shows that the major inputs to the VCR in the dorsal neck muscles are the contralateral anterior minus ipsilateral posterior canal pair and the horizontal canal pair. (Longus capitis is the only ventral neck muscle studied.)

While the above information describes VCR excitation, it does not provide any insight into the principles by which the brain has chosen a particular pattern of canal to muscle connections. An understanding of the VCR spatial organization requires not only a description of the semicircular canal inputs to the VCR, but also the output from the VCR, the unique pulling actions of the neck muscles that sum to produce the appropriately compensatory head torque.

We have described this output by making quantitative measurements of pulling strength and direction of many dorsal and ventral neck muscles in cats. Pulling

Figure 13.5.   Top: Average best excitation axis unit vectors for several neck muscles during the vestibulocollic reflex. Illustrated axes are for muscles on the right side of the cat. The axes are represented in a coordinate system that places the cat's head pitched 28° down from the stereotaxic position. (Reprinted from Baker et al., 1985.) Bottom: Estimated pulling directions and magnitudes for the same neck muscles, based on measurements of origins, insertions, and effective cross-sectional area. Abbreviations: B, biventer cervicis; C, complexus; L, longus capitis; M, rectus capitis major; O, obliquus capitis inferior; I, occipitoscapularis; S, splenius.

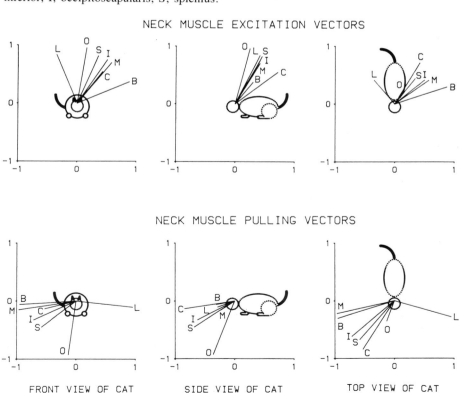

NECK MUSCLE EXCITATION VECTORS

NECK MUSCLE PULLING VECTORS

FRONT VIEW OF CAT   SIDE VIEW OF CAT   TOP VIEW OF CAT

Table 13.1. Semicircular Canal Inputs to Seven Major Neck Muscles during the Vestibulocollic Reflex

	LH − RH[a]	LA − RP[a]	LP − RA[a]
R. biventer	0.37	0.85	−0.39
R. complexus	0.54	0.81	0.22
R. rectus major	0.68	0.73	−0.07
R. occipitoscapularis	0.73	0.68	−0.01
R. splenius	0.79	0.60	0.12
R. obliquus	0.93	0.34	0.13
R. longus capitis	0.74	0.08	0.67

[a]LH − RH, Left horizontal minus right horizontal; LA − RP, left anterior minus right posterior; LP − RA, left posterior minus right anterior.

directions were determined by stereotaxic measurements of origins and insertions of the muscles. Strength of pull, determined by the cross-sectional area, was estimated as the mass of the muscle divided by its length. A torque vector was obtained by calculating the cross-product of the pulling strength vector from the insertion toward the origin and the vector from the estimated rotation axis to the insertion. Torque vectors for seven of the muscles are shown at the bottom of Figure 13.5, which represents the strength of pull by the length of the vector.

The vectors obtained generally supported statements in the literature describing the action of the neck muscles expected from their anatomy (Reighard and Jennings, 1963; Crouch, 1969). Biventer and the rectus capitis muscles primarily raise the head and longus capitis lowers it. Obliquus inferior rotates C1, which effectively turns the head from side to side. Complexus and splenius have pulling action in all three planes.

Given the six canal inputs to the VCR and the approximately 30 neck muscle forces that pull the head, there are many possible ways in which the VCR could make neural connections to produce correct compensatory head movements. The next chapter proposes a mathematical model of the VCR and the mechanisms by which its choice of neuromuscular outputs is made.

SUMMARY

This chapter explores the spatial (kinematic) properties of the vestibulocollic reflex (VCR) that enable it to compensate for perturbations of the head in three-dimensional space.

The analysis begins with the geometry of the three semicircular canals and two otolith organs, which determines how each receptor will respond to a movement having varying amounts of rotation about the yaw, pitch, and roll axes.

Responses of second-order vestibular neurons to the same rotations are then measured and analyzed to determine how these responses might result from convergent interaction of signals from canals and otolith organs.

Finally, electromyographic responses of neck muscles are recorded during three-dimensional head rotations and analyzed in the same way. Each muscle has a characteristic best rotation that activates it most strongly. Responses to high-frequency rotations about different axes decline with the cosine of the angle between that axis and the best axis. At lower frequencies of rotation some muscles exhibit more complex responses in which dynamic properties of the response shift with the rotation axis whereas response amplitude remains large.

Spatial properties of neck muscle responses are used to calculate which semi-circular canals provide input to each muscle. They can also be compared to the pulling direction of each muscle, determined from the geometry of its origin and insertion. Activation and pulling directions are quite different, a fact that will be examined theoretically in Chapter 14.

14

A Tensorial Model of
Neck Motor Activation

A. J. PELLIONISZ and B. W. PETERSON

The data presented in the previous chapter provide a detailed description of how the central nervous system organizes neck muscle activation in the context of a well-defined sensorimotor task—the vestibulocollic reflex (VCR). The fact that the geometrical alignments of both the sensory receptors (the 3 semicircular canals, Curthoys et al., 1977) and motor effectors (the 30 neck muscles, see Chapter 13 and Baker et al., 1984c) have been measured opens the possibility of modeling the VCR using the tensorial methodology described by Pellionisz and Llinás (1979) and Pellionisz (1984). This approach allows one to predict patterns of motor activation, such as those described in Figure 13.5, from the geometry of the receptors and effectors. This chapter describes the properties of the tensorial model of the VCR and shows that it predicts quite closely the actual VCR activation of the six neck muscles tested to date. The possibility of extending the model to other neck motor activities such as voluntary movement is also discussed. As an introduction to these issues, the next section will briefly discuss the conceptual problems presented by complex sensorimotor systems and review the rationale behind the development of the tensorial modeling approach.

CONCEPTUAL BASIS OF TENSORIAL MODELING

The problem faced by a sensorimotor system is to transform information about the environment, measured by a diverse set of sensors, into appropriate responses executed by multiple muscles acting in concert. When the spatial (kinematic) properties of the transformation are considered, the geometrical arrangements of sensors and muscles are critical, since they define the intrinsic biological coordinate frames in which the stimulus and response are expressed. The nervous system in turn must transform stimuli expressed in one frame into responses expressed in the other, perhaps by stages involving additional coordinate frames. The proposal by Pellionisz and Llinás (1979) that neuronal networks should be considered as tensors was based upon the conceptual definition that tensors are mathematical operators expressing the relationships among mathematical (vectorial) representations, in different frames of reference, of physical entities such as sensory events and the responses they generate (cf. Levi-Civita, 1926; Coburn, 1955). Tensorial operations that, for any particular frame of reference, take the form of matrices could thus express the stages of transformation of sensory stimulus to motor response.

Adoption of the tensorial concept and formalism emphasized an important difference between the representation of sensory input and motor output in their respective coordinate frames. The response of a sensor, such as a semicircular canal, to a stimulus is independent of the responses of other sensors and is proportional to the cosine of the angle between the sensor's axis of maximum sensitivity and the axis of the applied stimulus (or equivalently to the projection of the stimulus vector upon the sensor axis). Such projection-type representations are termed *covariant* in tensorial nomenclature (cf. Bickley and Gibson, 1962). On the other hand, the muscle activations that generate the response are not independent of one another, since the forces or torques they generate must sum in a parallelogram fashion to produce the desired movement. Such parallelogram-type representations are termed *contravariant*. The central nervous system (CNS) can thus be conceived of as a tensorial network that converts a covariant sensory input given in one frame into a contravariant motor output expressed in another frame (Pellionisz and Llinás, 1980).

Before constructing a tensorial model of the VCR, we must consider the conceptual problem raised by *overcompleteness* in motor systems. A motor system is overcomplete when the number of independent effectors (muscles) exceeds the number of controlled degrees of freedom of the appendage they control. As indicated in earlier chapters, it is difficult to be certain if the neck motor system is overcomplete in this most general sense. However, we can also consider the head–neck system to be *functionally overcomplete* in a given behavioral context when the number of muscles exceeds the number of *behaviorally relevant* degrees of freedom (three rotational angles of the head for the VCR). In this case we assume that the system does not independently control internal degrees of freedom (such as all angles of individual joints) as long as the required head movement is properly generated.

The difficulty posed by an overcomplete motor system is that it can produce the same movement using an infinite number of different patterns of muscle activation. Theory must then propose some type of optimality criterion that the system uses in "choosing" the particular pattern observed experimentally. The solution proposed by Pellionisz (1984) in the form of a tensorial modeling scheme utilizes the difference between covariant and contravariant representations of the desired movement, both expressed in the motor frame determined by the muscle geometry. The covariant presentation can always be found uniquely by projecting the movement vector upon each of the muscle axes. The problem is then to find an optimal contravarient representation. In a nonovercomplete system this is just the inverse of the covariant metric. In an overcomplete system the problem is not that such an inverse does not exist, but that there are an infinite number of inverses. Pellionisz (1983, 1984) hypothesized that the nervous system chooses an inverse equivalent to the Moore–Penrose generalized inverse of the covariant metric (Albert, 1972). This inverse has several attractive features. It minimizes the sum of squares of activity of the muscles during any movement. It may also be implemented by a network (matrix) that could plausibly be constructed by a developing nervous systems (Pellionisz and Llinás, 1985). As will be seen below, it is this choice of an optimal inverse that gives the VCR model its predictive power. Related models have been prepared for the vestibuloocular reflex (Simpson and Pellionisz, 1984) and voluntary arm movement system (Gielen and van Zuylen, 1986).

GENERATION OF A TENSORIAL MODEL OF THE VESTIBULOCOLLIC REFLEX

The sensorimotor frames of the vestibulocollic reflex in the cat are illustrated in Figure 14.1. As shown, the anterior, horizontal, and posterior (pairs of) semicircular canals constitute a three-dimensional nonorthogonal frame in which head movements are physically *measured* as the orthogonal projections (covariant components) of the head movement. In turn, the compensatory head movement is physically *generated* in the 30-axis motor frame, as a result of the sum of the (contravariant) motor vector components. Having such a dual relationship with a given physical entity, the vestibulocollic reflex is a primary sensorimotor system. Moreover, in this case both the 10-fold overcompleteness of the transformation (from 3 components to 30) and the nonorthogonality of the frames (particularly that of the motor axes) are self-evident.

The proposed theoretical solution is based on the three-step scheme of sensorimotor tensor transformation shown in Figure 14.2. The task is (1) to change the sensory frame into motor, (2) to change the measured, covariant type vector to an executable contravariant version, and (3) to increase dimensions from 3 to 30. The three steps of the transformation do not accomplish these goals one-by-one. The central, covariant embedding tensor accomplishes both (1) and (3) simply by projecting the 3 sensory (i subscripts) upon the 30 motor axes (p subscripts), which can be mathematically expressed as

$$c_{ip} = s_i \cdot m_p$$

where s and m are the coordinates of the (normalized) sensory and motor axes, respectively, and each matrix element of c_{ip} is the inner (scalar) product of the vectors of coordinates of the ith and pth axis.

The reason that the c_{ip} covariant embedding tensor is necessary but not sufficient in converting the covariant sensory reception vector s_r into contravariant motor execution m^e is that c_{ip} is a *projective* tensor. It turns a physical-type (contravariant) input vector into an output that is provided in its projection components (covariants). However, our case is the opposite; the available sensory input is covariant, whereas the output required is contravariant. This is why the other two conversions in the tensorial sensorimotor scheme are necessary; the sensory metric tensor g^{pr} (the small 3×3 matrix in Fig. 14.2) that converts covariant sensory reception into contravariant sensory perception, and motor metric g^{ie} (the large 30×30 matrix in Fig. 14.2) that turns covariant motor intention into contravariant motor execution. This general function of transforming covariant nonorthogonal

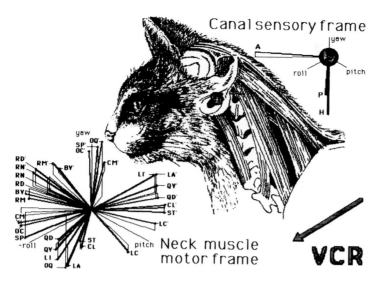

Figure 14.1. Illustration of the quantitatively established 3-axis vestibular frame of reference (data from Blanks et al., 1972) and the 30-axis collicular frame of reference (data from Peterson et al., 1985a). The heavy lines represent rotational axes of the head around which the semicircular canals measure changes in head angular orientation and axes around which the individual neck muscles generate head rotations. The vestibular apparatus and some representative neck muscles are visualized in the central schematic diagram, in which the cervical column is shown close to a vertical orientation (cf. Vidal et al., 1986). The task for tensor network theory is to explain how neuronal nets in the CNS accomplish the required overcomplete covariant-to-contravariant transformation of canal input to muscle output. A, P, and H refer to anterior, posterior, and horizontal canals, respectively. Abbreviations for muscles: BV, biventer; CL, cleidomastoid; CM, complexus; LA, longus atlantis; LC, longus capitis; LI, longissimus; OC, occipitoscapularis; OQ, obliquus capitis inferior; QD, obliquus capitis superior (dorsal division); QV, obliquus capitis superior (ventral division); RD, rectus capitis medialis; RM, rectus capitis major; RN, rectus capitis minor; SP, splenius; ST, sternomastoid. Primes indicate rotational axes of contractions of contralateral muscles.

versions into contravariant ones by a metric tensor can be accomplished for any given set of axes by a matrix of divergent–convergent neuronal connections among primary and secondary vestibular neurons and among brain stem premotor neurons and neck motoneurons (Markham and Curthoys, 1972; Baker et al., 1984b).

Mathematically, the required contravariant metric tensor $\mathbf{g}^{pr}$ can be established as the inverse of the covariant metric tensor $\mathbf{g}_{pr}$:

$$\mathbf{g}^{pr} = (\mathbf{g}_{pr})^{-1}$$

where $\mathbf{g}_{pr}$ is the inner (scalar) product of the vectors of coordinates of the (normalized) axes $\mathbf{s}_i$:

$$\mathbf{g}_{pr} = \mathbf{s}_i \mathbf{s}_i$$

Two important questions arise regarding such metric transformations: a math-

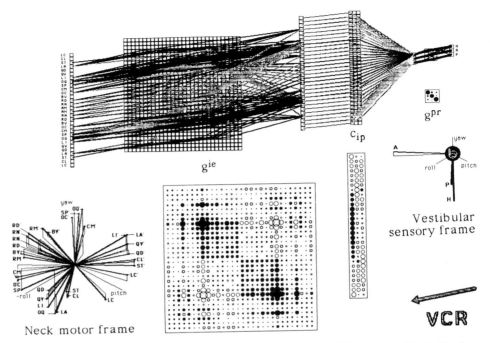

Figure 14.2.   Illustration of the tensor network model of the VCR in the cat (cf. Pellionisz and Peterson, 1985). The sensorimotor transformation occurs in three stages: $\mathbf{g}^{pr}$, sensory metric tensor, $\mathbf{c}_{ip}$, sensorimotor embedding tensor, and $\mathbf{g}^{ie}$, neck motor metric tensor. These general tensorial operations are expressed in the particular frames of reference of the VCR by matrices, which are here represented by patch diagrams in which positive and negative components are shown by filled and open circles whose surface area is proportional to the size of the component. The CNS can implement these matrices by neuronal networks as indicated in the upper part of the diagram. There the strengths of connectivities from H, A, P canals to the 30 neck muscles are represented by line shadings (black for excitation, grey for inhibition) and by line thickness proportional to the value of the interconnecting matrix element.

ematical and a biological one. First, even if such transformations are implemented by matrices corresponding to neuronal networks, the CNS does not arrive at them by mathematical computation, but by some unknown procedure feasible for a biological system. Second, at the level of pure mathematics, a problem occurs with *overcomplete* coordinate systems. In such cases $\mathbf{g}_{pr}$ is singular (its determinant is zero), thus $\mathbf{g}_{pr}$ has an infinite number of inverses. The question of how CNS neuronal networks can arrive at a unique covariant-to-contravariant transformation (even in case of overcompleteness) led to the proposal of a metaorganization principle and procedure that utilize the Moore–Penrose generalized inverse (Pellionisz, 1983, 1984; Pellionisz and Llinás, 1985). Biologically, the proposed solution is based on arriving at special vectors whose covariant and contravariant expressions have identical directions (so-called eigenvectors of the system) by a reverberative oscillatory procedure (muscle proprioception recurring as motoneuron output, setting up stabilizing tremors). These special activation vectors would imprint a matrix of neural connections that could serve as the proper coordination device (e.g., cerebellar neuronal circuit). Mathematically, a unique inverse of $\mathbf{g}^{ie}$ can be obtained from the outer (dyadic matrix) product (symbolized by $><$) of the eigenvectors $\mathbf{E}_m$, weighted by the inverses of the eigenvalues λ_m (the inverse is taken as 0 if $\lambda_m = 0$, cf. Albert, 1972):

$$\mathbf{g}^{ie} = \sum 1/\lambda_m (\mathbf{E}_m >< \mathbf{E}_m)$$

The tensor network model of the vestibulocollic reflex, based upon the above theoretical considerations, emerges from the preliminary data (presented in Chapter 13) in the form shown in Figure 14.2. Each of the three matrices in the model is represented by a box in which the size and sign of each matrix element are indicated by filled (positive) and open (negative) circles. Four columns represent canal inputs (H, A, P), motor nerve outputs (LC), and two intermediate neural stages. Once the model has been set up we can compare its properties to those of the VCR.

MODEL PROPERTIES

The model attempts to predict semicircular canal actions upon neck muscles. It therefore deals with the high-frequency VCR responses described in Chapter 13. One feature of those responses is that they vary sinusoidally with the angle between the animal and the stimulus axis. Semicircular canals are known to respond in this way (Estes et al., 1975). Since the three matrices of the model perform simple spatial transformations, they do not alter this sinusoidal behavior. The model therefore predicts such behavior at the neck motor output and at all intermediate stages.

The other key feature of the VCR data was that muscles were maximally activated by rotations in planes other than their pulling planes. This feature turns out to be the consequence of the nonorthogonality of the muscle axes. As shown in Figure 14.3, it can be demonstrated in a simple two axis, 135° coordinate frame. As illustrated, the contravariant activation of the muscle lying along the 0° axis is 1.0 if the desired movement is along that axis. Generation of the same sized movement in a direction that is *different* from the 0° axis (perpendicular to the second axis, i.e., at 45° with respect to the muscle being measured), however, requires a 1.4 unit activation of that muscle in order to produce forces that produce the correct parallelogram sum.

Although the divergence of activation and pulling directions is to be expected according to the above analysis, the actual activation directions that were consistently chosen in the five cats from the infinite number of possible directions must reflect an algorithm employed by the VCR to resolve the overcompleteness of the VCR system. How closely does this algorithm resemble the Moore–Penrose generalized inverse incorporated in the model? To answer this question the model's responses to the same stimuli used in the experiments were calculated and used to produce predicted activation vectors, which are plotted with the label $-\mathbf{M}$ in

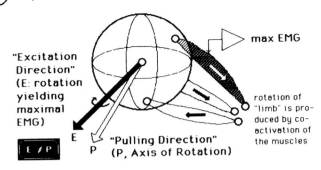

① Experiment   Pulling & Excitation Directions Differ

"Excitation
Direction"
(E: rotation
yielding
maximal
EMG)

max EMG

rotation of
"limb" is pro-
duced by co-
activation of
the muscles

E ≠ P

E
P

"Pulling Direction"
(P, Axis of Rotation)

② Theory: in Non-Orthogonal Frames this Difference is
   Expected and its Magnitude can be Calculated

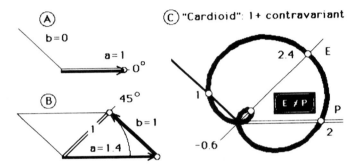

(A)

b = 0
a = 1   0°

(B)

45°
1   b = 1
a = 1.4

(C) "Cardioid": 1 + contravariant

2.4   E
1
E ≠ P   P
-0.6   2

Figure 14.3.   Difference between anatomical pulling directions and maximal excitation directions of a neck muscle (1) and its geometrical explanation (2). (1) If an appendage, such as the head, is rotated by coactivation of (neck) muscles, the rotation axis (pulling direction) of each muscle can be determined by anatomical measurements of the points of origin, insertion, and center of rotation (cf. Fig. 13.5). As also illustrated in Figure 13.5, axes of head movements that are accompanied by maximal activation of each muscle (**E**) are typically not aligned with the pulling directions (**P**). (2) The observed divergence between **P** and **E** can be explained by using the distinction between covariant (projection) and contravariant (parallelogram) representations in nonorthogonal coordinate systems. In the frame illustrated, in which two muscle axes are at an angle of 135°, a unitary displacement in the direction of axis a is generated by muscle activation $a = 1$, $b = 0$ (2A). However, as shown in inset 2B, a unitary displacement in the 45° direction (deviating from the axis direction itself) requires muscle activation of $a = 1.4$, $b = 1$ for the parallelogram sum of a and b to generate the required unitary displacement. The relationship of the contravariant component to the displacement direction can be visualized in a "cardioid" diagram in which $1 + a$ is plotted against displacement direction in polar coordinates. The plot in 2C clearly shows that activation of a reaches its maximum value not for displacements along its own axis but rather for displacements at an angle of 45° with respect to that axis. Thus, contrary to our intuitions that have been honed for orthogonal systems, in nonorthogonal coordinate frames the pulling directions and optimal activation directions of muscles can be expected (and predicted) to differ by large angles from one another.

Figure 14.4. As shown, these predictions are always rotated away from the muscle pulling directions (**P**) in the direction of the measured VCR responses (−**V**) and are typically quite close to the latter. Differences between −**V** and −**M** are small enough to be accounted for by the variability in existing measurements of the pulling directions (upon which the model is based) and of the actual responses. *Thus a tensorial model based solely upon the anatomy of the canals and neck muscles is able to predict with remarkable accuracy the spatial properties of the VCR.*

The successful approximation of overall input/output properties of the VCR (measured in six muscles) should be regarded as only an initial stage of the modeling effort (see also Pellionisz and Peterson, 1985). More muscles need to be tested and the experiments generalized to other species. The VCR model also predicts neural signals at intermediate stages of the sensorimotor transformation. These should be compared with actual neural recordings and the model altered if necessary to incorporate the actual coordinate frames found in the CNS. Finally, the model can be generalized to predict neck motor responses to visual, somatosensory, or other inputs. The tensorial method should therefore be useful in advancing and testing hypotheses concerning neural processes that generate volun-

Figure 14.4.   Comparison of pulling directions (**P**), maximal excitation directions during VCR (**V**), and model predictions of VCR direction (**M**) for four neck muscles in decerebrate cats. As in Figure 13.5, pulling and optimal response axes are indicated by unit vectors aligned with the axis. Vectors indicated by **P** are as in Figure 13.5. Vectors **V** and **M** are plotted with their signs reversed to facilitate comparison of them with the pulling directions. Assuming that the VCR generates attempted head movements in the direction opposite to the rotation applied by the turntable, the reversed vectors −**V** and −**M** therefore indicate the direction of head motion for which each muscle is maximally activated. Whereas the angles between **P** and −**V** in the muscles illustrated ranged from 18° to 31°, model predictions were within 4° to 10° of −**V**.

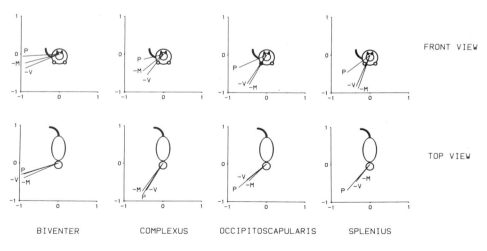

BIVENTER   COMPLEXUS   OCCIPITOSCAPULARIS   SPLENIUS

P = PULLING DIRECTION   V = VESTIBULAR RESPONSE   M = MODEL PREDICTION

tary tracking or orienting head movements, which involve motor patterns that differ from those observed in the VCR (see Chapter 2).

SUMMARY

This chapter describes a tensorial model of the VCR that predicts the muscle activation patterns that are generated when a cat is rotated in three-dimensional space.

The treatment begins with a description of two types of representation in nonorthogonal coordinate frames: covariant (sensory or projection type) representations and contravariant (motor or parallelogram type) representations. The issue of overcompleteness that occurs when the number of muscles exceeds the number of degrees of freedom of movement is also discussed. In overcomplete systems an infinite number of motor patterns can be used to generate a movement.

The VCR model has three transformation stages consisting of matrices that represent tensorial operations. Stage 1, a 3×3 matrix representing the vestibular metric tensor, converts vestibular sensory input from covariant to contravariant form. Stage 2, a 3×30 matrix representing the sensorimotor embedding tensor, converts the signals from vestibular to neck motor coordinate frames. Stage 3, a 30×30 matrix representing the neck motor metric tensor, converts the neck motor command from covariant to contravariant form. Because the system is overcomplete (30 muscles generating head movements in 3 rotational degrees of freedom), an infinite number of stage 3 matrices could be chosen. The model incorporates the matrix corresponding to the Moore–Penrose generalized inverse of the covariant motor metric.

Choosing the Moore–Penrose inverse for stage 3 causes the model to predict a particular pattern of neck muscle activation in response to vestibular stimulation. Comparison of this predicted pattern with the experimentally measured patterns presented in Chapter 13 indicates that the model is quite effective at reproducing the spatial properties of the VCR.

15

Cerebellar Pathways Contributing
to Head Movement

N. HIRAI

The classical experiments demonstrating the cerebellar involvement in the control of the tonus of the neck muscles were made in the cat by Pollock and Davis (1927). In the usual decerebrate animal, barring subtentorial hemorrhage, opistotonus of the head (an attitude in which the head is bent extremely dorsally) is not clear (Bazzet and Penfield, 1922). However, it becomes conspicuous (Fig. 15.1A) with additional removal of the cerebellum or with ligation of both carotid and basilar arteries (anemic decerebration), which renders either the cerebellar anterior lobe or the whole cerebellum anemic depending on the level of the ligation, together with ischemic damage of the cerebrum (Pollock and Davis, 1927). These authors stated that "Immediately following removal of the cerebellum, the head assumed an attitude of extreme opistotonos" and "The degree of opistotonos we have described in decerebro-cerebellate animals has never been observed by us in ordinary decerebrate animals." However, after destruction of the labyrinth in such animals, the opistotonus disappears entirely. At this time, if the head is suspended and then released, it drops into a position of flexion, and the forelegs are flexed in all joints while the rigidity in the hindlegs is strengthened, probably due to the tonic neck reflexes (Fig. 15.1B). From these findings, Pollock and Davis (1927) concluded that "the cerebellum as a whole inhibits tonic labyrinthine reflexes which are responsible . . . for the extreme opistotonos."

Tonic fits, characterized by extension of the limbs and opistotonus just as in decerebrocerebellate animals, are sometimes seen, particularly in children with midline cerebellar tumor. Jackson (1907) reported such a case and called this the "cerebellar attitude" (Fig. 15.1C). Because tumors within the cerebellum are usually associated with hydrocephalus, which leads to increased intracranial pressure, this kind of fit is now regarded as due to dysfunction of the brain stem or forebrain, or both, rather than to cerebellar damage itself (Walton, 1977). It is possible that coincidental damage of the cerebellum and the other structures is responsible for genesis of fits, just as it causes opistotonus in decerebrocerebellate animals.

Hypotonia of the extensor muscles has usually been observed in primates, including humans, in association with dysfunction of the cerebellum alone (Holmes, 1917; Crosby et al., 1966). In subprimates, the development of extensor rigidity

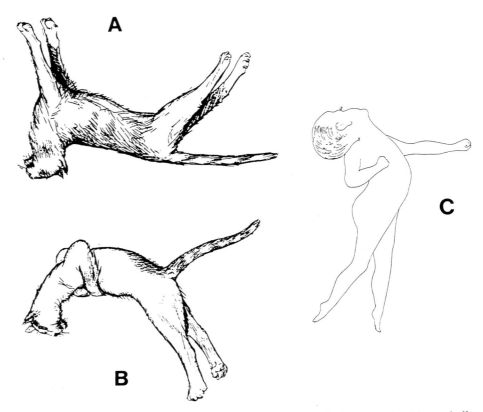

Figure 15.1.   Postures of decerebrocerebellate animals and of a patient with cerebellar tumors. (A) Opistotonus due to removal of the cerebellum in a decerebrate animal. Even when placed up-side-down, marked retraction of the head persisted (Pollock and Davis, 1927). (B) Posture of a suspended anemic decerebrate animal after destruction of the labyrinths (Pollock and Davis, 1927). (C) Attitude during the cerebellar seizure in a patient with midline cerebellar tumor (Jackson, 1907).

after decerebellation may be explained by interruption of the tonic inhibitory influence of the cerebellar anterior lobe vermis on vestibulospinal tract (VST) and fastigial nucleus neurons, as will be described later. On the other hand, destruction limited to the paravermal cortex causes flexion of the ipsilateral extremities (Yu, 1972). Because the vermal part of the primate cerebellum becomes shallow upon expansion of the hemisphere, lesions in the cerebellar anterior lobe of the primate rarely involve the vermis alone and may extend laterally to regions related to flexion. For these reasons, hypotonia rather than hypertonia of the extensor muscles probably predominates after cerebellar lesions in primates. This seems to hold true for tonus of the neck muscles. Holmes (1917) examined about 40 patients with cerebellar lesions due to gunshot injury in the war, but observed no hyperactivity of neck muscles. Instead, the patients rotated their heads toward the opposite side because of hypoactivity of the muscles that would normally be controlled from the injured side. Thus, when damaged bilaterally, "each patient had difficulty in holding his head in any attitude if it was unsupported, and in sitting up if unaided" (Holmes, 1917). He also observed in one patient "the failure of his head and eyes to move simultaneously when he looks to one or the other side," suggesting cerebellar participation in the control of eye–head coordination as well.

In spite of these classical observations, few investigations have been made into the cerebellar involvement in head movement. This chapter considers fundamental aspects of cerebellar relations to head movement: neck afferent inputs to the cerebellum and cerebellar influence on neck muscle activity.

NECK AFFERENT INPUTS TO THE CEREBELLUM

The classical, generally accepted sensory and motor maps of the body in the cerebellar anterior lobe, lobules I–V of Larsell (1953), and lobule VI were found to be an anteroposterior arrangement in the order of tail (lobule I; the lingula), hindlimb (lobules II–III; the centralis), forelimb (lobules IV–V; the clumen), and face (lobule VI; the declive or simplex) (cf. Dow, 1970). In the course of stimulation experiments to define the somatotopy of the cerebellum, Hampson et al. (1946) located the neck area in lobule VI in agreement with the concept advanced by Bolk (1906) on the basis of comparative anatomical observations. However, regions related to head movement are not restricted to lobule VI, as will be seen.

Berthoz and Llinás (1974) were the first to record neck-related mossy- and climbing-fiber responses in lobules V and VI, with the mossy-fiber responses most prominent in the ipsilateral vermal zone of lobule V. They not only confirmed previous data showing that lobule VI received various afferent inputs from the face and head (i.e., trigeminal, extraocular, visual, labyrinthine, and neck), but also extended the data by showing convergence of these afferent inputs on single Purkinje cells in the pars intermedia of this lobule via the inferior olive nucleus (Berthoz and Llinás, 1974).

The vestibulocerebellum is another main projection area of neck afferent inputs. Electrical stimulation of neck afferents induces both mossy- and climbing-fiber responses in the flocculus (Wilson et al., 1975a). On the other hand, in the nodulus (Precht et al., 1976) and in the lateral part of the uvula (Schwarz and Milne, 1976), neck afferents yield only mossy-fiber responses. Recently, lobule I, which together with the nodulus, uvula, and flocculus constitutes the "vestibular floor" (Ingvar, 1928), has been found to receive profound neck afferent inputs via mossy-fibers (Hirai et al., 1984a; Hirai, 1987).

When natural stimuli are applied to the neck, responses are widespread in the cerebellum. In the decerebrate and immobilized cat, Pompeiano and his colleagues extensively studied response characteristics of cerebellar neurons to neck rotations about the longitudinal axis by moving the body with the head fixed. The areas surveyed and the proportions of responsive neurons in the populations sampled were the anterior lobe vermis (35%; Denoth et al., 1979a), the intermediate cortex (65%; Boyle and Pompeiano, 1980a), the cortex of the lateral hemisphere (52%; Chan et al., 1982), the rostral part of the fastigial nucleus (38%; Stanojević, 1981), the interpositus nucleus (58%; Boyle and Pompeiano, 1980a), and the dentate nucleus (47%; Chan et al., 1982). Although both climbing- and mossy-fiber responses could be recorded in the cortex, their analyses were mainly of responses relayed through mossy-fibers. Most of the neurons responded, with directional selectivity, to the position of the neck angular displacements, and some responded to velocity. The predominant response of the Purkinje cells and nuclear cells in the intermediate zone and vermal cortex was excitation during side-down neck rotation (i.e., the body rotated with the head fixed in space in such a way that the shoulder of the recording side moved toward the vertex) and inhibition when rotation was in the other direction (Denoth et al., 1979a; Boyle and Pompeiano, 1980a). Neurons that also responded to this manipulation, predominantly in opposite direction, were found in the rostral fastigial nucleus (Stanojević, 1981).

Joint receptors are the most likely candidates for producing the above responses, since the skin was denervated, the dorsal neck muscles were disconnected from the vertebrae and lambdoidal ridge, and ventral rami of the first three cervical nerves were crushed in these preparations. However, the following reports suggest that neck muscle afferents may also participate in producing responses in the cerebellum. Many precerebellar neurons responded to electrical stimulation of neck muscle afferents. These include neurons in the lateral reticular nucleus (Group II; Coulter et al., 1977), in the central cervical nucleus (Groups I and II; Hirai et al., 1984b), and in the cuneate nucleus (Group I; Murakami and Kato, 1983). Neurons in Group x of the vestibular nucleus also relay neck afferent inputs to the cerebellum (Wilson et al., 1976), although the relevant receptors have not been identified. Thus, it is necessary to examine how inputs from neck muscle afferents are integrated with those from joint receptors in the cerebellum or in precerebellar neurons.

The labyrinth is a detector of head displacement in space and is closely related to the cerebellum phylogenetically. Anatomical and physiological studies have traced projections of labyrinthine inputs to a wide area of the cerebellum beyond the so-called vestibulocerebellum (cf. Kotchabhakdi and Walberg, 1978). Details of this have been described by Wilson and Melvill-Jones (1979) and Ito (1984). Hence, interactions between vestibular and neck inputs in the cerebellum will now be dealt with. In brief, most areas that receive neck afferent inputs also receive vestibular afferent projections. These areas include the flocculus (Wilson et al., 1975a), the lateral part of the uvula (Schwarz and Milne, 1976), the cerebellar nuclei (Boyle and Pompeiano, 1980a; Stanojević, 1981; Chan et al., 1982), the cerebellar cortices of the anterior lobe (Denoth et al., 1979a; Chan et al., 1982), and lobules I–II (Hirai, 1987) and V–VI (Berthoz and Llinás, 1974). Combined stimulation of the neck and labyrinth by sinusoidal rotation of the head about the longitudinal axis at 0.026 Hz indicates that 20–30% of the neurons in the cortices of the anterior lobe and the cerebellar nuclei receive convergent but reciprocal inputs from both receptors (Boyle and Pompeiano, 1980a; Chan et al., 1982; Denoth et al., 1980). When a neuron responds with excitation during side-down rotation of the neck, it tends to respond with inhibition during whole body rotation (thus stimulating the labyrinthine receptors alone) toward the recording side, and vice versa. Such individual stimulation of the neck or labyrinthine receptors can be combined simultaneously when the head is rotated toward the recording side while the body remains stationary. At this time, the total response closely corresponds to what is predicted by vectorial summation of the individual responses that tend to antagonize each other. These results seem to be in line with the idea of von Holst and Mittelstaedt (1950) that tonic neck and labyrinthine reflexes cancel each other in the extremities, so an animal is able to move his head freely without affecting the balance of muscle tone.

CEREBELLAR INFLUENCE ON NECK MUSCLE ACTIVITY

Extensive experiments to correlate stimulation of various areas of the cerebellar cortex with head movement were made by Mussen (1927, 1930, 1931). The following is a summary of his description of mapping experiments that involved stimulation of cerebellum in cats with their heads free to move. Stimulation of the anterior lobe vermis (the centralis) yielded contraction of the posterior neck muscles, whereas the anterior neck muscles were contracted by stimulation of the posterior lobe (the pyramis). When the middle lobe (lobules VI–VII) was stimulated, the head rotated toward the side stimulated with either the anterior or posterior direction depending on the electrode location; when the anterolateral (or posterolateral) part of the middle lobe was stimulated, the head flexed backward (or forward) and to the side stimulated. He also did corroborative lesion experiments (Mussen, 1931). When the posterior lobe was destroyed, the head pulled far backward, whereas destruction of the anterior lobe produced a tendency for the head to fall forward. The destruction of the left half of the middle lobe led to positioning of the head to the right. Thus, the head position after destruction of a lobe was just opposite to that caused by stimulation of the corresponding area. From these observations, he concluded that the anterior and posterior lobes regulate forward and backward balance, respectively, whereas the middle lobe is concerned with lateral flexion of the head, and the normal cerebellum always acts as a whole to coordinate the activity of neck muscles (Mussen 1931).

A concept completely opposite to that of Mussen was proposed by Clark (1939), who based his view on stimulation of the anterior and posterior vermes of unanesthetized, freely moving cats. Upon stimulation of the anterior lobe, just rostral to the primary fissure, the head went down toward the floor, whereas the effects of stimulation of points behind the primary fissure were the reverse. Upon termination of the stimulation, the head suddenly returned toward the original position in a poststimulus rebound, i.e., it moved in the direction described by Mussen. Clark therefore claimed that the description by Mussen was of the rebound phenomenon. However, it seems unlikely that Mussen was merely observing the rebound phenomenon, since the direction of lateral head flexion during stimulation of the middle lobe was agreed on by both authors. Some points should be considered when discussing their discrepancy. Contradictory effects of stimulation of the same point on muscle activity have sometimes been reported for the cerebellum, depending on stimulus frequency and strength (Nulsen et al., 1948; Moruzzi, 1950) and, in the unrestrained animal, depending also on initial posture (Chambers, 1947) as well as head position (Koella 1953). Moreover, intracellular recordings have revealed that stimulation of the cerebellar cortex frequently induces direct excitation of VST neurons (Ito et al., 1969; Fukuda et al., 1972;

Hirai and Uchino 1984; Hirai, 1987), although the outputs of the cerebellar cortex (Purkinje cells) should be inhibitory (Ito and Yoshida, 1964). This must be regarded as an artificial effect due to axon reflex of excitatory cerebellar afferents via collaterals. Because of these contradictions, stimulating experiments can lead to diverse results unless well controlled.

These disadvantages of stimulating experiments can be partly overcome by lesion experiments, which should reveal functional deficits related to the specific region. However, there is also contradiction among the results of lesion experiments. Mussen's results showing that anterior lobe destruction induces forward falling of the head agrees with results of Ferrier (1886) and Ingvar (1923), but are inconsistent with the general understanding that opistotonus of the head appears after anterior lobe lesions (see next section). Sprague and Chambers (1953) claimed that lesion of the pyramis resulted in ventriflexion of the head, i.e., the reverse of Mussen's observation. No explanation of these conflicts has come forth. However, it should be mentioned that a tendency to fall back, or some opistotonus following posterior lobe lesions in the monkey, dog, and cat, has been reported by several investigators (Ferrier, 1886; Rothmann, 1913; Ingvar, 1923; Chambers and Sprague, 1955b; Crosby et al., 1966), although the relevant lobules seem to be more posterior (lobules IX and X) than Mussen reported (lobule VIII). This will also be considered further in the next section; it is sufficient to say here that the middle part of the anterior and posterior vermis may be related to head movement in a sagittal plane around the frontal axis (cf. Botterell and Fulton, 1938).

There is general agreement on the direction of the lateral flexion of the head (ipsilaterally) when the middle lobe is stimulated. It is also agreed that such head movement is accompanied by conjugate eye movement in the same direction (Ferrier, 1886; Mussen, 1927; Clark, 1939; Chambers and Sprague, 1955a). As described, this area receives teleceptive and labyrinthine inputs as well as proprioceptive inputs from the eye and neck, all of which are indispensable information for visually triggered head movement or for the orienting reflex. Moreover, correlation of Purkinje cell activity in this area with the eye movement has been reported (Llinás and Wolfe, 1977; Suzuki et al., 1981). Thus, this area might be expected to be involved in eye–head coordination. Ritchie (1976) examined this in the monkey by lesion of lobules VI–VII and observed dysmetric saccadic eye movement but no disorder of head movement. However, because gaze control is disordered in patients with cerebellar ataxia (Shimizu et al., 1981; cf. Holmes, 1917), these lobules are still an attractive area for further study of eye–head coordination.

In closely controlled stimulation mapping experiments in the cerebellar nuclei of the baboon, Rispal-Padel et al. (1982) found that the effective foci for producing head movement are in the ventral part of the posterior interpositus nucleus and in the mediodorsal zone of the dentate nucleus. Although stimulation of the interpositus nucleus evoked head movement alone, head movement induced by stimulation of the dentate nucleus was usually accompanied by hand movement. Thus, it might be suggested that the dentate nuclei are involved in initiating head and hand coordinated movement. If so, convergent sensory inputs from the neck and forelimbs to some dentate neurons (Chan et al., 1982) might provide feedback signals of movements in process. Wilson et al. (1978b) revealed direct excitatory connection of neurons in the rostral fastigial nucleus with contralateral neck muscle motoneurons by detailed stimulating and lesion experiments in the cat.

OPISTOTONUS, VESTIBULOCOLLIC NEURONS, AND CEREBELLUM

As suggested by Sherrington (1897) and demonstrated experimentally by Pollack and Davis (1927), one mechanism for enhancement of the rigidity that follows decerebellation is the release of the tonic labyrinthine reflex from inhibition by the cerebellum. VST neurons in the lateral vestibular nucleus, which exert an excitatory influence on extensor muscle motoneurons (Lund and Pompeiano, 1968; Grillner et al., 1970), receive both direct projections from Purkinje cells in the B-zone and indirect projections from the A-zone through the fastigial nucleus (cf. Oscarsson, 1979). Because Purkinje cells are inhibitory in nature, decortication of the anterior lobe vermis increases the activity of VST neurons, thus in turn overdriving the activity of the extensor muscles. Inhibitory influence from the A-zone to reticulospinal neurons through the fastigial nucleus should also be considered. These neural linkages have been amply corroborated (Pompeiano, 1974; Wilson and Melvill-Jones, 1979; Ito, 1984). Indeed, upon stimulation of the anterior lobe vermis of the cerebellar cortex, hyperpolarizing membrane potentials without appreciable change in membrane resistance could be recorded from the extensor hindlimb muscle motoneurons (Terzuolo, 1959; Llinás, 1964). This membrane potential change may be a result of reduction of the sustained background activity that normally impinges on motoneurons (disfacilitation).

A mechanism for producing opistotonus of the head has been explained by an analogy. In line with the early observation that stimuli to the anterior lobe caused relaxation of decerebrate rigidity in the neck of the monkey (Sherrington, 1897), opistotonus has been observed following destruction of the anterior lobe (Rothmann, 1913; Pollock and Davis, 1927; Sprague and Chambers, 1953; Chambers and Sprague, 1955b; Battini et al., 1957). Even bilateral localized lesion in the rostrolateral part of the fastigial nucleus is sufficient to develop opistotonus (Battini and Pompeiano, 1958), probably due to interruption of corticovestibular fibers (Pompeiano, 1974). Indeed, about 80% of those VST neurons that terminate in the upper cervical segments (vestibulocollic, VC, neurons) were inhibited by stimulation of the anterior lobe vermis (Akaike, 1983a).

In most of the studies described above, precise sites of lesions and stimulation of the cerebellum were not identified, so the question of which lobules in the anterior lobe are responsible for suppressing the activity of VC neurons or for producing the opistotonus has not been answered (Fig. 15.2B). Recently, experiments utilizing microstimulation were made to explore this problem (Hirai, 1987). Lobules I and II were chosen for study, because anatomical and physiological experiments had revealed that lobules I and II receive almost all of the projections from spinocerebellar tract neurons that originate in the central cervical nucleus (Wiksten, 1979; Matsushita and Okado, 1981; Hirai et al., 1984a) and relay neck afferent inputs (Hirai et al., 1978, 1984a,b). In addition, lobule I receives projections of primary vestibular afferents (Ingvar, 1918; Brodal and Høvik, 1964; Carpenter et al., 1972; Hirai, 1983). Thus, these lobules seem to be the sensory

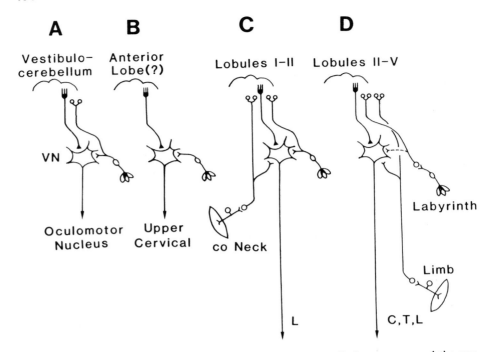

Figure 15.2.   Diagrams of relations of cerebellar corticovestibular neurons and the vestibular reflex arcs. (A) Secondary vestibuloocular neurons are specifically inhibited from the vestibulocerebellum. (B) Most of vestibulocollic neurons receive inhibition from an unspecified anterior lobe vermis. (C) Vestibulospinal neurons that send their axons to the lower thoracic or more caudal segments (L) and receive excitatory neck afferent inputs from the contralateral side are inhibited from lobules I–II. (D) Vestibulospinal neurons that receive no excitatory neck afferent inputs but probably receive afferent inputs from the limbs are inhibited from anterior lobe vermis except lobule I. Some may also receive labyrinthine inputs. This group includes neurons that send their axons to cervical (C), thoracic (T), or lumbar (L) segments. VN, Vestibular nuclear neurons.

areas for the neck or the vestibular organ, or both. If this is so, VC neurons would be expected to receive an inhibitory influence from these areas by analogy with the somatotopic organization of the fore- and hindlimb areas between the cerebellum and the vestibular nucleus (Fig. 15.2D: cf. Fanardjian and Sarkissian, 1980). Contrary to this expectation, however, these lobules exerted inhibitory influence on VST neurons sending axons to the lower thoracic or lumbar segments, but rarely to VC neurons (Hirai, 1987). Most of these inhibited VST neurons had another common feature. They received convergent excitatory inputs from the labyrinth and contralateral neck afferents, and may thus be common relay neurons of the vestibulospinal and neck reflexes (Fig. 15.2C). Because some VST neurons with long descending axons usually give off collaterals to the more rostral segments (Abzug et al., 1974) or even to the upper cervical segments (Rapaport et al., 1977), these lobules may be related to the interaction of the neck and vestibulospinal reflexes acting on rather wide portions of the body, but not the neck proper. Other lobules should be investigated as areas related to VC neurons.

In this connection, the vestibulocerebellum does not exert direct inhibition on VST neurons, in contrast with vestibuloocular neurons (Fig. 15.2A: Fukuda et al., 1972; Akaike et al., 1973b; Precht et al., 1976). Even vestibular neurons conjoining the vestibuloocular and vestibulocollic reflexes by way of bifurcating axons are free of floccular inhibition (Hirai and Uchino, 1984). However, as described, ablation of lobules IX and X (the uvula and nodulus) results in dorsiflexion of the head. When the lesion is unilateral, the head is rotated with the occiput toward the opposite side, which is the reverse of the attitude seen after unilateral labyrinthectomy (Dow, 1938). These results suggest that the vestibulocerebellum in the vermal part is related to VC neurons, probably indirectly through the fastigial nucleus. Moreover, it has been suggested that the nodulus and uvula are important in eye–head coordination. Igarashi et al. (1983) demonstrated alteration in the properties of eye–head coordination during optokinetic and vestibular stimulation after uvulonodulectomy in the monkey.

Sherrington (1906) regarded the cerebellum as the "head ganglion" in the sense of a chief coordination center of the body. However, the studies described above were made by the stimulation or lesion experiments, and thus the question of how the "head ganglion" controls the execution of the head movements still remains open. To resolve this matter, another useful and promising approach should be attempted, i.e., to correlate neuronal activity in the cerebellum with a particular aspect of head movement, for future developments in this field.

SUMMARY

Experiments dating back to the beginning of the century have described a diverse variety of changes in neck motor tone and head position following lesions or electrical stimulation of the cerebellar cortex or deep nuclei. This chapter examines some of the possible neuronal substrates of these changes.

Pathways are described that relay neck afferent input to lobules I, V, VI, IX, and X and to the flocculus via both mossy- and climbing-fibers.

Most of the cerebellar regions that receive neck input also receive input from the vestibular labyrinth. Neuronal recordings indicate that signals from the two sources tend to cancel when the head is rotated on a fixed trunk.

The cerebellum may act on neck motoneurons via a variety of pathways that either increase or decrease muscle activity. Figure 15.2 suggests some neuronal circuits that may play a role in head position control.

16

Eye–Head Coordination in Gaze Control

D. GUITTON

INTRODUCTION: THE OCULOCENTRIC VIEW

It is only within the last 5 years that research on coordinated eye–head-orienting movements has actually been concerned with the nature of the head movement itself. Prior explanations of how eyes and head are coordinated were based on an elegant model suggested by Bizzi and colleagues (Bizzi et al., 1971, 1972a; Dichgans et al., 1973; Morasso et al., 1973; Bizzi, 1981) which was essentially "oculocentric" in nature. This proposed motor strategy operated as illustrated in Figure 16.1 (Morasso et al., 1973). A monkey began the task with eyes and head initially aligned on a fixation point situated straight ahead. A target appeared unexpectedly 30° to the monkey's right. In Figure 16.1A the monkey's head was unexpectedly prevented from moving by a mechanical brake applied to a shaft to which the head was held. In Figure 16.1B the monkey performed a normal head-free gaze shift. Gaze (G) is computed by adding eye position relative to the head (E) to head position relative to space (H). Soon after target onset a saccadic eye movement was triggered as the head accelerated more slowly. In this example, by the time that G was on target the head had contributed little to the overall gaze shift. In much larger gaze shifts this is not the case, as we shall see below. Once the visual axis was on target, the G trace remained constant in spite of head motion. This was due to the eye rotating back toward the orbital center with a velocity that exactly opposed the head velocity.

To visual inspection the G traces in Figure 16.1A and B appear identical and numerical comparisons confirmed this observation (Morasso et al., 1973) and led to the conclusion that gaze trajectory was *not affected* by suddenly preventing head motion. These findings implied that in the head-free condition, the ocular saccade was being attenuated by an amount equal to the head's contribution to the gaze shift. Indeed, saccade amplitude, velocity, and duration decreased in the head-free condition. One mechanism for mediating this effect would be for vestibular and/or neck proprioceptive "copies" of head motion to "subtract" from the saccade generator signal. In an elegant experiment, Dichgans et al. (1973) surgically eliminated the semicircular canal input in monkeys and observed that the saccades with the head fixed and free were identical so that in the head-free condition, the gaze overshot the target. Furthermore, after the saccade had ter-

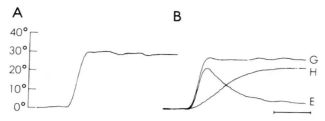

Figure 16.1.   Comparison of eye saccades and gaze in monkey. (A) Eye saccade to a suddenly appearing target with head fixed. (B) Coordinated eye saccade (*E*) and head movement (*H*) to the same target with head free. Gaze movement (*G*) represents the sum of *E* and *H*. Note remarkable similarity of eye saccade in (A) and gaze trajectory in (B) as well as reduced saccade amplitude in (B). Time calibration, 100 msec. (From Morasso et al., 1973)

minated, gaze was not stabilized by an ocular motion that compensated for the ongoing head rotation. Taken together these data implied that programming of a saccadic eye movement is identical, irrespective of whether or not the head is to move. If the head does move, the vestibularly induced compensatory eye movement is added linearly to the saccade signal. Thus, saccade velocity and amplitude are reduced by amounts equal to the velocity and amplitude of the head movement. This vestibuloocular reflex–saccade interaction hypothesis has been called the "addition" hypothesis (Robinson and Zee, 1981) or "linear summation" hypothesis (Laurutis and Robinson, 1986).

RELATIVE ONSET TIMES OF EYE AND HEAD MOVEMENTS

Experiments have shown that saccadic eye and head movements may be initiated at quite different times relative to one another. Variations in eye–head latency have been shown to be dependent on the subject's "set," or on target amplitude, predictability, and visibility (Bizzi et al., 1972a; Funk and Anderson, 1977; Barnes, 1979; Zangemeister and Stark, 1982a,b; Guitton and Volle, 1987). In gaze shifts to targets of unpredictable location (within the subject's oculomotor range, OMR[1]) and onset time, the eye typically precedes the head by about 40 msec. However, when target position and timing are predictable, the eye lags the head. According to Zangmeister and Stark (1982b) this is because the head starts earlier in the predictable target condition whereas the eye latency relative to target onset remains approximately constant. There is only partial agreement on this point in the literature (Barnes, 1979; Gresty, 1974). Zangmeister and Stark (1982b) also state that, within any one experimental condition, changes in eye and head latencies covary.

These observations suggest that the motor signals driving the eye and head systems are loosely coupled at least in terms of their onset times. From the point of view of the oculocentric motor strategy this does not pose a problem since head movement does not influence gaze and therefore only the eye movement is assumed to be programmed for target acquisition.

PROBLEMS WITH THE OCULOCENTRIC VIEW
OF EYE–HEAD COORDINATION

In spite of the elegance of the mechanisms proposed by Bizzi and colleagues, at least three important problems emerge. The first relates to how targets can be acquired when their eccentricity lies *beyond* the subject's oculomotor range (OMR), the second pertains to how saccades and vestibulooocular reflex (VOR) signals interact, and the third concerns the role of vestibularly induced quick phases in gaze control. These questions are discussed in the ensuing sections.

TRAJECTORIES DURING ACQUISITION OF TARGETS LYING WITHIN
AND BEYOND THE OCULOMOTOR RANGE

In order to shift the gaze to targets that lie beyond the OMR with single-step, saccade-like gaze shifts, the oculocentric strategy requires that the brain program saccades that are too large to be physically possible. An alternative view suggests that gaze shifts of amplitude greater than the OMR cannot be made as single steps. Multiple-step gaze shifts of overall amplitude greater than the OMR are generated by the cat, monkey, and human, but, particularly in the highly motivated subject, the most frequent response is the single-step saccade-like gaze displacement (Gresty, 1974; Barnes, 1979; Fuller et al., 1983; Guitton et al., 1984a; Laurutis and Robinson, 1986; Tomlinson and Bahra, 1986a; Guitton and Volle, 1987).

Figure 16.2 shows examples of single-step gaze displacements to targets within and beyond the OMR in cats (Fig. 16-2A–C) and humans (Fig. 16.2D–F). The *E*, *H*, and *G* traces show classic trajectories, qualitatively similar to those of the original monkey data (e.g., Fig. 16.1B). Close comparison of small and large gaze shifts does reveal quantitative differences that are not illustrated here. In general, small gaze shifts (less than approximately 10° in cat, 20° in monkey, and 30° in humans) have "bell-shaped" velocity profiles. Larger single-step gaze shifts have velocity profiles that are either flat-topped or more complex in shape (Guitton et al., 1984a; Tomlinson and Bahra, 1986a; Guitton and Volle, 1987).

LIMITS TO SACCADE AMPLITUDE DURING GAZE SHIFTS TO TARGETS
BEYOND THE OMR

Under the oculocentric hypothesis, execution of a large single-step gaze shift would involve programming of an eye saccade to a point outside the OMR. However, Figure 16.3A and B indicates that minimizing head motion in large gaze displacements resulted in an eye saccade in both cat and human that stopped quite short of the limits of the OMR. The relationships ("main sequences," e.g., Bahill et al., 1975; Baloh et al., 1975) between maximum velocity and amplitude and between duration and amplitude for these saccades were independent of whether they were made with the head fixed voluntarily or unexpectedly prevented from moving by a brake. This implied an identical motor program in both conditions.

These observations are expressed more quantitatively in Figure 16.4. The

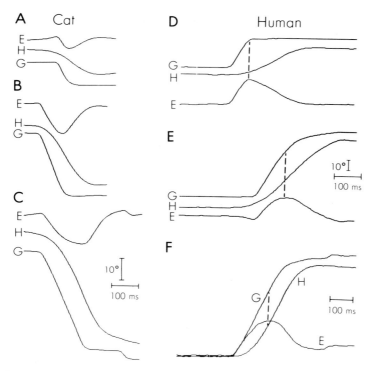

Figure 16.2.   Examples of "single-step" gaze shifts using coordinated eye–head movements in cat (A–C) and human (D–F). (A, D) Gaze shifts of 10° and 40°, respectively;
target within the oculomotor range (OMR). (B, C, E, F) Gaze shifts of 30°, 45°, 80°, and
120°, respectively; target outside OMR. Eye movements are measured with the search coil
technique. In "human" data, a vertical dashed line is drawn above the eye saccade's point
of maximum displacement. Note in (E) and (F) that the G trace continues well beyond
this point.

abscissa represents the target offset, the angle (say, T) through which the subject
intended to displace his gaze. The ordinate is the amplitude of the eye saccade
that resulted when head motion was prevented. If, as predicted by the oculocentric
strategy, preventing head motion revealed a saccadic eye movement of amplitude
equal to target offset angle, then all points would lie on or near the dashed line
oriented at 45°, for target offsets less than the OMR, and along the OMR limit
for larger target offsets. For the human subject (Fig. 16.4B) the experimental
points lie on or near the dashed line up to about $T = 50°$, after which the amplitude
of the saccade remained approximately constant at 45–47° whereas the OMR in
this subject equalled 60°.

    Similar results were obtained in the cat (Fig. 16.4A). All points lie on or
near the dashed line for about $T < 12°$. For $T = 30°$ and 50°, the points depart
from the line and attain an average amplitude of only about 12°. They do not
cluster at or even near the limits of the cat's OMR. These data imply that the
limit to saccade amplitude is imposed neurally, not mechanically. Analogous results based on observations of saccade amplitude distribution in large gaze shifts

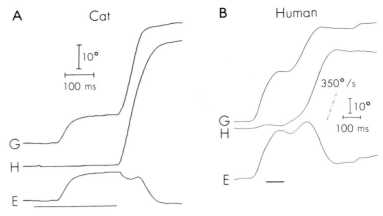

Figure 16.3.   Examples of visually triggered orienting eye–head movements in which a brake unexpectedly prevented or minimized head rotation during the eye saccade. (A) Attempted 50° gaze shift in cat. Saccade of about 10° does not attain limits of OMR (= ±25°). (B) Attempted 80° gaze shift in human subject. Saccade of 34° does not attain limits of OMR (= ±54°). When head is released in (A) the initial "compensatory" ocular rotation does not stabilize gaze. This is followed by a new rapid eye movement which brings gaze rapidly and *accurately* onto target. The same phenomenon occurs when the head is released in (B), except that gaze is initially stabilized by compensatory eye rotation. The slope of the inclined dash–dot line in (B) indicates 350°/sec. In humans a head velocity beyond this value exceeds the VOR's linear response (Pulaski et al., 1981). Horizontal bar beneath *E* trace indicates when brake was on.

without head brakes suggested that monkeys limit saccades to an amplitude of about 40° (Tomlinson and Bahra, 1986a,b).

The experiments showing that the central nervous system limits saccade amplitude and yet can program single-step gaze shifts greater than this limit suggest that the hypotheses underlying the oculocentric motor organization are incorrect. Further evidence for this is that the linear summation hypothesis is either invalid or too labile to be relied upon for gaze accuracy and that gaze accuracy is excellent, when linear summation is absent, even when head motion is perturbed unexpectedly. These points will be considered below.

INFLUENCE OF HEAD MOTION ON THE SACCADE TRAJECTORY:
THE LINEAR SUMMATION HYPOTHESIS

The manner in which the saccade signal is attenuated by head motion is of considerable interest. One way of experimentally investigating this problem is to brake the head suddenly and unexpectedly *during* the saccade. In this condition, visual feedback is too slow to modulate the saccade and neck proprioceptive influences are negligible (Bizzi, 1981). Thus, according to the linear summation hypothesis this experimental manipulation should suddenly remove the influence of the VOR on the pulse generator and the saccade, in principle, should accelerate within 10–20 msec.

Both Fuller et al. (1983) and Guitton et al. (1984b) used a brake to interrupt the motion of a cat's head for short periods during eye–head orienting gaze shifts. Braking could be timed to occur at different points in the eye trajectory. The former authors braked the head only during those rapid eye movements that occurred in and about the middle portion of large gaze shifts and concluded that no VOR–saccade interaction existed. Visual inspection and comparison of the E, H, and G traces suggested to them that there *was* interaction during the first saccade. Guitton et al. (1984b) braked the head during the first saccade and indeed reported VOR–saccade interaction (Fig. 16.5A). A change in eye velocity compensated for the change in head velocity so as to leave the trajectory of the initial gaze saccade unaltered. Blakemore and Donaghy (1980) applied motor-driven, unexpected head movements during saccades made by cats whose heads were otherwise held fixed. These perturbations caused changes in eye velocity compatible with linear summation, with the consequence that gaze trajectories were essentially unaffected by the head perturbation.

Tomlinson and Bahra (1986b) performed similar experiments in monkeys. A monkey's head was perturbed by a torque motor with the advantage that the head could either be decelerated or accelerated during the saccade. They concluded that there was no VOR–saccade interaction when the gaze shift was approximately >40°, but for smaller gaze shifts, particularly <10°, the VOR and saccade signals clearly interacted. There was a transition zone between 40° and 10° within which

Figure 16.4. The effect on saccade amplitude of unexpectedly preventing head motion. The dashed line oriented at 45° indicates where saccade amplitude equals target offset angle. The horizontal dashed line shows the limits to ocular motility defined as the oculomotor range (OMR). (A) Filled circles indicate saccade amplitude when cat head motion is unexpectedly prevented for the duration of the saccade. (B) Open circles joined by a dotted line show analogous data for a human subject. Vertical lines on each point indicate the standard deviation.

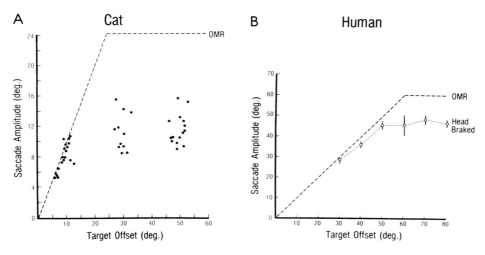

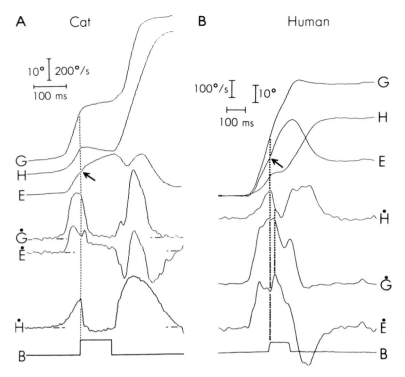

Figure 16.5.   Linear summation present. Examples of eye–head movements in which head motion in cat (A) and human (B) subjects was suddenly interrupted by a brake during a saccade. Leftward vertical dotted line plus arrow on E trace show where eye accelerates when head decelerates. See also velocity traces. The gaze trace remains relatively unaffected by the brake as can be seen by a normal "bell-shaped" velocity profile in (A) and constant velocity between the two vertical dotted lines in (B). The trace labeled B indicates when brake was on. $\dot{G}$, $\dot{H}$, and $\dot{E}$, gaze, head, and eye velocities.

the VOR operated with a gain less than unity. They also reported that linear summation was absent only in the plane of the gaze shift but that the VOR slow phase remained functional in the orthogonal direction.

Laurutis and Robinson (1986) mechanically perturbed head movements during head-fixed and head-free gaze shifts in two human subjects. For gaze shift amplitudes >40° they concluded that head perturbations did not affect the eye saccade trajectory, but for smaller movements the results were less clear.

Analogous experiments by Guitton and Volle (1987) in four human subjects yielded results in which VOR–saccade interaction was much more variable. In two subjects a sudden and unexpected head deceleration yielded no concomitant acceleration of the eye for gaze shift amplitudes ranging between 20° and 120° (Fig. 16.6) and, as expected, in these two subjects the maximum saccadic eye velocity ($\dot{E}_{max}$) was independent of head velocity. There was evidence in these two subjects that VOR–saccade interaction depended on gaze error—the angle between current gaze and desired gaze positions—since for small gaze errors (about <20°) the linear summation hypothesis became valid. By comparison in a third subject, a head perturbation consistently caused an oppositely directed change in eye velocity (Fig. 16.5B) during the entire gaze shift, at least for the gaze amplitude range tested (20° to 80°). Responses in a fourth subject were variable and appeared to be task dependent: gaze shifts to unpredictable targets showed VOR–saccade interaction whereas gaze shifts to targets of known predictable amplitude showed no interaction.

The results of Guitton and Volle (1987) do not support the strong conclusion of Laurutis and Robinson (1986) that linear summation is absent for human gaze shifts >40°. Their results favor a more temperate view suggesting considerable variability in the interaction between the VOR and saccade signals.

The neurophysiological mechanisms that permit a head velocity signal to affect a saccade signal are unclear. Two important inputs to ocular motoneurons come from vestibuloocular relay neurons that receive head velocity signals from semicircular canals and thus form the middle portion of the three neuron arc of the VOR, and from burst neurons in the reticular formation, whose activity produces the rapid muscle contractions during saccades (for review see Fuchs et al., 1985). The failure of linear summation is compatible with evidence that vestibuloocular relay neurons pause during saccades (e.g., see King et al., 1976; Pola and Robinson, 1978; Tomlinson and Robinson, 1984). However, other evidence supporting linear summation suggests that the frequency of some burst neurons may be modulated by a head velocity signal, thus allowing canal signals to alter the saccade trajectory (Whittington et al., 1984). To complicate matters, the discharge rate of motoneurons during saccades may also be influenced by certain cells in the vestibular nuclei that burst during all saccades, whereas others burst and pause for ipsilateral and contralateral saccades, respectively (Fuchs and Kimm, 1975; Pola and Robinson, 1978; Tomlinson and Robinson, 1984). Thus the burst signal responsible for driving a rapid eye movement may result from the complex interplay between signals from different sources impinging on ipsilateral and con-

Figure 16.6.   Linear summation absent. Examples of human eye–head movements in which the head motion was suddenly interrupted by a brake. The horizontal bar beneath each *E* trace indicates when the brake was on. The brake-induced stop and start of head motion was associated with similar changes in the gaze trajectory whereas the eye trajectory remained uninfluenced by the head perturbation. In (B) the eye remained relatively immobile at about 25° in the orbit, far from the OMR limits at 52°.

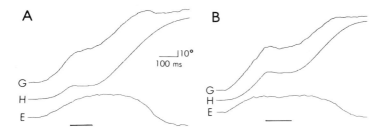

tralateral motoneurons and at this stage in our knowledge it is impossible to clearly link the behavioral observations to the physiology.

THE GAZE FEEDBACK HYPOTHESIS

The data for humans, monkey, and cat, summarized above, show that the mechanisms responsible for controlling eye–head movements are far more complex than originally proposed by Bizzi and colleagues. The observations vary and the question that arises is whether there are unifying features permitting a generalized scheme of the gaze control system in humans, monkey, and cat.

First there is general agreement that the oculocentric strategy—involving both linear summation and the coding of a saccade whose amplitude equals target offset angle—is valid for gaze shifts of $<10°$ in humans, monkey, and cat. Second, for larger gaze shifts the linear summation hypothesis appears to break down although the precise "transition" point may be highly variable, even between individuals of one species or in one individual from day to day. Third, in those gaze shifts in which linear summation is initially absent there is clearly a time, within the gaze shift, at which the VOR signal again becomes functional in the classic sense and stabilizes the visual axis in space. This reactivation of the VOR occurs when gaze position error—the difference between current and desired gaze positions—approaches or equals zero, i.e., when gaze is on or near the target.

Since the predictions of the oculocentric hypothesis—linear summation and saccade amplitude equal to target offset angle—have not been upheld experimentally, it is necessary to develop a substitute scheme. Quite clearly a mechanism that focuses on the control of *both* the eye and head systems is required.

Such an alternative mechanism was first proposed to explain results of collicular stimulation in the cat (Guitton et al., 1980; Roucoux et al., 1980a,b), which revealed orienting mechanisms very similar to those now described in normal humans, monkey, and cat. This hypothesis was based on the principle of gaze feedback: an internal copy of actual gaze position is obtained by summing internal copies of eye and head positions. This sum is then subtracted from desired gaze position to yield a gaze position error signal, which drives the oculomotor and head motor machineries. The principle that gaze itself is the controlled variable has been reiterated by others (Fuller et al., 1983; Guitton et al., 1984a; Tomlinson and Bahra, 1986b; Pélisson and Prablanc, 1986, 1987; Guitton and Volle, 1987) and in a more quantitative formulation by Laurutis and Robinson (1986). Their model is based on the observation that linear summation does not occur between the VOR and saccade signals but does not predict a maximum, neurally determined, ocular deviation in the orbit. A gaze feedback schematic that includes an eye position saturation element has been presented for cat and humans (Guitton et al., 1984a; Guitton and Volle, 1987) and is given in Figure 16.7 in a more simplified form. This diagram should be viewed as a picture summary of how a number of complex processes are linked; it is not a model for computer simulation.

On the left, desired gaze position G_D (corresponding to target position in space) is compared to current gaze (corresponding to the position of the visual

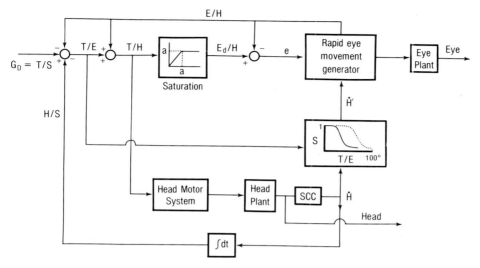

Figure 16.7. Schematic representation of a gaze feedback system which calculates gaze error (T/E) by subtracting current eye position relative to space (E/S) from target position relative to space (T/S). T/E is then converted to target position relative to head (T/H), which drives the head motor system and also determines an eye position relative to head (E_d/H) which is no greater than the level set by the saturation element. E_d/H drives the saccadic oculomotor system in the same manner as Robinson's (1975) local feedback model. Head velocity $(\dot{H})$ obtained from the semicircular canals (SCC) is attenuated by a gain element such that $\dot{H}' = S\dot{H}$. S is subject dependent and also depends on T/E. $\dot{H}'$ interacts with the saccade generator as in the linear summation hypothesis.

axis in space, $G = E/H + H/S$) to yield gaze position error or an internal representation of target position relative to the eye (T/E). Note here that head position relative to space H/S is conveniently assumed to be obtained by integration of the semicircular canal signal. This is purely speculative and may be incorrect due to high head velocities that could drive the canals to saturation (Pulaski et al., 1981; for discussion of this point in eye–head coordination, see Tomlinson and Bahra, 1986b; Guitton and Volle, 1987). The quantity T/E is assumed to be converted first to target position relative to the head (T/H) and then passed through a saturation element in which, based on head-braking experiments, the quantity a is assigned values of $45°$, $35°$, and $15°$ approximately in humans, monkeys, and cats, respectively. The output of this element yields desired eye position relative to the head (E_d/H). This quantity is then compared to current eye position relative to the head (E/H) in the manner of the classic local feedback model for the oculomotor system (for review, see Fuchs et al., 1985). The rapid eye movement generator is driven until $e = E_d/H - E/H = 0$. The influence of head velocity on eye movement is shown schematically as a "diminished" head velocity signal $(\dot{H}')$ that influences the rapid eye movement generator. The value of $\dot{H}'$ is dependent on current gaze error (T/E) which is assumed[2] to influence S in the equation $\dot{H}' = S\dot{H}$.

THE ROLE OF VESTIBULARLY DRIVEN QUICK PHASES IN EYE–HEAD COORDINATION

When the head is *passively* displaced there ensues, after a short delay, a rapid eye movement in the direction of head rotation (Melvill-Jones, 1964; Barnes, 1979). This eye movement is driven by signals originating in the semicircular canals and is known as the quick phase of vestibular nystagmus.

As we saw in a previous section the rapid eye movements that accompany target-triggered orienting gaze shifts can vary considerably in their onset time relative to head motion. For gaze shifts in which the eye lags the head, e.g., to predictable targets, Barnes (1979) first suggested that the rapid eye movement is a vestibularly driven quick phase. This idea was based primarily on the observation that when the passively induced head trajectory resembled an active head rotation, the resulting passive gaze trajectory was very similar to the gaze trajectory generated actively. Barnes (1979) proposed that "the vestibulo-ocular reflex provides an estimate of future head position, thus allowing the more rapidly moving eye to anticipate the head movement, and aid the process of visual search." To test this hypothesis it would be necessary to unexpectedly and totally prevent head motion in gaze shifts to predictable targets in which the eye lags the head consistently. In humans this has not been done.

Cats have rapid eye movements whose onsets usually lag the head movement (Fuller et al., 1983; Guitton et al., 1984a). When head motion is unexpectedly prevented in the cat a saccade is still present (Fig. 16.2). This would not happen if the rapid eye movement, as proposed by Barnes, was vestibularly induced. However, in large gaze shifts the cat's eye frequently moves with a series of closely spaced—often almost coalesced—rapid displacements (Fuller et al., 1983; Guitton et al., 1984a). Guitton et al. (1984a) proposed that those following the first main saccade are quick phases since they are dependent on head motion, never appearing in the head-braked condition. Of considerable interest is that these combinations of visually triggered saccades and putative quick phases generate very accurate gaze shifts (see next section).

Further evidence for the role of quick phases in human gaze control has been provided by Segal and Katsarkas (1986) and Guitton and Volle (1987).

GAZE ACCURACY

The need for the central nervous system (CNS) to monitor both eye and head positions in gaze shifts to targets situated beyond the ocular position saturation suggests that these movements might be less accurate than gaze shifts to targets attainable by an eye movement alone.

The experimental evidence does not suggest an important degradation in gaze accuracy when target eccentricity increases. Barnes (1979), Gresty (1974), and Guitton and Volle (1987) found that the mean error at the end of the first single-step gaze saccade made both in the light and in the dark to a remembered location was generally considerably less than the 10% value usually given for the accuracy of saccades made head fixed. Barnes (1979) found that accuracy worsens as head velocity decreases. Most remarkably, when head motion is perturbed the accuracy of gaze[3] is not strongly affected (Laurutis and Robinson, 1986; Guitton and Volle, 1987; R. D. Tomlinson, private communication).

SUMMARY

Recent experimental findings on how gaze is controlled using coordinated eye–head movements require that the "oculocentric" view of this system be reexamined. Evidence suggests that visually triggered saccades, VOR slow phases and quick phases may be used synergistically to attain a desired target. To control precisely the position of the visual axis, it is suggested that eye and head positions are monitored by corollary discharges that calculate an internal representation of current gaze position. This is compared to desired gaze position to yield an internal signal specifying gaze position error. Recordings of the activity of tectoreticulospinal neurons indicate that these collicular output cells carry such a gaze position error signal (Munoz and Guitton, 1985, 1986; cf. chapter 18).

Acknowledgments
The author was supported by the Fonds de la Recherche en Santé du Québec and the Medical Research Council of Canada.

Notes

1. The rotational limits of the eye are called the oculomotor range (OMR). In humans the OMR extends about $\pm55°$ from the central gaze position (Guitton and Volle, 1987), which is about the same as in the rhesus monkey (Tomlinson and Bahra, 1986a). By comparison, in cat, the OMR is small, being limited to about $\pm25°$ (Guitton et al., 1980). The eye–head movement mechanisms in cats, monkeys, and humans have been studied extensively and they are interesting to compare, particularly with the cat, since its OMR is so small.

2. Gaze is normally stabilized when the visual axis is on target and this is expressed in the schematic by making $S = 1$ when $T/E = 0°$. For humans and monkeys, data suggest in general that $S = 0$ when $T/E > 40°$. It seems reasonable to suppose a smooth transition from $S = 0$ to 1 as T/E decreases from 40° to 0° and a hypothetical curve is shown in the box showing the relationship between S and T/E. Note that the results of Guitton and Volle (1987) for human subjects showed considerable intersubject variability in VOR–saccade interaction. In the box this is permitted by simply shifting the curve to a new location such as that shown by the dotted profile. Data for cat are not as simply expressed since S appears to go from 1 to 0 and back to 1 as a T/E goes from a large value (say 80°) to 0°.

3. Excellent gaze accuracy implies, in the gaze feedback model, an extremely reliable monitoring by the nervous system of current head (H) and eye (E) positions. E is thought to be provided by corollary discharges (Fuchs et al., 1985). The fact that brake-induced head perturbations do not alter gaze accuracy suggests it is not the head motor program, per se, that furnishes H but rather that it is calculated from information provided by sensors, notably the semicircular canals and neck muscle proprioceptors. The respective role of these systems is still to be determined.

17

Control of Head Movement During Visual Orientation

A. ROUCOUX AND M. CROMMELINCK

Earlier chapters have discussed the crucial role of the head movement system in producing the required orientation and stabilization of the telereceptors, such as eyes, ears, and vibrissae, that are contained in the head. Without accurate control of head position these receptors could not function effectively since their spatial coverage is usually restricted to a portion of the surrounding space. For vision, this problem is particularly acute because only a very narrow part of the visual field can be captured on the fovea. The neck plays an important role in the orientation of the gaze. However, this role is complicated by the potential for movement of the eye in the orbit, and thus the problem of eye–head coordination becomes central in the study of gaze. This chapter addresses two aspects of this problem: the coupling of central motor commands sent to extraocular and neck muscles and the role of the superior colliculus in generating gaze shifts produced by combinations of eye and head movement.

HEAD–EYE MOTOR COUPLING IN VARIOUS SPECIES

Phylogenetically older species usually orient their gaze by means of a rotation of the whole body. Insects do not have mobile eyes, but some, such as the blowfly (Land, 1975), possess a certain degree of neck mobility. Whereas the hover fly looks around by means of body movements, the bowfly uses head movements (up to 15°). In insects having a fovea (some flies or spiders), movements that orient the body are very similar to saccades.

Fishes have mobile eyes and their orienting behavior involves combined eye movements and body turns. Easter et al. (1974) demonstrated a strong coupling of eye saccades and body turns in the goldfish.

In the frog, whose head is more mobile than that of the fish, Dieringer et al. (1982) have shown that fast eye movements and fast resetting head movements are coupled in an obligatory fashion during optokinetic stimulation (rotation of the visual surround) or vestibular stimulation (whole body rotation). With its head immobile or fixed, the frog never makes an eye saccade: saccades are present only in association with a head movement.

Dunlap and Mowrer (1931) analyzed the curious alternating slow and rapid head movements that many birds execute when walking. They demonstrated that this nystagmuslike head movement pattern was of optokinetic origin. Birds also scan their environment with the help of head saccades, which are very similar to eye saccades. Every head saccade is accompanied by a flick of the nictitating membrane across the eye, a phenomenon comparable to the saccadic suppression observed in man. Huizinga and Van der Meulen (1951) observed, in the pigeon, a predominance of head nystagmus over ocular nystagmus during vestibular and optokinetic stimulation.

The guinea pig has a very mobile head. During optokinetic or vestibular stimulation, anticompensatory eye saccades (quick phases) are synchronized with steplike anticompensatory movements of the head (Gresty, 1975). This pattern of coupled eye and head movements resembles the voluntary gaze shifts observed in this species and seems universal for all head movements that are not passive.

Collewijn (1977) extensively described eye and head movements in freely moving rabbits. In contrast with the restrained rabbit, which makes few spontaneous eye movements, the free rabbit displays an active oculomotor behavior. Many saccades are initiated while the head is stationary and are accompanied by a head rotation of the same amplitude. Typically eye and head movement starts simultaneously. Other saccades are observed when the head is already moving. No eye saccades are observed without an accompanying head movement. Fuller (1980b, 1981) studied the coordination of eye movements with head torque or head movement in rabbits with head fixed or free. When the head is fixed, voluntary saccades are accompanied by rapid shifts in head torque. During vestibular stimulation, fast and slow phases of the eye are reflected in the torque signal. With head free, the linkage between eye and head movement is less clearly observed for vestibular nystagmus. However, large (more than 15°) spontaneous head movements are accompanied by two or more eye saccades associated with a sudden increase in head velocity. Fuller reports that spontaneous eye saccades can occur in rabbits with their heads fixed. This would be the first level in the phylogenetic scale at which eye saccades are generated independently of head movements, a behavior that is likely to be related to the appearance of a pseudofovea.

The cat possesses a better differentiated foveal region, the area centralis, and readily generates eye saccades when its head is restrained. With head free, almost all saccades larger than 4° are accompanied by head rotation. Blakemore and Donaghy (1980) reported that head movement typically started at a variable delay after the beginning of the eye movement (most frequently 30 msec). In contrast Guitton et al. (1984a) and Roucoux and Crommelinck (1980) reported that the great majority of saccades in their cats lagged behind the head movement. Guitton et al. (1984a) also observed that for rapid gaze displacements greater than 30°, the pattern of movements is often characterized by a series of rapid eye movements in the same direction. In these cases, head trajectories exhibit repetitive small accelerations associated with eye saccades. They also noted that, on average, an eye–head movement terminates with the head aligned on target and, therefore, with the eyes centered.

In alert rhesus monkeys with their heads fixed, Lestienne et al. (1984) demonstrated that the horizontal component of eye movement is highly correlated with head torque and neck muscle EMG during pursuit, spontaneous saccades, and vestibular nystagmus. They also observed a phasic pause in neck EMG (particularly in the splenius) during contralaterally directed eye saccades, which began 10 to 20 msec before the initiation of the saccade.

The first authors to study extensively eye and head coupling and coordination in the rhesus monkey were Bizzi et al. (1971, 1972a,b), who described two modes of eye–head coordination. In response to an unexpected target, their monkeys made a saccadic eye movement and, after a latency of 25 to 40 msec, a head movement in the same direction. They called this behavior "triggered mode." EMG records showed that the neck muscles were activated first, followed 20 msec later by the eye muscles. The apparent lag in the appearance of head movement was attributed to the greater inertia of the head. The neck muscle activity consisted of a burst of activity in all the agonist muscles followed by a 20 to 30 msec pause. The activity of antagonist muscles was suppressed during the agonist burst. Amplitude and duration of that burst depended on the starting position and amplitude of the head movement.

After a series of repetitions, the monkey learned the location at which to expect a target and made "predictive" movements. In this case, the head began to move well before the eye saccade was initiated (150 to 200 msec). The EMG pattern was different: the agonist muscles exhibited a gradual increase of activity that was mirrored by a decrease of activity in the antagonists. These observations suggest that quite different neural mechanisms may underlie the initiation of triggered and predictive gaze shifts.

Kubo et al. (1981) studied eye and head movements evoked by optokinetic or vestibular stimulation in squirrel monkeys. They showed that such stimulation may elicit a head nystagmus that has quick phases that are almost always associated with the quick phase of eye nystagmus. The authors compare this head nystagmus with that of guinea pigs, pigeons, or chickens.

In humans, a number of investigators described the coupling of eye and head movements during visual orientation: the whole pattern is very similar to that described in the monkey. Outerbridge and Melvill-Jones (1971) demonstrated that head nystagmus can be induced in humans by rotational stimulation. The occurrence of a saccadic flick of the head is almost always accompanied by a particularly large saccade, suggesting that the generation of eye and head saccades is closely related. Gresty (1974) emphasized differences in the head movement component of visually triggered gaze shifts depending upon whether the target is illuminated continuously or flashed for only 40 msec. The proportion of the gaze shift accomplished by the head movement was significantly larger in the condition in which a target was flashed, suggesting that visual feedback may play a role in controlling the head movement, at least in its terminal stages. Barnes (1979) presents interesting observations concerning the latency of the eye movement with respect to head acceleration. The eye precedes the head when the total gaze displacement is less than 50°. Beyond this amplitude, the eye lags behind the head proportionally to the increase in amplitude. This author reports that the total head displacement covers 80% of the target offset, regardless of whether the target was flashed or illuminated continuously. Barnes proposes that, for small target offsets, up to 45°, the control of the eye saccade would be mediated by retinal error and, for larger offsets, the eye saccade would be generated by the system that is responsible for head–eye coordination in the dark, i.e., the vestibular quick phase generator. Zangemeister and Stark (1982a,b) analyzed further the relative latencies of eye and head motor activation. Their EMG recordings from splenius and sternocleidomastoid muscles show equal latency in control signals sent to the eye and head. Variable delays between the onset of the movements themselves would be due to biomechanical properties of the head.

This review reveals that the coupling between eye and head movement is a universal process throughout the phylogenetic scale. In species in which the eye or the neck is not mobile, a similar process involves eye and body, head and body, or any mobile appendage supporting the eye (this is the case in some arthropods). Coupling occurs during voluntary visual orienting behavior as well as during reflexes that stabilize images on the retina (vestibular and optokinetic slow phases). It is of interest to note that these reflexes also contain anticompensatory saccadic movements involving eye and head, which serve to reorient eye and head in the direction of the movement of the rest of the body. Their function is thus to destabilize gaze: they correspond to periods of inactivation of the stabilizing reflexes. Robinson (1981) proposes that orienting saccades tied to a head movement and quick phases share many similarities and are probably functionally identical. The most phylogenetically advanced vertebrates have the faculty of moving the eye alone, thereby decoupling eye and head. This capacity is apparently linked to the presence of a functional area centralis or fovea. As opposed to "afoveate" saccades, Robinson calls these "foveate" saccades. Roucoux et al. (1981) proposed that this saccade, unlike the quick phase, is added to the slow phases of the stabilizing reflexes, so that the accompanying head movement does not contribute to the overall gaze shift, being treated instead as a perturbation whose effect is nulled by a compensatory vestibuloocular eye movement.

PATTERNS OF MUSCLE ACTIVATION DURING GAZE SHIFTS

Recent studies of the coupling of eye and head movements in cats have involved electromyographic recording from multiple muscles or compartments within muscles. Roucoux et al. (1982) and Vidal et al. (1982) reported that, in head-fixed cats, the EMG activity of a series of neck muscles was correlated with horizontal eye position. Not only does this muscular activity mimic spontaneous eye movements, but also eye movements during vestibular or optokinetic nystagmus. Wilson et al. (1983) studied this eye position-related activity in the splenius muscle and showed that the different compartments of this muscle behave similarly, suggesting that the whole muscle receives a common central descending signal.

To define the spatial properties of the eye position signal in the neck muscles Roucoux et al. (1985) observed cats trained to fixate suddenly appearing visual targets. The EMG activity of seven pairs of neck muscles was recorded together with eye and head movements. The heads of the animals were either fixed or left

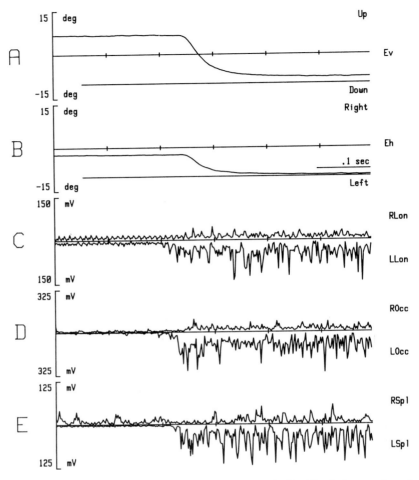

Figure 17.1.   Rectified and integrated EMG activity (C, D, E) of three pairs of neck muscles (longissimus, Lon; obliquus capitis cranialis, Occ; splenius, Spl) recorded in a head fixed cat trained to fixate visual targets (the occurrence and position of the target are indicated by a horizontal line in (A) and (B) together with vertical and horizontal position of the eye: Ev, Eh). Eye position is recorded by the coil technique.

free. Figure 17.1 illustrates the activity of three pairs of muscles recorded in a cat foveating a visual target situated at 10° downward and to the left while the head was held fixed. The three left muscles show a sharp increase of their discharge, which begins about 30 msec before saccade onset, attains a stable level even before the eye starts moving and goes on as long as fixation is maintained. No clear phasic discharge related to the saccade can be seen. The right muscles show a similar behavior, at a much lower level. Note also that the relative amplitude of the obliquus capitis discharge is much higher than that of the two other muscles. The three muscles thus show a certain degree of cocontraction, probably related to the downward component of the eye movement, as well as a stronger activation of the left muscles, related to the leftward horizontal component. All the analyzed muscles behaved in a comparable way, although some were preferentially activated by upward eye deviations (rectus capitis, biventer) or downward eye deviations (splenius, obliquus capitis cranialis, longissimus). However, all of them were sensitive to variable extents to lateral deviations. Figure 17.2 illustrates the mean tonic level obtained for at least five fixations along the horizontal or the vertical meridians for the obliquus capitis. Each muscle of the pair discharges for ipsilateral deviations of the eye in a reciprocal, push–pull manner. When the eye is in its primary position, both muscles are activated. Both muscles discharge together proportionally to the downward deviation of the eye. In case of nonvisually guided movements, the latency between the EMG modulation and the eye movement is much larger (200 to 300 msec), suggesting a decoupling of eye and neck once no visual target is present.

The same muscles have also been recorded in the head-free condition. Figure 17.3 shows the activity of the same three muscles as in Figure 17.1 during a combined eye–head movement toward a visual target situated 20° down and to the right. The gaze shift is typical: movement of the eyes starts simultaneously with the head movement and is followed, once gaze comes close to the target, by a backward compensatory eye movement lasting until the head movement stops. The head attains a velocity of 200°/sec. Each right muscle discharges phasically during the acceleration phase of the head, with a typical latency of 30 msec with respect to the onset of the head movement. In this particular case, the tonic level of discharge makes it difficult to obtain a precise estimate of the latency. The end of this phasic discharge corresponds to the acquisition of the target, as if this pulse was controlled by gaze position. The peak discharge occurs early in the head movement and is synchronous with the peak acceleration of the head.

The peak phasic discharge has been correlated with direction, amplitude, and starting head position for the different muscles. Each muscle is characterized by a direction for which the phasic discharge is maximal: this is illustrated in Figure 17.4. Along these preferential directions, however, amplitude and starting position influence the discharge. The larger the amplitude, the higher the burst; the more ipsilateral the initial position, with respect to the muscle, the larger the intensity. Some muscles have specific properties. For instance, during horizontal movements, the ipsilateral splenius has a short phasic burst occurring at the time of peak acceleration, whereas the contralateral splenius exhibits a "braking" burst, at the end of the head movement. For downward movements, the complexus shows a clear inhibition followed by a braking burst. The rectus major, whose preferential direction is about 60 to 80° upward, shows a clear bilateral braking pulse for downward movements of the head.

Since the above descriptions are based upon preliminary observations, it is premature to specify more precisely the functional peculiarities of each muscle. One further comment can be made, however, on the relation between neck muscle activity and maintained deviation of the head from its primary position. For small head deviations, tonic discharges are hardly seen. When head eccentricity in-

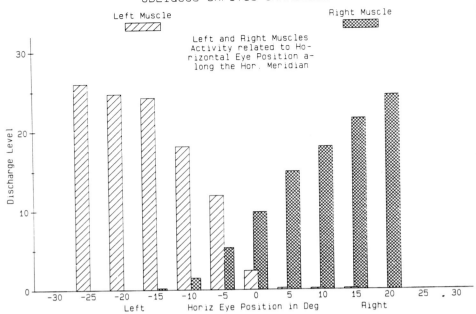

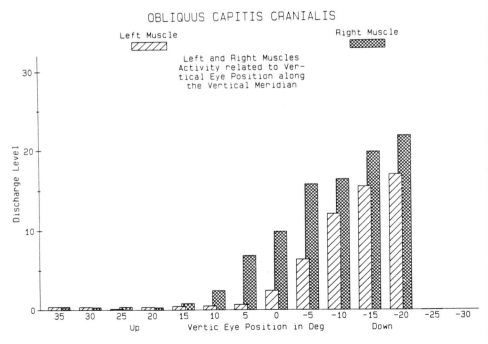

Figure 17.2. Mean tonic discharge of the obliquus capitis muscles as function of horizontal (A) and vertical (B) eye position in the head fixed trained cat. The level of the EMG is in arbitrary units.

214

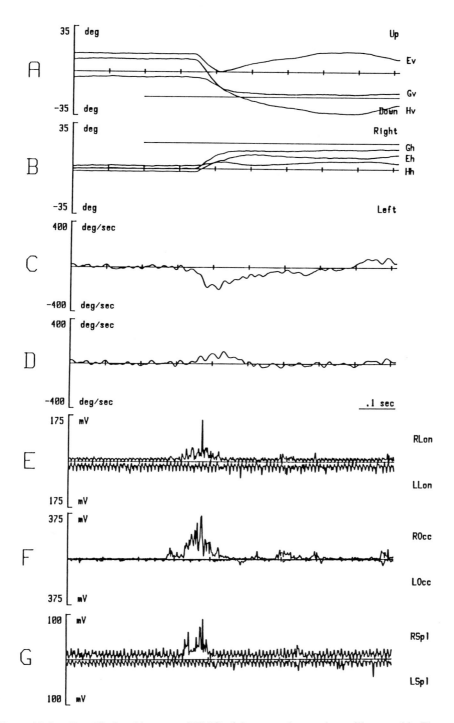

Figure 17.3.   Rectified and integrated EMG of the same three pairs as illustrated in Figure 17.1 (E, F, G) recorded in a head free trained cat. In (A) vertical eye, head, and gaze positions (Ev, Hv, Gv). In (B) horizontal positions (Eh, Hh, Gh). In (C and D) head vertical and horizontal velocity. Eye and head are recorded with the coil technique.

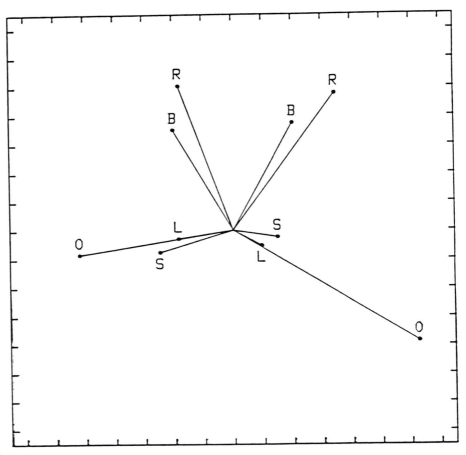

Figure 17.4.   Resultant of the phasic burst intensity as a function of head movement orientation but not of starting position or amplitude calculated, for each muscle, on 252
movements. The absolute values of the integrated EMG have been used, permitting some
evaluation of the relative contribution of each muscle. R, rectus capitis major; S, splenius;
L, longissimus; O, obliquus capitis cranialis; B, biventer cervicis.

creases, several muscles show a sustained activity composed of EMG bursts emit-
ted at a regular frequency. An increase of the deviation along a muscle's preferential direction results in larger bursts at a higher frequency. This phenomenon
is particularly common in splenius, complexus, and obliquus.

    Compared to the head-fixed paradigm, the behavior of the muscles in the
more natural situation with the head free is quite different. Neck muscles show
high tonic levels of activity related to eye position when the head is fixed, whereas
they mostly discharge phasically in relation with head acceleration when the head
is free. However, the "preferential directions" of the muscles are comparable,
suggesting that the eye position signal seen with head fixed reflects a functional
eye–head coupling, whose timing and amplitude, but not spatial properties, are

altered when the head is free to move. This fact will be discussed later in this chapter.

ROLE OF THE SUPERIOR COLLICULUS IN GENERATING EYE AND HEAD MOVEMENTS

It had long been known that electrical stimulation of the cat's superior colliculus evokes conjugate eye and head movements, the direction of which depends on the site of stimulation (Adamuk, 1870). Godlowski (1938) and Hess et al. (1946) reproduced these findings and showed that the orienting pattern is very similar to the natural behavior of the animal.

Other species were also studied: a particularly spectacular example has been offered by Schapiro and Goodman (1969), who stimulated the optic tectum of the alligator and evoked circling movements and forward progression depending on the stimulated region. Ewert (1967) electrically stimulated the optic tectum in toads and showed that turning movements can be released that are variously oriented in space depending on electrode location in the structure. This behavior is very similar to natural orienting movements toward prey.

Schaefer (1970) studied both the cat and the rabbit. In the rabbit, he reports that stimulation of the superior colliculus, particularly its caudal part, evokes brief orienting evoked responses involving only the head and eyes. Gaze is directed toward that region of the visual field corresponding to the position of the electrode on the retinotectal map. If stimulation is prolonged, body turning occurs. Results in the cat are very similar; the speed of the evoked head movement, however, is higher when more caudal zones of superior colliculus are stimulated, and gaze is brought to more eccentric positions (Schaefer, 1970; Syka and Radil-Weiss, 1971).

Straschill and Rieger (1973) recorded eye movements evoked by stimulation of the cat's superior colliculus. They were the first to report "goal-directed" evoked saccades in which the eyes reach the same final position in the orbit, irrespective of initial eye position. They interpret this response as forming part of an orienting system involving combined eye and head movements. Roucoux and Crommelinck (1976), also stimulating deep layers of the cat's colliculus, distinguished two zones on the basis of the organization of the evoked saccades. In the *rostral zone,* which receives projections of the central retina, saccades evoked at a given site are all nearly identical, irrespective of eye starting position: they are retinotopically coded. In the *caudal zone,* corresponding to the peripheral retina, saccades evoked at a particular point always bring the eye to a given position in the orbit irrespective of its initial position, very similar to the evoked saccades described by Straschill and Rieger. The transition between the two zones corresponds to 25° of eccentricity on the retina.

The two zones of the colliculus also differ in the way in which they activate the head movement system. With the head free, a brief pulse applied to the *rostral zone* does not elicit a head movement. With the head fixed, however, longer stimulus trains applied to this zone can lead to activation of neck muscles. In the case of the biventer muscle, illustrated in Figure 17.5, this activation occurs when the staircase of saccades elicited by the stimulus causes the eyes to move past the midline to the side of the muscle whose activity is being recorded. In Figure

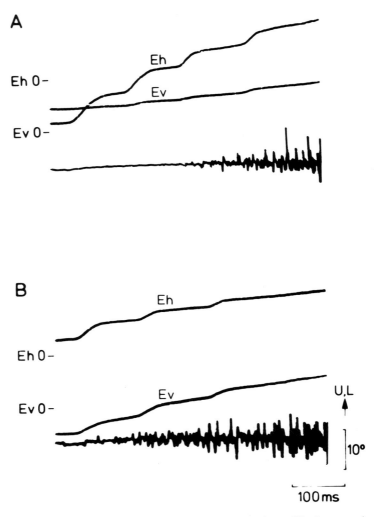

Figure 17.5.   The left biventer EMG evoked by right superior colliculus rostral zone electrical stimulation in the head fixed cat depends on initial eye position. Eh, Ev, Horizontal and vertical eye position. EvO, EhO, Primary eye position. U, L, Up, left. The stimulus starts at the beginning of the trace and lasts 400 msec.

17.5A, in which the eyes started on the opposite side, muscle activation is delayed. In Figure 17.5B, the saccades start past the midline and the muscle discharges almost at the time of application of the stimulus. There is therefore a linear relationship between EMG latency and initial eye position in the orbit.

In other neck muscles, such as splenius and obliquus capitis, which have a "preferential direction" not too far from the horizontal, rostral collicular stimulation may evoke a weak phasic discharge even when the eyes are deviated to the opposite side. As illustrated in Figure 17.6, however, amplitude of the response is modulated by initial eye position: responses are fairly weak when the accompanying saccade starts on the right and increase rather abruptly as soon as eye positions greater than 6° to the left are attained.

In the *caudal zone* head movements are evoked even by a brief pulse of stimulation. Figure 17.7 shows the activity of the left biventer cervicis evoked by a stimulation in the caudal part of the right colliculus. The pattern of evoked saccades is illustrated in the upper left corner: these saccades bring the eye within a rather limited zone in the orbit (craniocentric coding). The dotted line represents the boundary of the oculomotor range. The saccades are numbered and their time course illustrated in the rest of the figure, along with the corresponding biventer activity. Whatever the starting position of the eye, a short latency burst (7 msec) can be seen followed by a period of relative silence and, with a latency of 50 msec, by a second intense discharge lasting as long as the stimulus. This pattern is, on the average, constant for a given stimulation site and this observation is valid for most neck muscles studied.

The patterns of EMG activation described above can be related to the pattern of head movements observed by Roucoux et al. (1980a,b) and Harris (1980) following microstimulation of superior colliculus in cats with the head free. When the stimulus is delivered in the anterior colliculus, a slow contraversive head movement is evoked if the stimulus is long enough to bring the eye beyond a position threshold, often situated a few degrees from the primary position. Saccades accompanying this head movement are reduced in amplitude by the vestibular slow phase signal. In contrast, head movements evoked from the posterior colliculus are also contraversive but have a large amplitude, a high velocity (saccadelike), and a short and constant latency (25–30 msec), and the synchronous saccade is not modified by the vestibular slow phase. The direction and amplitude of these movements are in accordance with the retinal map. When they stimulated the very caudal regions of the colliculus, Roucoux et al. (1980a,b) observed head movements combined with centering eye movements. The head movements were saccadic and brought the head's axis to a particular position in space by means of either contraversive or ipsiversive movements. This movement pattern was not seen by Harris (1980), but its occurrence has recently been confirmed by McIlwain (1986).

The role of the cat's superior colliculus in generating head movements is supported by observations of neurons within the deeper layers of the colliculus that discharge prior to head movements (Straschill and Schick, 1977; Harris, 1980). Munoz and Guitton (1985) recorded antidromically identified tectospinal cells in head free cats. These cells can be visually activated and discharge for a given amplitude and direction of head rotation provided that the animal was "aroused" by the target. The anatomical and physiological properties of the tectospinal or tectoreticular cells are discussed in Chapter 18.

In the rhesus monkey, the existing data suggest that the superior colliculus is not directly involved in generation of orienting head movements. Stryker and Schiller (1975) showed that head movements accompanying saccades evoked by electrical stimulation are extremely variable in size and latency and mostly appear when the eye reaches extreme deviations. Robinson and Jarvis (1974) failed to find neurons whose discharge was related to head movement or position; they

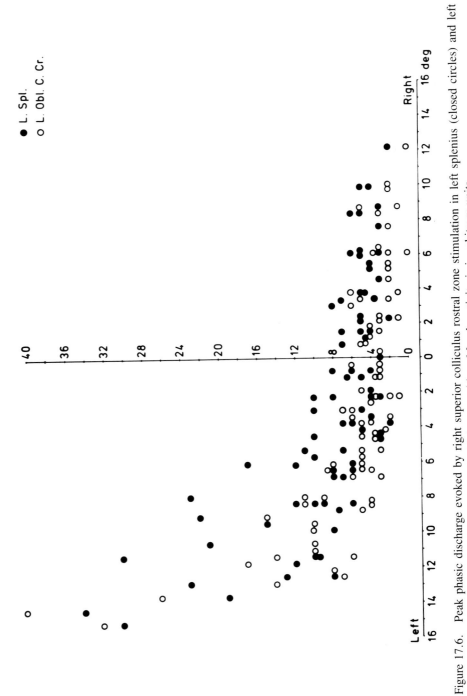

Figure 17.6. Peak phasic discharge evoked by right superior colliculus rostral zone stimulation in left splenius (closed circles) and left obliquus capitis (open circles) as a function of initial eye position. Muscle activity is in arbitrary units.

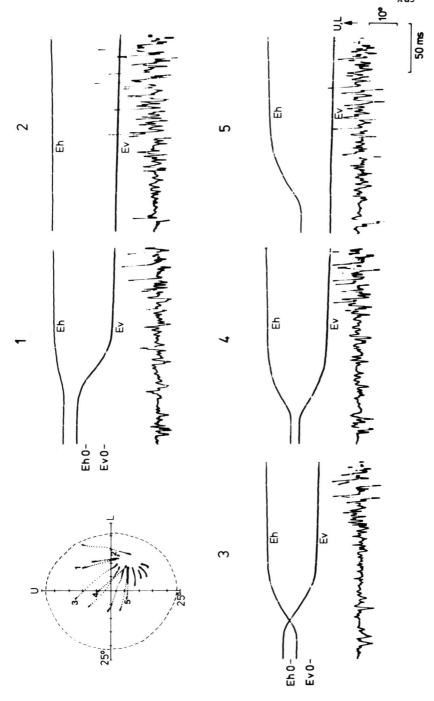

Figure 17.7. The left biventer EMG evoked by the right superior colliculus caudal zone in the head fixed cat does not depend on initial eye position. Abbreviations are the same as in Figure 17.5.

221

concluded that primary superior colliculus is not the site for the generation of orienting head movements.

A TENTATIVE SYNTHESIS

Careful consideration of the mode of operation of visual orientation in the cat reveals a number of general principles, which may aid in understanding the gaze behavior of other species. As far as vision is concerned, the cat occupies an intermediate position among the vertebrates: compared to man or monkey, its fovea is not as well developed and its eye mobility is more limited. Unlike the rabbit, frog, or fish, the cat exhibits an area centralis and "foveate" saccades. Curiously, the functional organization of the cat's colliculus is double. The rostral part receives a retinal projection covering the cat's oculomotor range (25° on either side) and appears implicated in the generation of "foveate" saccades and not in head orientation: it would correspond to the entire monkey colliculus. This is the "retinocentric" colliculus. The caudal part is connected to the peripheral retina, outside the oculomotor range, and seems involved in the elaboration of combined eye–head movements: it would correspond to the entire rabbit or frog colliculus. This is the "craniocentric" colliculus.

How may we integrate the presence of an eye position signal in the neck muscles with this scheme? The answer may reside in the following consideration: every signal of retinal origin destined to move the head must be recoded from retinocentric to craniocentric coordinates. This recoding is achieved by the addition of eye position in the orbit to the retinal error, exactly the two factors that influence neck EMG activity during stimulation of the rostral colliculus. How is it then that the output from the caudal colliculus to the neck is independent of eye position? Probably, as the organization of evoked eye saccades suggests, the output layers of the caudal colliculus are already recoded in a head frame of reference, a fact that again emphasizes the unique role of the caudal colliculus in head motor control.

SUMMARY

The direction of gaze is determined by the orientation of the eyes in the head and of the head in space. This chapter explores how extraocular and neck motor commands are coordinated to produce accurate gaze shifts and examines the role of the superior colliculus in producing these motor commands.

The first section describes the coupling between eye and head movements in various species. In lower vertebrates all eye movements are accompanied by turning of the head or body, whereas primates often make eye movements without head turns. The cat lies between these extremes: eye movements less than 4° are made in isolation, whereas larger gaze shifts are made by a combined eye–head movement. In eye–head movements to unexpected targets the neck muscles are typically activated about 20 msec before eye muscles.

The second section describes how the patterns of neck muscle activation during an eye–head gaze shift depends upon the final gaze position. Each muscle has a preferential direction for which it is activated most strongly. Activation is tonic if the head is prevented from moving, whereas complex phasic activation of agonist and antagonist muscles occurs during active head turns.

The third section reviews the role of the superior colliculus in generating eye and head movements. In lower species stimulation of the colliculus elicits linked eye and head turns. A similar pattern is evoked by stimulation of the caudal region of the cat's colliculus, which is related to eye movements of more than 25°. Stimulation of the rostral colliculus in cat and of the entire monkey colliculus elicits stereotyped eye movements that are accompanied by a head movement only when they drive the eyes past the midline toward the edge of the orbit. These results appear to relate to an evolution of collicular function that accompanies the development of a fovea.

18

The Role of the Tectoreticulospinal System in the Control of Head Movement

A. GRANTYN and A. BERTHOZ

Active head movements can serve different biological purposes, and their repertoire is extemely rich, particularly in higher vetebrates. The mammalian superior colliculus (SC)[1] is more often viewed as a subcortical structure participating in sensorimotor transformations during orientation toward objects in the contralateral space. However, there is also evidence that the SC may contribute to other types of behavior, such as aversive reactions of the escape-avoidance type that, according to the direction with respect to the triggering sensory stimulus, are the opposite of orienting reactions (Schaefer, 1970; Kilpatrick et al., 1982; Sahibzada et al., 1986). The present review will not be concerned with processing in the intracollicular circuits that leads to a selection of a behaviorally appropriate motor pattern. We shall summarize only the available data bearing on the neural organization of tectal output related to the execution of contraversive, orienting patterns that include, of course, head movements. The substrate of this output is the crossed tectobulbospinal tract (TbsT) and its parallel connections with the spinal cord through the brain stem reticular formation (RF). This chapter will show that the contribution of the SC to the control of head movements depends on additional signal processing in the reticular circuits and, hence, the tectospinal and the reticulospinal systems should be considered as a functional entity.

THE SUPERIOR COLLICULUS AND THE TECTOBULBOSPINAL TRACT

The first indication that pathways originating in the SC participate in the control of head movement came from observations of motor patterns induced by collicular stimulation. Results of these experiments are reviewed in Chapter 17. Two factors should be kept in mind when analyzing the neural organization of tectal efferent pathways. (1) The contribution of the SC to the control of head movement is not the same in different species. It appears to decrease with the development of foveal vision and the acquisition of a larger range of eye movements. As indicated in Chapter 17, the SC of the cat has a dual organization, transitional between foveate and afoveate species. (2) Studies in freely moving animals all emphasize the fact that stimulation of the SC results in "synergically coordinated 'compact' motor performance" (Hess et al., 1946). The sequence of eye, pinna, head, trunk, and limb movements resembles naturally occurring contraversive movements during orienting. Hence, the contribution of the SC to the control of head movement should be considered in the context of coordination of motor synergies.

The Tectobulbospinal Tract (TbsT)

The crossed tectobulbospinal tract has traditionally been considered to be the pathway that transmits excitatory SC influences to neck and eye motoneurons engaged in contralaterally directed orienting movements. Such movements induced by stimulation of the SC do not depend on its ascending pathways, since they persist in decorticated and decerebrated animals (Faulkner and Hyde, 1958; Schaefer, 1970). The crossed nature of the pathway is obvious from the observation that stimulation of the SC activates neck muscles on the contralateral side. Although the SC has several efferent systems that cross the midline (Edwards, 1977), physiological evidence is in favor of the TbsT, which is the only rapidly conducting, direct pathway to the upper cervical segments. For example, Hess et al. (1946) observed jerklike eye and head movements after each stimulus pulse during low-frequency stimulation of the deep SC layers. They concluded that "The innervation pattern organized in the tectum . . . is transmitted to corresponding effectors by the tectospinal tract to motor nuclei subserving eye and neck muscles." The shortest latencies of EMG responses in dorsal neck muscles, of the order of 5 msec (Guitton et al., 1980; Peterson and Fukushima, 1982), are compatible with monosynaptic transmission to motoneurons if the time required for temporal summation of EPSPs is taken into account.

The Tectospinal Component of the TbsT

Projection of the TbsT to upper cervical segments and cervical enlargement has been demonstrated in many species, e.g., monkeys (Harting, 1977; Castiglioni et al., 1978), cats (Rasmussen, 1936; Altman and Carpenter, 1961; Nyberg-Hansen, 1964; Petras, 1967), and rats (Waldron and Gwyn, 1969; Petrovicky, 1976). Its presence has been denied in the rabbit (Holstege and Collewijn, 1982). It seems that the presence or absence of a direct tectospinal connection cannot be simply related to different modes of head movement control by the SC of foveate and afoveate animals, as discussed in Chapter 17. All studies agree that only a small number of fibers reaches the spinal cord. The loss of fibers in the predorsal bundle (FprD) begins at the level of the abducens nucleus (Abd-N) and proceeds rapidly toward the rostral pole of the inferior olive (Rasmussen, 1936). Although the actual fraction of fibers in the TbsT that extends to the spinal cord has not been reported, comparison of numbers of SC neurons labeled after horseradish peroxidase (HRP) injections in the second cervical segment and in the pontobulbar tegmentum (Kawamura and Hashikawa, 1978) indicates that this fraction is on the order of 20%. Thus a great majority of tectal neurons projecting in the TbsT are "tectobulbar."

In cats, the control of head movement by the caudal SC (beginning with retinal eccentricities of more than 25°) appears to be more direct, as compared to its anterior zone (see Chapter 17). However, as shown in Figure 18.1, there is no obvious rostrocaudal gradient of cell density, i.e., the caudal parts of the SC representing visual periphery do not contain more neurons descending directly to the spinal cord (Huerta and Harting, 1982; Murray and Coulter, 1982). Thus functional differences between the zones are not reflected in the degree of development of the tectospinal connection, and the idea that the role of the TbsT is to assure rapid orienting movements of the head is incorrect, if this connection is considered

Figure 18.1. Density gradients, with respect to the retinotectal map, of tectospinal neurons projecting to the first cervical segment. The representation of the contralateral visual hemifield on the dorsal view of the SC is adopted after Feldon et al. (1970). VM, HM, Vertical and horizontal meridians, respectively. Numbers indicate vertical and horizontal eccentricities in degrees. The dashed line and oblique arrows mark the transition between the anterior (retinocentric) and intermediate (craniocentric) zones (see Chapter 17). Open columns are proportional to the numbers of cells located within corresponding segments oriented approximately in parallel with horizontal isoeccentricity lines. Shaded columns are the same for segments oriented in parallel to horizontal meridian. Calculation of cell numbers is based on the distribution, in the horizontal plane, of retrogradely labeled neurons after HRP injection into the gray matter of C1 (Huerta and Harting, 1982, Fig. 13). Note greater cell numbers in the anterior zone and in the lower quadrant.

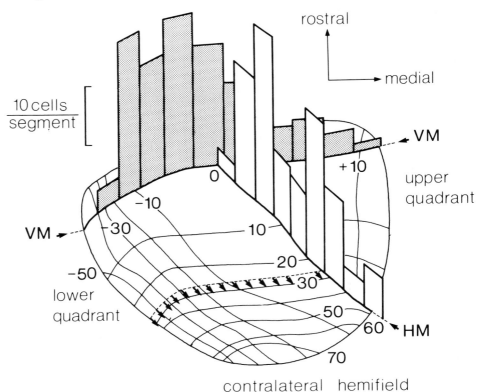

in isolation. In addition, the weakness of monosynaptic tectal input to neck motoneurons has been demonstrated by intracellular recording (Anderson et al., 1971). This study indicated that tectal excitation of neck motoneurons is due mainly to the transmission through the brain stem RF.

Pontobulbar Terminations of the TbsT

Rhombencephalic projections through the TbsT (FprD) are directed mainly to the medial pontobulbar RF. The distribution of terminals is not quite uniform. Terminations in the caudal medulla, beginning from the rostral pole of the inferior olive, are quite sparce [Altman and Carpenter, 1961 (cat); Harting, 1977 (monkey); Holstege and Collewijn, 1982 (rabbit)]. As shown in Figure 18.4A, in the pons and medulla there are two regions of denser terminations (Kawamura et al., 1974; Huerta and Harting, 1982): at midpontine level [rostral nucleus reticularis pontis caudalis (R.p.c.)] and just posterior to the Abd-N [junction of R.p.c. and nucleus reticularis gigantocellularis (R.Gc.)]. Terminal fields are limited to the dorsal one-half to two-thirds of the medial reticular nuclei. Edwards and Henkel (1978) reported particularly dense terminations ventrally to the Abd-N. According to Kawamura et al. (1974), the regions of enhanced tectoreticular projections coincide with the main sites of origin of reticulospinal tracts. Outside the reticular core FprD fibers establish connections with the following structures: all the precerebellar nuclei (Kawamura et al., 1974; Frankfurter et al., 1976; Harting, 1977; Hess, 1982; Holstege and Collewijn, 1982; Huerta and Harting, 1982), the nucleus prepositus hypoglossi (Grantyn and Grantyn, 1982; Huerta and Harting, 1982), the abducens (Edwards and Henkel, 1978; Grantyn and Grantyn, 1976, 1982), and facial motor nuclei (Holstege and Collewijn, 1982; Huerta and Harting, 1982).

The general idea that each of the identified connections may originate from separate groups of efferent neurons, presumably different in function, has not yet been proven experimentally for neurons projecting in the FprD. Morphological data are available only for thick FprD axons (6–10 μm) originating from large neurons, most of which project to the spinal cord (Grantyn and Grantyn, 1982; Grantyn and Berthoz, 1985). As shown by intracellular HRP tracing, these neurons establish collateral connections with most, if not all, of the previously described targets of the FprD (Fig. 18.2A). It can be concluded that "purely" tectospinal neurons do not exist. All signals transmitted to the spinal cord by tectospinal axons are also distributed to the RF and other rhombencephalic structures through the collaterals of tectoreticulospinal neurons (TRSN). Since direct tectomotoneuronal connections are weak, the activity generated in parallel transreticular circuits is probably essential for the control of neck motoneurons.

Mesodiencephalic Targets of Tectoreticulospinal Neurons

Studies using anterograde degeneration and autoradiographic tracing ascribed most of the tectal connections in the rostral brain stem to fiber systems other than the TbsT. However, tracings based on intracellular HRP injections, due to their better resolution, revealed extensive mesodiencephalic collateral connections of neurons

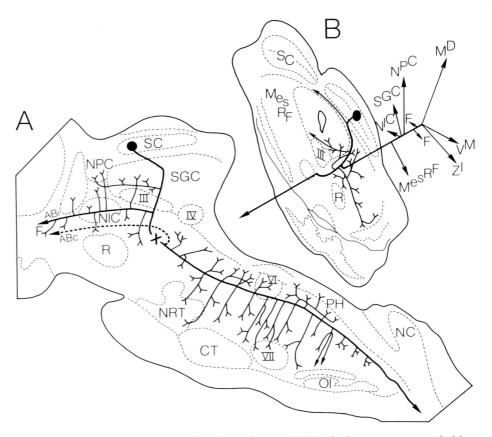

Figure 18.2. Presently known connections of tectoreticulospinal neurons as revealed by intracellular HRP injections (Grantyn and Grantyn, 1982; Grantyn et al., 1982; Grantyn and Berthoz, 1985; Moschovakis and Karabelas, 1985) and mapping by antidromic stimulation (Chevalier and Deniau, 1984). (A) Representation in the parasagittal plane. The site of decussation is marked by X. ABi, the ipsilateral main ascending branch; ABc, the occasionally observed contralateral main ascending branch. Its secondary branching, symmetrical to ABi, is not entered in the drawing. Arrows indicate continuation of branches suggested but not proven by intracellular HRP tracing. (B) Representation of midbrain collaterals in the frontal plane and rostral connections of the main ascending branch. Connections to thalamic nuclei and zona incerta are entered based on the results of antidromic mapping. See list of abbreviations (note 1) for anatomical notations.

projecting in the FprD and to the spinal cord (Grantyn and Grantyn, 1982; Grantyn et al., 1982; Moschovakis and Karabelas, 1985). All neurons issue at least one "main ascending branch" passing through the medial midbrain tegmentum into the parafascicular complex of the thalamus (Fig. 18.2A and B). Collaterals of this branch and of the main descending axon before its decussation distribute terminals to the mesencephalic RF, the supraoculomotor central gray, the interstitial nucleus of Cajal (NIC), the region of the rostral interstitial nucleus of the medial longitudinal fasciculus, and the nucleus of posterior commissure. The highest density of terminations is in the medial RF, throughout its dorsoventral extent. Connections with the lateral RF, including the paralemniscal region, are weaker. Thalamic connections of the "main ascending branches" could not be followed with intracellular HRP. Using antidromic stimulation, Chevalier and Deniau (1984) proved that they project to the zona incerta and to the intralaminar, mediodorsal, and ventral medial nuclei of the thalamus. Thus, TRSNs appear to contact virtually all the target areas of other fiber systems linking the deep subdivision of the SC with the mesodiencephalic structures. Since some of these structures are implicated in the control of head movements (see below), the rostral brain stem, as well as the pontobulbar tegmentum, should be considered as the origin of pathways acting in parallel with the TbsT.

Activity of Collicular Neurons in Relation to Head Movements

Recordings of signals carried by neurons in the SC have provided important insights concerning its role in generating head movements. This section reviews two sets of studies, one involving recordings from neurons whose projections were not identified and one in which only identified tectoreticulospinal neurons were studied.

Unidentified Neurons

Working on monkeys, Robinson and Jarvis (1974) failed to find neurons whose discharges were correlated with head movements. It was concluded that "the primate superior colliculus is related to the generation of eye movements and is not the site of generation of head movements or the integration of head and eye movements." Data in the cat are quite limited and not consistent. Straschill and Schick (1977) recorded neurons activated selectively with active head movements in the deeper SC layers. A majority of them were of a phasic-tonic type, exhibiting activity related to both velocity and position of the head. A few were of either phasic or tonic type. Microstimulation at sites of recording from head-related units resulted in contraversive head movements. The authors regard ". . . the deeper layers of the colliculus superior as a premotor center of spinal neck muscle motoneurons." In contrast, Harris (1980) found only a few deeper layer neurons (4 out of 99) discharging with head but not eye movements. They were of the phasic type, with discharges much shorter than the duration of head movement. However, the two studies agree that neurons related to head or to eye movements represent separate populations.

Identified Tectoreticulospinal Neurons

Grantyn and Berthoz (1983, 1985) studied the activity of TRSN axons during orienting toward visual targets in cats with fixed heads. They identified a class of "visuomotor" TRSNs that are activated by moving visual stimuli even in the absence of motor orienting. These visual responses are directionally tuned. Burst discharges are enhanced if a visual stimulus elicits orienting saccades. Activity is particularly strong when both stimulus and eye movements coincide with the neuron's preferred direction. However, TRSNs do not discharge with saccades of the same direction and amplitude when the animal spontaneously scans a homoge-

neous visual background. Novel, three-dimensional objects elicit the strongest firing when they are moved in the appropriate direction and are followed by orienting
saccades terminating in the contralateral hemifield. Usually, during such gaze shifts
there is a strong activation of contralateral neck muscles acting predominantly in
the horizontal plane (Vidal et al., 1982). After the initial EMG burst, muscle
activity slowly declines to a new steady-state level that is proportional to ipsilateral eye position during fixation (Fig. 18.3, 18.5). TRSN bursts begin before the
saccadic eye movement and the onset of the phasic neck EMG discharge. Typically, the bursts are of short duration and coincide with only the initial part of
phasic muscle contractions (Fig. 18.3). Grantyn and Berthoz did not observe TRSNs
with truly tonic activity and only a few with bursts corresponding to the total
duration of phasic EMG events.

The relatively short duration of bursts indicates that TRSNs can contribute
to the facilitation of neck motoneurons only during the initial part of phasic muscle
contractions. Signals needed to produce the complete pattern of motor response
must be generated in circuits acting in parallel with TRSNs. Another observation
to be emphasized is the conditional linkage between TRSN bursts and neck EMG.
For example, strong activity of "visuomotor" TRSNs is completely decoupled
from EMG when eyes are directed in the hemifield ipsilateral to the neuron (Fig.
18.3, events 3 and 7). Similarly, even intense bursting of the so-called "visual"
(Grantyn and Berthoz, 1985) TRSNs is never "translated" into neck muscle activity. The access of tectal efferent signals to the final common pathway is obviously under the control of gating or selective channeling mechanisms, which
remain to be studied.

These conclusions are in general agreement with the data obtained from TRSNs
in cats with their heads free to move (Munoz and Guitton, 1985 a,b). The generation of phasic TRSN discharges during contraversive gaze shifts is not obligatory. They are reliably present and show good correlation with head movement
when cats perform strongly motivated, high-velocity gaze shifts contingent on
reinforcement. Geometrically identical gaze shifts to the predicted position of an
invisible target are not associated with TRSN bursts. Such gaze shifts are usually
of lower velocity and it can be supposed that phasic discharges of TRSNs, when
present, contribute to the acceleration of the head. The results of Munoz and
Guitton (1985a) also provide a remarkable example of the decoupling of TRSN
activity from head movement and corresponding activity of neck muscles. TRSNs
generate a tonic discharge coding the gaze error when the animal is looking into
the ipsilateral (with respect to the SC) hemifield while preparing a contralateral
gaze shift. Obviously, the contralateral neck muscles are relaxed during this time
and the tonic TRSN signal seems to have no access to motor output. The functional significance of the directionally inverted tonic TRSN signal remains obscure.

MIDBRAIN SUBSTRATES OF HEAD MOVEMENT CONTROL

In parallel with the investigations of the role of the SC in controlling head movements, which have been described above, neuroanatomists and neurophysiologists
were investigating the role of structures in the mesencephalon in motor control.

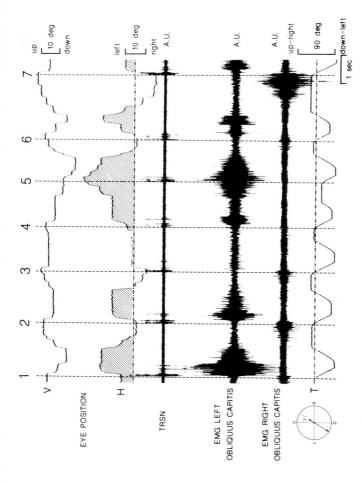

Figure 18.3. Activity of an identified tectoreticulospinal neuron located in the right SC during visuomotor behavior of an alert cat (A. Grantyn and A. Berthoz, unpublished). From top to bottom: vertical (V) and horizontal (H) eye position, spike activity of the neuron, EMG of left and right mm. obliquus capitis cranialis, and position of a visual target moving in oblique direction, as shown in the inset on the left. Amplitudes of electrical activity have no absolute calibration and are expressed in arbitrary units (A.U.). Vertical interrupted lines are drawn through the beginning of burst discharges of the TRSN. Note that the neuron is activated each time when the target departs to down-left. Bursts precede saccades matching approximately the direction of target movement. Coupling of neuronal activity with the left EMG is conditional on eye–head synergy: temporal coincidence of bursts with phasic muscle contractions is clear only during large gaze shifts to the left (events 1 and 5). With leftward gaze shifts terminating closer to the vertical meridian (e.g., events 3 and 6), the relationship becomes quite variable.

231

This section reviews evidence, based on studies employing electrical stimulation, neuroanatomical tracing of connections, and electrophysiological recordings, that several midbrain regions are involved in generating head movements.

Evidence from Stimulation Experiments

A contribution from the midbrain to the control of head movements was revealed by stimulation experiments as far back as 1930 (see Hinsey et al., 1930; Ingram et al., 1932). The typical evoked motor pattern is known as the "tegmental reaction" ("TeR"), which consists "of a flexion of the forelimb of the side stimulated, an extension of the contralateral forelimb, a curving of the neck and trunk in an arc concave on the side stimulated and a turning of the head toward the side stimulated" (Ingram et al., 1932). Ipsiversive head turning can, in some cases, be the only manifestation of the TeR. Mapping experiments indicated its origin in the central and lateral thirds of the mesencephalic reticular formation (MesRF). Ingram et al. (1932) regarded the TeR as a phylogenetically old pattern, absent in the motor repertoire of adult animals. Later studies in freely moving cats (Monnier, 1943, Hassler, 1956 a & b; Kuroki, 1958) and rats (Robinson, 1978) tended to indicate that stimulus-induced ipsiversive head turning, stepping, and circus movements do resemble naturally occurring coordinated performance. Hassler (1956a) judged that the TeR replicates anticompensatory adjustments of head and body during passive angular acceleration. He also suggested that the ipsiversive "substrate" of the central and lateral MesRF is the site of convergence of telencephalic and tectal contraversive systems that cross the midline within the midbrain.

When stimulation is applied to the medial third of the MesRF and, in particular, to the NIC, torsional and vertical components are added to ipsiversive head deviations (Westheimer and Blair, 1975; Hassler and Hess, 1954; Hassler, 1956 a & b). The possible role of the NIC and adjacent medial MesRF has been recently discussed by Fukushima (1986) whose review should be consulted for further details. Only two general conclusions should be mentioned here. (1) Torsional head deviations induced by NIC stimulation do not reflect the excitatory action of the interstitiospinal tract on neck motoneurons (Fukushima et al., 1979a) but rather the tonic inhibitory action of the NIC on pontobulbar structures exerting facilitatory control of neck muscle tonus (Fukushima et al., 1985). The underlying pathways are not yet elucidated. (2) Vertical components of head movement might be mediated by NIC-spinal and MesRF-spinal systems. This supposition is based on the assumption that medial midbrain structures containing neurons related to the control of vertical eye movements (Büttner et al., 1977; King et al., 1981) are also engaged in the control of head movement. Whether this reasoning by analogy is correct remains to be determined by recordings from midbrain neurons during attempted or actually executed head movements.

Relationship of Tectal Efferents to Sites of Origin of Mesencephalic Descending Projections

The NIC projects ipsilaterally in the interstitiospinal tract, which reaches lumbosacral segments of the spinal cord (Nyberg-Hansen, 1966; Carpenter et al.,

1970; Mabuchi and Kusama, 1970). About one-third of NIC spinal fibers terminate in the upper cervical segments (C1–4) (Fukushima et al., 1981). The NIC receives a modest tectal projection (Altman and Carpenter, 1961; Niimi et al., 1970; Edwards and Henkel, 1978; Harting et al., 1980) which includes collaterals of TRSN (see above, Fig. 18.2). Electrophysiological studies (Fukushima et al., 1981; Grantyn et al., 1982) showed that a small fraction of NIC neurons (about 5%) receive monosynaptic excitatory input from the SC. Disynaptic and polysynaptic responses, mediated through the MesRF, are observed more frequently and the strength of this relayed effect is much higher. Hence, the NIC is obviously one of the targets of the tectoreticulospinal system. Descending pathways originating in the NIC can be regarded as a parallel channel dealing with the control of torsional and vertical head movements.

The MesRF is another source of direct projections to the spinal cord terminating in or passing through the upper cervical segments (Carpenter et al., 1970; Mabuchi and Kusama, 1970; Kuypers and Maisky, 1975; Castiglioni et al., 1978; Tohyama et al., 1979b; Fukushima et al., 1980a; Holstege and Kuypers, 1982; Huerta and Harting, 1982; Zuk et al., 1982; Jones and Yang, 1985). Stimulation experiments suggested functional gradients within the MesRF with respect to the control of head movements. It seems justified to distinguish between the medial MesRF containing torsional and vertical "substrates" and the central and lateral MesRF related predominantly to movements in the horizontal plane.

Connectivity patterns of *medial MesRF* spinal neurons bordering the NIC laterally, dorsolaterally, and rostrally are essentially the same as for the NIC proper (Carpenter et al., 1970; Mabuchi and Kusama, 1970). Fukushima et al. (1980b) concluded that they should be regarded as "belonging" to the NIC, the only distinction between the two populations being the lower responsiveness of MesRF neurons to vestibular stimulation (Fukushima et al., 1980 a,b). This may suggest a predominance of other inputs. Indeed, intracellular HRP data show that terminations of TRSNs in the MesRF adjacent to the NIC are much denser than in the NIC itself. Cortical input to medial MesRF spinal neurons has also been demonstrated (King et al., 1980; Fukushima et al., 1981). As a working hypothesis, it seems reasonable to regard the medial MesRF spinal system as functionally identical with the NIC and serving as a potential link between tectal output (TRSN) and premotor structures controlling vertical and/or torsional head movements.

As discussed above, *the central and lateral MesRF* was considered basically as a "substrate" of ipsiversive head movements. Since these regions receive projections mainly through ipsilateral collaterals of TRSNs and, in turn, project almost exclusively to the ipsilateral spinal cord, it appears that their action would be opposite to that of the crossed TbsT. Huerta and Harting (1982) proposed that the ipsilateral MesRF spinal system may be inhibitory. However, there is some evidence that the MesRF contains a mixture of ipsiversive and contraversive "substrates." Bender et al. (1964), Skultety (1962), and Westheimer and Blair (1975) observed contraversive head turns from some stimulation points. In rats, the ratio between contraversive and ipsiversive responses is 2:3 (Robinson, 1978). Cohen et al. (1981, 1982) reported that stimulation of the central MesRF, which receives ipsilateral SC input, results in contraversive saccades. Crossed MesRF spinal projections are quite weak (Castiglioni et al., 1978; Tohyama et al., 1979a; Huerta and Harting, 1982; Jones and Yang, 1985). On the other hand, anterograde tracing reveals a strong contingent of fibers crossing in the ventral tegmental decussation and terminating in the pontobulbar tegmentum where they may possibly contact the cells of origin of reticulospinal tracts (Edwards, 1975). It may be supposed that TRSNs selectively contact those central MesRF neurons that establish direct or indirect crossed connections with the spinal cord and thus act synergically with the TbsT. However, in the absence of direct experimental evidence, several alternative hypotheses are possible.

CONTROL OF HEAD MOVEMENTS BY THE PONTOBULBAR RETICULAR FORMATION

As previously discussed, signals carried by tectoreticulospinal neurons lack certain features required to produce the actually observed patterns of neck muscle activity during orienting reactions. Moreover, head movements are often performed in the absence of TRSN discharges. Other structures must thus provide additional components to the neck premotor signal and, in certain conditions, be able to create this signal independently of the SC. This section reviews evidence that the medial pontobulbar RF plays a key role in both tectal and nontectal control of head movements. The reticular nuclei that will be considered below include nucleus reticularis pontis oralis (R.p.o.) and caudalis (R.p.c.), nucleus reticularis gigantocellularis (R.Gc.), nucleus reticularis paramedianus (R.pm.), and nucleus reticularis ventralis (R.v.).

Evidence from Stimulation and Lesion Experiments

Based on his review of stimulation and lesion experiments, Monnier (1943) considered the pontobulbar RF as a final motor pathway for execution of ipsiversive and, due to decussations in the midbrain, also contraversive motor reactions initiated at different levels of the "extrapyramidal" system: premotor cortex, basal ganglia, and tectum. More recent evidence can be summarized as follows.

1. The RF exerts generalized tonic facilitatory and inhibitory influences on the spinal segmental apparatus (Magoun and Rhines, 1946; Niemer and Magoun, 1947). The presence of facilitatory tonic control of neck muscles is revealed by a contralateral head deviation that appears after unilateral lesions of the medial pontine (Bender et al., 1964; Sirkin et al., 1980) and rostral bulbar RF (Monnier, 1943). The facilitatory reticular region extends from the midbrain to the rostral medulla, and the inhibitory region is limited to the caudal medulla and invades, more rostrally, the ventral part of R.Gc. (Magoun and Rhines, 1946; Ito et al., 1970).

2. Unilateral stimulation of the pontobulbar RF elicits ipsilateral deviations of the head, predominantly in the horizontal plane. In the older literature (Ingram et al., 1932; Monnier, 1943; Sprague and Chambers, 1954), turning of the head was considered a component of ipsiversive motor synergies involving also the body and the limbs ("tegmental reaction"). Any par-

ticular regions related in a more specific way to head movement *per se* were not revealed.

The Sites of Origin of Reticulospinal Tracts

Morphological Evidence
The anatomy and physiology of the reticulospinal systems are treated in a number of recent reviews (Wilson and Peterson, 1981; Fukushima et al., 1979b; Huerta and Harting, 1982; Peterson, 1984) and will not be covered in detail here. Chapter 11 discusses four medial pontobulbar reticular nuclei (R.p.o., R.p.c., R.Gc., and R.v.) that are especially important in neck motor control and describes their ipsilateral (RSTi), medial (RSTm), and contralateral (RSTc) descending projections. The focus in Chapter 11 is upon the role of these nuclei and pathways in vestibulocollic reflexes. The same regions receive projections from the SC and other structures involved in orienting reactions. They therefore form the focus of the following discussion of the role of the RF in the control of head movements initiated in the supratentorial structures.

According to Tohyama et al. (1979a) (Fig. 18.4B), the rostral R.p.o. contains few, if any, "neck-related" reticulospinal neurons (RSN). Moderate numbers are present in the caudal R.p.o. and rostral R.p.c., anterior to the Abd-N. Just posterior to the Abd-N, the density abruptly increases, is maintained on a high level through the rostral half of the R.Gc., and decreases again toward its caudal pole. In the caudal medulla (R.pm./R.v.), the numbers of cells are moderate. This rostrocaudal profile of distribution has been confirmed by Huerta and Harting (1982), except that they report a new increment of density toward the bulbospinal junction (Fig. 18.4C).

This discrepancy is not important in the present context, since tectal projection to the caudal-most medulla is quite weak. There is only one region of overlap between the increased density of tectal terminations and a higher concentration of "neck-related" RSNs, namely, in the R.Gc. (Fig. 18.4, compare A with B and C).

In the R.Gc., "neck-related" RSNs are about equally distributed between the dorsal (gigantocellular) and ventral (magnocellular) subdivisions corresponding, respectively, to the gigantocellular and magnocellular tegmental fields (FTG and FTM) of Berman (1968). Collicular projection through the FprD is limited almost exclusively to the FTG (Kawamura et al., 1974; Huerta and Harting, 1982) and, hence, to the site of origin of RSTm (Tohyama et al., 1979a). The caudal pontine zone of increased density of tectoreticular terminations also contains predominantly RSTm neurons (Torvik and Brodal, 1957; Tohyama et al., 1979a).

In the pontine RF rostral to the abducens nucleus, numbers of RSNs projecting to contralateral upper cervical segments are extremely low (Fig. 18.4B and C). With respect to the bulbar RF, the profiles of rostrocaudal distribution derived from the data of Tohyama et al. (1979a) and Huerta and Harting (1982) do not show much correspondence (Fig. 18.4, compare B and C), due, possibly, to injections in different segments. Peterson's data (1977) are in better agreement with the data of Tohyama et al. (1979a).

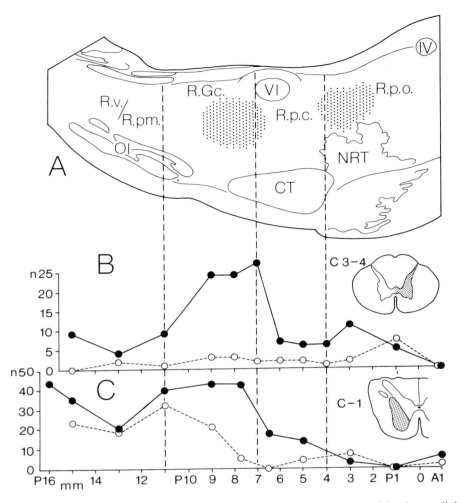

Figure 18.4. Rostrocaudal distribution of reticulospinal neurons located in the medial pontobulbar reticular formation and projecting to the gray matter of the upper cervical segments. (A) A parasagittal scheme of the lower brain stem indicating the approximate extent of the medial reticular nuclei. Dotted areas correspond to the zones of increased density of predorsal bundle terminations, according to Kawamura and co-workers (1974). (B) Numbers of RSNs (ordinate) in frontal sections at different rostrocaudal locations (abscissa) retrogradely labeled with HRP after injection in the gray matter of C3–4 (inset). Filled symbols, ipsilaterally projecting neurons; open symbols, contralaterally projecting neurons. Cell counts are based on Fig. 7 of Tohyama and co-workers (1979a). (C) The same representation for RSNs labeled after HRP injection in the gray matter of C1 (inset). Cell counts are based on Fig. 7 of Huerta and Harting (1982). Note overlap between the zones of increased density of tectal projection and of "neck-related" RSNs in the rostral R.Gc. See list of abbreviations (note 1) for anatomical notations.

236

Electrophysiological Evidence

Microstimulation of the medial RF revealed strong excitatory monosynaptic connections with ipsilateral motoneurons of dorsal neck muscles (Peterson et al., 1978). Contralaterally, the effects are about two times weaker. In agreement with the anatomy, the probability of eliciting monosynaptic EPSPs from the rostral pons (R.p.o.) is close to zero. Starting from the R.p.c., it increases in the caudal direction, due both to increasing density of "neck-related" RSNs and to costimulation of fibers originating at more rostral levels.

The origin of the inhibitory reticulomotoneuronal connections is entirely within the bulbar RF (Peterson et al., 1978). It occupies the dorsal R.Gc. (FTG) between Abd-N and the rostral pole of the hypoglossal nucleus and, more caudally, the whole dorsoventral extent of the R.pm./R.v. The inhibitory zone thus lies within the borders of the excitatory zone. The monosynaptic inhibitory projection is much stronger ipsilaterally than contralaterally. Obviously, the terminations of tectal neurons projecting in the FprD (TRSN) can potentially contact at least four different groups of "neck-related" RSNs: ipsilateral, contralateral, excitatory, and inhibitory. Such connections may be appropriate, e.g., for bilateral activation of synergistic muscles in producing vertical components of head movement and for different schemes of reciprocal innervation.

It should be stressed that the zones of overlap between TbsT terminations and sites of origin of RSTm contain far fewer "neck-related" RSNs than neurons projecting to cervical enlargement and thoracic and lumbar spinal cord (Peterson et al., 1975b). A majority of the latter group of RSNs with long descending axons appears to establish collateral connections with cervical segments (Peterson et al., 1975b). They could thus participate in polysegmental coordination of fully developed motor responses to tectal or reticular stimulation. Studies of monosynaptic connectivity (Peterson, 1977; Peterson et al., 1979) indicated that polysegmental actions of the medial RF are directed mainly to axial (neck and back) motoneurons. However, lesion experiments suggest that the medial reticulospinal system can also control the activity of proximal limb segments (Lawrence and Kuypers, 1968; Kuypers and Huisman, 1982).

Synaptic Inputs to RSNs Located Within the Innervation Domain of the TbsT (TRSN)

Tectal Input

The pioneering studies of Peterson et al. (1971, 1974) demonstrated a high efficacy of collicular input to RSNs. It was shown that 74% of RSNs can be excited by contralateral SC stimulation, 38–47% of the responses being monosynaptic. Responses to ipsilateral stimulation were also excitatory, but they were tentatively ascribed to activation of the MesRF bordering the deep SC layers. Later it was shown that 50% of reticular neurons located in vicinity of the Abd-N display an asymmetric pattern of response which could be appropriate for transmission of reciprocally organized synaptic input to ocular motoneurons (Grantyn and Grantyn, 1976; Grantyn et al., 1977). These neurons received monosynaptic EPSPs from the contralateral and disynaptic or polysynaptic IPSPs or no input from the ipsilateral SC. Intracellular labeling with HRP (Grantyn et al., 1980) revealed that a majority of these neurons are RSNs establishing a collateral connection with the Abd-N (see below). A recent study on a large sample of RSNs (Peterson and Fukushima, 1982) indicated that neurons with asymmetrically organized SC input can be encountered throughout the R.p.c. and the dorsal G.gc., with the highest concentration around the Abd-N. A majority of them (about 80%) project in the RSTm and their discharges induced by collicular stimualtion are well correlated with the EMG response of ipsilateral neck muscles.

Nontectal Inputs
It seems obvious that RSNs, especially those projecting in the RSTm, are a substrate for transmission of tectal influences upon neck motoneurons. At the same time, the term "relay neuron" cannot be strictly applied to these neurons, since they receive convergent inputs from a number of nontectal structures. Among them are the cerebral cortex (Magni and Willis, 1964; Peterson and Felpel, 1971; Peterson et al., 1974; Pilyavsky, 1974; Alstermark et al., 1983a), the deep cerebellar and vestibular nuclei (Eccles et al., 1975; Peterson and Abzug, 1975), the mesencephalic reticular formation (Mancia et al., 1971; Alstermark et al., 1983b), and the spinal cord (Ito et al., 1970; Udo and Mano, 1970). A particularly high degree of convergence should be expected for excitatory cortical and tectal inputs, since the former activate over 90% and the latter activate over 74% of RSNs (Peterson et al., 1971). The weighting of different inputs on functionally identified RSNs has not been studied. Nevertheless, it can be predicted that tectal signals impinging on RSNs will be qualitatively modified due to interaction with signals from other structures.

Head Movement Related Activity of Medial Reticular Neurons

This section reviews the emerging evidence that reticulospinal neurons transmit activity related to orienting movements of the eyes, head, and body. Initial evidence came from recordings of the activity of unidentified reticular neurons in alert animals. More recently it has been possible to show that signals related to head movement are present on reticulospinal neurons identified by electrophysiological tests and by intracellular straining techniques.

Unidentified Neurons
The firing rate of RF neurons situated in vicinity of the Abd-N has been correlated with the EMG activity of neck muscles during attempted head movements in alert cats with fixed heads (Berthoz et al., 1982; Vidal et al., 1983). Four of 13 neurons were tonically active. During periods of eccentric fixation, their firing rate showed a closer correlation with the ipsilateral neck EMG than with eye position. The remaining cells displayed, in addition to tonic activity, burstlike discharge components synchronous with ipsilateral saccades and associated phasic neck muscle contractions. Correlation of the firing rate was equally good with eye and neck components of the motor synergy. It was tentatively suggested that these neurons correspond to RSNs receiving asymmetric SC input and projecting both to the Abd-N and the spinal cord.

   Working in freely moving cats, Siegel and Tomaszewski (1983) reported that units related to ipsilateral head movements represent an important fraction (19%) of the neurons in the medial pontobulbar RF. Most of them are encountered close to the Abd-N but, in general, they are distributed throughout the medial RF, from rostral pons to caudal medulla. Typically, these neurons discharge before and during head movement and only a few maintain tonic discharge during static head deviations.

Identified Reticulospinal Neurons
Recently, Grantyn and Berthoz studied antidromically identified RSN axons in alert cats with fixed heads (Grantyn et al., 1985; Berthoz and Grantyn, 1986; Grantyn and Berthoz, 1987). Only those RSNs located in the caudal pontine RF and receiving monosynaptic excitatory input from the contralateral SC are considered here. As shown in Figure 18.5, these neurons generate bursts of activity in association with ipsilateral saccades and neck muscle contractions. The instantaneous frequency profiles may show close correspondence to the time course of phasic EMG components (e.g., Fig. 18.5, b1, b4, and b5). However, sustained EMG activity has no correlate in neuronal firing. RSN bursts appear to be linked to saccadic eye movements only when the latter are accompanied by an attempted head movement (eye–head synergy). Thus, RSNs are not activated with ipsiversive saccades terminating in the contralateral (with respct to RSN) hemifield. Under this condition there is no neck muscle activity on the side of the RSN. Thus these RSNs can be described as a type of neuron that generates phasic and decaying tonic discharges that are related primarily to the phasic component of

Figure 18.5.   Activity of an identified pontine RSN located on the right side and receiving monosynaptic excitatory input from the left SC. From top to bottom: vertical (V) and horizontal (H) eye position (shaded area indicates when the eyes are deviated ipsilaterally, with respect to RSN), firing rate of the neuron, and rectified and integrated EMG of the right m. longissimus capitis. Note close correspondence between the frequency profiles of neuronal activity and phasic, but not tonic, components of the EMG. Note also that RSN discharge is dissociated from eye movement during the later part of event b3. (From Grantyn and Berthoz, 1987.)

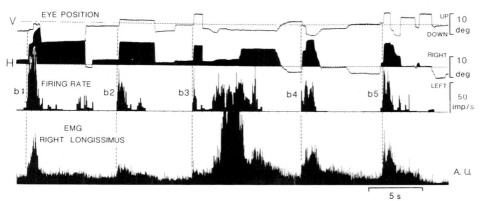

the ipsilateral neck EMG. A strong tonic bias appears only with large eccentric eye deviations to the ipsilateral side (Grantyn and Berthoz, 1987). There is also a conditional coupling to ipsiversive saccades, in the case of orienting eye–neck synergies. Descriptively, these cells can be called "eye–neck RSNs" (EN-RSN).

EN-RSN receive monosynaptic excitatory input from the contralateral SC which must be mediated by the TRSNs described earlier in this chapter. However, in identical behavioral situations, the activity of presynaptic (TRSN) and postsynaptic (EN-RSN) elements of the tectoreticulospinal "pathway" shows obvious differences. For example, TRSNs do not discharge during spontaneous gaze shifts when the animal is scanning homogeneous or familiar environment (Grantyn and Berthoz, 1983, 1985; Munoz and Guitton, 1985). Since EN-RSNs do discharge under this condition, they must derive excitatory input from other structures, possibly nontectal. A separate input must also be postulated to explain the prolonged decay of firing rate after the initial burst, since a vast majority of TRSNs generate discharges of much shorter duration. It also appears that inhibitory inputs may act upon EN-RSNs to prevent their coactivation with TRSNs. This occurs, e.g., when TRSNs are activated by visual stimuli not used as targets for orienting, a condition under which EN-RSNs remain silent. These examples suffice to illustrate the transformations of tectal signals at the interface with EN-RSNs. As shown below, the "original" and "transformed" signals may converge and interact not only in spinal segments but also in the lower brain stem.

Morphology of Pontine RSNs Related to Eye–Neck Synergies (EN-RSN)

Axonal branching of two neurons whose activity in the alert animal proved that they belonged to the group of EN-RSNs has been reconstructed after intraaxonal HRP injections (Grantyn et al., 1985; Berthoz and Grantyn 1986; Grantyn et al., 1987). As shown in Figure 18.6, they are typical members of the class of extensively branched RSNs (Scheibel and Scheibel, 1958; Grantyn et al., 1980). The location of the cell bodies corresponds, as discussed above, to the rostral zone of enhanced tectoreticular terminations and to the origin of RSTm.

EN-RSNs establish collateral connections with the medial bulbar RF (Fig. 18.6, light shading), in particular, with the dorsal R.Gc. (FTG). It is in this region that one observes a strong overlap between the direct tectoreticular and second-order, tectopontobulbar connections. Another site of overlap of TRSN and EN-RSN terminal fields is the nucleus prepositus hypoglossi (PH). Both groups of neurons generate signals related to gaze velocity (Berthoz et al., 1986; Grantyn and Berthoz, 1987), which could participate in the process of neural integration and synthesis of gaze-related tonic signals in the PH and related structures (Lopez-Barneo et al., 1982; McCrea and Baker, 1985). EN-RSNs also supply with terminals the Abd-N and the facial nuclei which are, at the same time, the targets of TRSNs. The cooperative action of the TRSNs and pontine RSNs in coordination of motor synergies involving eye, head, and pinna movements is quite likely, at least on morphological criteria.

EN-RSNs establish ipsilateral connections that are not shared by TRSNs,

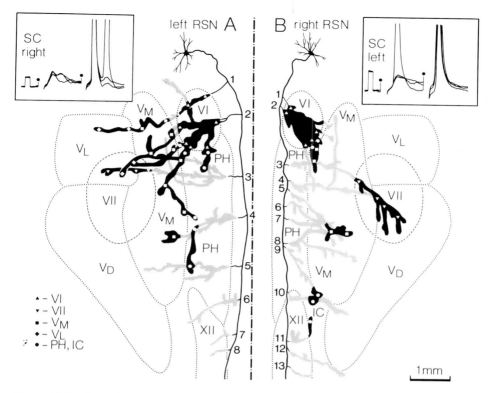

Figure 18.6. Location and axonal morphology of two neurons identified as "eye–neck" RSNs according to their activity during orienting reactions of an alert cat. Insets show monosynaptic responses to stimulation of the contralateral SC (calibration pulses are 0.5 msec, 1 mV). Collaterals are reconstructed after intraaxonal HRP injection and represented in the projection on the horizontal plane. Midline is marked by a dash-dotted line; rostral is up. Domains of terminations and/or preterminal branching are indicated by shading. Light shading: domains limited to the reticular formation. Heavy shading: domains engaging the "nonreticular" nuclei. White symbols mark parts of collaterals branching in different nuclei, as indicated by the key on the lower left. See list of abbreviations (note 1) for anatomical notations.

namely, with the lateral and medial vestibular nuclei (V_L, V_M). Connection with the V_L can be interpreted as an additional channel acting, potentially, in parallel with the tectoreticulospinal system. In any case, excitatory action of the V_L on motoneurons of ipsilateral neck extensor muscles (Wilson and Yoshida, 1969b) would be synergistic with EN-RSNs. Functional interpretation of the connection with V_M whose action on ipsilateral neck motoneurons is inhibitory (Wilson and Yoshida, 1969a), i.e., antagonistic to EN-RSNs, is less straightforward. By analogy with the oculomotor system, one could suppose that EN-RSNs activate local inhibitory neurons and thus contribute to the suppression of the compensatory vestibuloocular reflex during active head movements.

CONCLUSIONS

In summary, there is no doubt that the mammalian SC and its descending pathways participate in the control of head movements. The positive evidence is derived mainly from stimulation and lesion experiments and from hodological studies that indicated "appropriate" connections of the SC with the spinal cord and the sites of origin of reticulospinal tracts. It must be noted, on the other hand, that the knowledge of *how* the SC controls head movements is rather rudimentary. Even in the cat, the best studied species, the data on neuronal activity in relation to head movements are scanty and in many points contradictory. The latter may be explained, at least in part, by the fact that contribution of the SC to execution of qualitatively similar movements may vary depending on behavioral situation.

Signals generated by SC neurons with identified projection in the predorsal bundle and to the spinal cord (TRSN) have begun to be studied only recently. One important observation is the conditional linkage of phasic TRSN discharges to contraversive head movements. It is obvious that the latter can be performed without activation of TRSNs and, on the other hand, burst activity of TRSNs is often not "translated" in movement. Clear temporal correlations of TRSN bursts with contractions of contralateral neck muscles are observed only with high-velocity gaze shifts, when the head is free to move, and with gaze shifts attaining large eccentricity, under the "head fixed" condition. Even then, bursts of TRSNs are too short to account either for the whole duration of phasic components or for tonic components of muscle activity. It seems safe to conclude that in no case can the spike trains generated by TRSNs and conducted to the upper cervical segments depolarize neck motoneurons above the threshold for rhythmic firing. However, in cooperation with other structures, excitatory output from the SC may contribute to faster recruiting and frequency build up of motoneurons and, hence, increase the velocity of head movements. Axonal branching of TRSNs in the lower brain stem suggests that further transformation and, probably, enhancement of tectal signals take place at the interface with reticulospinal neurons (RSN) that, in turn, form cascadelike interconnections defined by Lorente de No (1938) as "multiple chains."

RSNs receiving monosynaptic input from the SC and discharging in relationship to neck muscle activity have only recently been studied. The transformation of the tectal signal by these "relay" neurons is evident. The most typical transformation observed in the discharge pattern of the group of RSNs presently analyzed is the appearance of a decaying tonic component that is absent in the vast majority of "presynaptic" TRSNs. The correlation between the profile of neuronal firing rate and the time course of the initial part of neck muscle activity is thus considerably improved. This is only one example demonstrating that the neck muscle-related discharge of RSNs that receive monosynaptic collicular projection is also controlled by, and may sometimes be completely dominated, by nontectal inputs. The axonal branching of neck-related RSNs in the pons and medulla is extensive and overlaps considerably the zones of termination of TRSN collaterals. In fact, axonal ramifications of these two types of neurons are a constituent component of the general network of the reticular core (Scheibel and

Scheibel, 1958). According to the presently available morphophysiological evidence, it is in this network that final, functionally adequate premotor signals for neck motoneurons are elaborated through interactions between neurons bearing partial signals. The role of the SC in the control of head movement would be to feed its partial signal into the reticular network where it can be treated facultatively, i.e., either utilized in the formation of motor pattern in parallel with other inputs or rejected.

SUMMARY

This chapter examines the role of the superior colliculus and related brain stem structures in generating rapid, orienting head movements. In each section data obtained from experiments involving electrical stimulation, anatomical tracing of connections, and recording of neuronal activity are reviewed.

The first describes the projections of neurons in the superior colliculus to the brain stem and spinal cord via the tectobulbospinal tract. The termination sites of these highly branched neurons include the mesencephalic, pontine, and medullary reticular formation, the parafascicular complex of the thalamus, the interstitial nucleus of Cajal, the nucleus of the posterior commissure, the prepositus hypoglossi nucleus, the spinal ventral horn, and neck, facial, and extraocular motor nuclei. Recordings from tectoreticulospinal neurons reveal short bursts of activity related to visual stimuli and to visually elicited orienting behavior. The greatest activity is observed when a novel, arousing visual target moves in the neuron's on direction and the animal makes a combined eye–head movement to follow the target. The activity of these neurons is not closely locked to neck muscle activation since neuronal discharge coincides only with the initial phase of EMG activation during orienting and visually elicited discharge may occur in the absence of orienting movements.

The second section discusses the role of two midbrain structures, the interstitial nucleus of Cajal (NIC) and the mesencephalic reticular formation (MRF) in head movement control. The NIC receives tectal and cerebral cortical inputs, projects to spinal and extraocular motor nuclei as well as other brain stem structures, and appears to be related to vertical head movements. The medial MRF resembles the NIC, whereas the lateral MRF plays a role in generating ipsiversive horizontal head movements.

The third section describes the role of reticulospinal neurons (RSNs) located in the medial pontomedullary reticular formation in generating head movement. These neurons establish excitatory or inhibitory connections with neck motoneurons and receive inputs from many sources including the superior colliculus, cerebral cortex, vestibular nuclei, and spinal cord. The superior colliculus projects particularly strongly to medial RSNs, which have divergent projections not only to the neck but also to extraocular, facial, and limb motor nuclei and to other premotor brain stem nuclei. The discharge of these RSNs is more closely related to the activity of neck muscles, which indicates that they represent a later stage in the neck motor control network than tectoreticulospinal neurons.

Notes

1. *Abbreviations*: Abd-N, abducens nucleus; CT, trapezoid body; EMG, electromyogram; EPSP, excitatory postsynaptic potential; F, fields of Forel; FprD, predorsal bundle; FTG, gigantocellular tegmental field; FTM, magnocellular tegmental field; HRP, horseradish peroxidase; IC, nucleus intercalatus Staderini; MD, mediodorsal thalamic nucleus; MesRF, mesencephalic reticular formation; NC, cuneate nucleus; NIC, interstitial nucleus of Cajal; NPC, nucleus of posterior commissure; NRT, nucleus reticularis tegmenti pontis; OI, inferior olive; PH, nucleus prepositus hypoglossi; R, red nucleus; RF, reticular formation; R.Gc., nucleus reticularis gigantocellularis; R.p.c., nucleus reticularis pontis caudalis; R.pm., nucleus reticularis paramedianus; R.p.o., nucleus reticularis pontis oralis; RSN, reticulospinal neuron; RSTc, RSTi, RSTm, contralateral, ipsilateral, and medial reticulospinal tracts, respectively; R.v., nucleus reticularis ventralis; SC, superior colliculus; SGC, central gray substance; TbsT, tectobulbospinal tract; TeR, "tegmental reaction"; TRSN, tectoreticulospinal neuron; VM, ventromedial thalamic nucleus; V_D, V_L, V_M, descending, lateral, and medial vestibular nuclei, respectively; ZI, zona incerta; III, IV, VI, VII, XII, oculomotor, trochlear, abducens, facial, and hypoglossal nuclei, respectively.

19

Head Movement Models, Optimal Control Theory, and Clinical Application

L. STARK, W. H. ZANGEMEISTER, and B. HANNAFORD

This chapter concludes the discussion of modeling of the head–neck system that was introduced in Chapter 2 and continued in Chapter 12. Chapter 12 dealt with models of head stabilization in which the emphasis is upon relatively automatic responses to external perturbations. The emphasis in this chapter is upon modeling of voluntary head movements in normal subjects and in patients with neurological disorders. The goal of the work described here is to construct models whose elements will represent the actions of different components of the neural and biomechanical system that generates head movements in order to increase understanding of how those components interact in controlling head movement in normal and pathological situations.

A key to realizing the goal described above is to construct models that are homeomorphic (Bellman, 1965). Homeomorphic models are those whose elements correspond to the anatomical, physiological, biomechanical, and neural elements of the experimental system. They typically have more parameters than the less realistic phenomenological or input/output model. This added complexity is offset, however, by the modeler's ability to define or constrain some of the parameters to values that have been measured for components of living systems such as muscle strengths, tendon compliances, etc. As the remainder of the chapter will show, the homeomorphic approach has allowed those modeling voluntary head movements to examine questions about the roles of specific components of the head–neck system in the generation of normal movements or in pathological conditions such as torticollis.

A problem that faces both experimental and theoretical studies of voluntary head movements is that these movements can vary tremendously depending upon the intention of the subject. The approach that is taken here to limit this variability is to study movements that are made "as fast as possible." The movements that are made under this constraint can then be investigated using the powerful techniques of time optimal control theory developed by Bellman (1965) and Pontryagin et al. (1962). As described below, these techniques have been utilized to develop and experimentally investigate sixth-order nonlinear homeomorphic models of the eye and head movement systems. They have been particularly useful in understanding the role of the triphasic motor commands observed in neck muscle EMG during head movements. They have also shed light on why these patterns change in disorders such as torticollis.

FAST HEAD MOVEMENT CONTROL

This section begins by introducing homeomorphic dynamic models, recalling points raised initially in Chapter 2. These models are then used to simulate eye and head movements, which have a number of features in common. Finally, modeling techniques are used to investigate the roles of different components of muscle EMG activity and the neural mechanisms that generate them.

Modeling Dynamic Physiological Systems

Complex dynamic systems, such as those responsible for head and eye movements, are modeled by a multistep analytical process in which a formal structure is given to our knowledge of the dynamics and statics of each relevant tissue, organ, or structure. The first step involves the identification of anatomical structures relevant to the movement. In the case of head movement, these are the neck muscles, tendons, supporting ligaments, intervertebral discs, and the skull and its contents, etc. To simplify modeling, structures that are redundant in the context of the behavior being modeled can be combined into equivalent structures in the model. For example, in horizontal rotation, the left splenius and right sternocleidomastoid act synergistically and are modeled as a single entity.

Once the appropriate structures are identified, constitutive relations must be defined for each structure. The constitutive relation is the fundamental physical principle operating in the element. If more than one physical principle is at work, the physiological structure must be split into separate elements for modeling. For example, a tendon may be modeled as an elastic element. In the linear case, (see Chapter 2 for elaboration) the constitutive relation is

$$F(x) = kx$$

where x is length, $F(x)$ is the force as a function of length, and k is a parameter specifying the stiffness of the tendon. If the mass of the tendon is significant, another element must be included in the model having the constitutive relation

$$F(x) = ma$$

where a is acceleration, the second derivative of the tendon's position, and m is a parameter specifying the mass of the tendon. In the case of head movement, the mass of the skull is so much greater than that of the tendons that the latter can be safely neglected.

Once all of the model components have been characterized, their interaction as a complete system is studied through the identification of a set of state variables—a minimal set of positions, velocities, forces, etc. that completely characterize the dynamic state of the system. To compute the dynamics of the state variables, the constitutive relations of the individual components must be combined into a set of state equations. This complex process has been formalized for a wide class of dynamic systems in the bond graph method (Paynter, 1961; Rosenberg and Karnoop, 1983). The state equations can be expressed in the matrix form

$$\mathbf{x} = A\dot{\mathbf{x}} + B\mathbf{u}$$

where $\mathbf{x}$ is a vector containing the state variables, $\dot{\mathbf{x}}$ is their time derivative, $\mathbf{u}$ is a vector of the model inputs (external forces or neurological control signals), and A and B are matrices of coefficents simply obtained from the state equations. This equation then says that the rate of change of the state variables depends upon the current state of the system and upon the external forces and neural inputs acting upon the system.

At this point, the model can easily be expressed as a computer program that can calculate the state of the system ($\mathbf{x}$) as a function of time.

Modeling Eye and Head Movement

Both the eye and head can be modeled approximately as rigid spheres rotating about their centers of mass. In either case the model (Zangemeister et al., 1981a,b; Hannaford, 1985; Hannaford et al., 1986b) (Fig. 19.1, upper left) consists of a linear mechanical system with defined inertia, viscosity, and stiffness (J_p, B_p, K_p, upper center) representing the eyeball or skull, which is connected to two identical muscle models that represent the agonist and antagonist muscle for the movement (lower left and lower right). Different forces, lever arms, parameter values, and velocities apply when modeling neck versus extraocular muscles. In horizontal eye rotation, the two in-plane extraocular muscles act as agonist and antagonist. In head rotation, the agonist and antagonist muscle components of the model each represent the combined action of several muscles.

The muscle models consist of elements representing the biophysical properties of muscle. The contractile element (box: left and right) represents the excitation, activation, and force generation process by a simple system having first-order dynamics. Tissues such as the muscle sheath, which constitute the passive length–tension properties of muscle, are represented by the parallel elastic element, K_p (left and right). The incremental length–tension properties of the molecular cross bridges and the muscle tendons are lumped into the series elastic element, K_s (left and right). The active length–tension relationship is assumed to be constant over the range of muscle lengths present in the movements under study. Finally, each muscle has a viscous element that represents the force–velocity behavior of muscle (Hill, 1938). This viscosity is a function of velocity; an important nonlinearity required to accurately simulate the hyperbolic form of the length–tension relationship. The equations used are derived from Hill's in Lehman and Stark (1979).

The inputs to the model are nervous excitation signals representing a product of firing rate and recruitment. Note that because of the dynamics of the contractile element, the input signal represents only a commanded level of force production. The actual muscle force is a function of the excitation signal *and* the muscle state.

The considerable difference between the dynamics of head and eye rotation

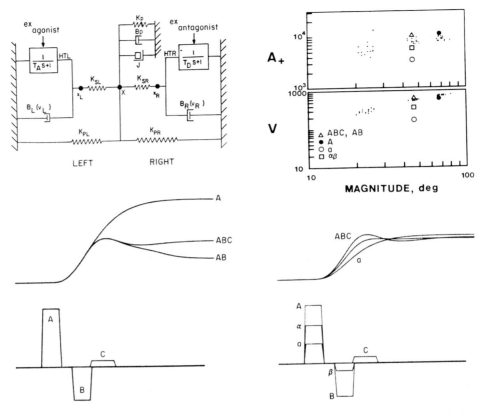

Figure 19.1   Simulation of fast head movements with a three-pulse (PABC) control signal. Sixth-order, nonlinear model of neck muscles and skull for single degree of freedom (horizontal rotation) (upper right). When driven by the three-pulse control signal (lower left panel, trace ABC), this model accurately simulates the recorded dynamics of one subject's 40° time-optimal head movements. Removal of control signal pulses (traces AB and A) reveals their dynamic functions (clamping final position, pulse C, and truncating movement, pulse B). When pulse heights are recomputed to preserve the correct final position (lower right panel), addition of control signal pulses results in a reduction of the time required to reach the neighborhood of the target. The partial main sequence diagram (upper right) shows that addition and modulation of control signal pulses (as in lower right panel) results in vertical displacement (open symbols). Pulse removal (as in lower left panel) causes a horizontal shift giving dynamics characteristic of larger movements. (Figure modified from Hannaford and Stark, 1985.) *Main sequence* (upper right). Key movement parameters from the simulated movements are abstracted in this figure, which plots peak positive head acceleration (A_+) and velocity (V) against movement amplitude. Points in each of the plots, representing previously described simulated movements, appear in horizontal and vertical rows. In the horizontal rows the movement magnitude varies, but the movement dynamic parameters, A_+ and V, are relatively constant as pulses are subtracted from the simulated control, but movement parameters vary as pulses are subtracted and the heights of the remaining ones are varied.

is reflected in the different parameter values used in the model (Table 19.1). The inertia of the head is approximately 10^4 times that of the eye. The elasticity of supporting structures, K_p, is of the same order of magnitude. The large differences in the parameters of the eye and head movement biomechanical systems (plants) require neurological control signals with different timing and magnitude.

The relative timing of eye and head movements and of the EMG activity that produces them is influenced not only by the biomechanical factors listed in Table 19.1 but also by neural control strategies selected by brain stem or higher level neural circuitry. Four classes of gaze shifts can be defined as shown in Table 19.2 (Zangemeister and Stark, 1982b,d). Table 19.3 gives the frequency with which these classes occur when normal subjects and patients with various neurological disorders attempt to make rapid gaze shifts (Zangemeister et al., 1982a, 1986; Zangemeister and Stark, 1982c, Zangemeister and Mueller-Jensen, 1985). Neurological disorders may be associated with abnormalities of the periphery, of primary brain stem control networks, or of higher neural networks. As observed by many investigators (Bartz, 1965; Sugi and Wakakuwa, 1970; Bizzi et al., 1972b; Dichgans et al., 1974; Zee, 1977; Guitton et al., 1982), these abnormalities introduce longer, more variable time lags into generation of eye and head movements, which in turn alter the distribution of gaze classes as shown in Table 19.3.

Fast-Head Movements: EMG's and Head Model

Homeomorphic dynamic models can be used to study both the properties of the movement itself and the muscle activation commands that produce it. When head movements are made as quickly as possible, their velocities range up to 600°–700°/sec. EMG activation patterns recorded from neck muscles have a three-burst or "triphasic" pattern consisting of an initial burst in the agonist muscle followed by a burst in the antagonist during which agonist activity is suppressed and then by a final burst in the agonist muscle. The head movement model can be used (Hannaford, 1985; Hannaford and Stark, 1985) to determine the roles of the three

Table 19.1. Parameter Values Used in Modeling Eye and Head Movements

Parameter	Units	Definition	Eye	Head	Scaling factor
J	g-sec^2/deg	Inertia	4.3×10^{-5}	1.8×10^{-1}	10^4
B	g-sec/deg	Viscosity	1.5×10^{-2}	2.0	10^2
K_p	g/deg	Parallel elasticity	1.5	2.0	1
K_{sl}	g/deg	Series elasticity	1.8	40.0	10^1
F_{max}	g	Maximum muscle force	100.0(10°)	600.0(10°) 2000.0(40°)	10^1
F_{min}	g	Minimum muscle force	2.0	2.0	1
T_a	sec	Activation time constant	4.0×10^{-3}	5.0×10^{-2}	10^1
T_d	sec	Deactivation time constant	8.0×10^{-3}	5.0×10^{-2}	(10^1)

Table 19.2. Gaze Types Defined by Latency [Eye Minus Head Latency (msec)]

Type	EMG	Position
I	0^a	$+50^b$
II	<0	$<50^c$
IIIa	$0-150$	$50-200$
IIIb	$150-500$	$200-500$
IV	>500	$>550^d$

^{a}Synchronous EMG.

^{b}Due to dynamic lag of head movement.

^{c}"Z—zip" due to anticipated CEM (compensatory eye movement) before reflex VOR.

^{d}HM complete before EMG saccade starts.

pulses (two in the agonist, one in the antagonist) in controlling the dynamics of fast movements. The control signal used as input to the model is based upon the patterns of EMG recorded during fast movements (Fig. 19.2). The role of each pulse is revealed by "ablation" experiments in which simulations are performed with particular pulses missing from the triphasic control signal. Without PC, the second agonist pulse, the final position of the head drifts back to the starting position (see trace AB in Fig. 19.1) due to the energy stored in the antagonist muscle. Because of this role in holding the final position, PC can be labeled the "clamping pulse." When PB, the antagonist burst, is removed as well, the resulting head movement goes approximately twice as far as intended, at which point it is stopped by passive forces. Thus, PB can be labeled the "braking pulse" because it controls and limits the movement amplitude. PA, the "action pulse," initiates the movement and determines its initial acceleration and, to a large extent, its peak velocity.

In further "pulse ablation" simulations, one or more pulses were removed after which the amplitudes of the remaining pulses were recomputed to keep final

Table 19.3. Frequency of Occurrence of the Four Gaze Types in Normal Subjects as Compared to Seven Groups of Patients with Different Neurological Diseases

	Gaze types			
Diagnosis	I Synchronous eye neck EMG (%)	II Late head movement (%)	III Early head movement (%)	IV Late eye saccade and early head movement
Normal	34	4	43	19
Parkinson	49	33	18	0
Cerebellar	44	2	46	8
Homonymous hemianopsia	52	25	21	2
Oculomotor apraxia	0	0	77	33
Spinocerebellar atrophy	11	0	58	23
Progressive supranuclear palsy	5	10	70	15
Labyrinthine defective	52	0	46	2

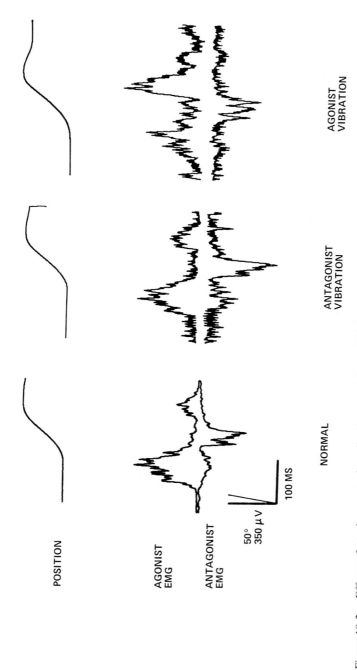

Figure 19.2. Effects of continuous tendon vibration on triphasic EMG control signal. Subjects have multiple practice movements in which to adapt control strategy to altered proprioception. Ipsilateral vibration increases the area of late bursts of EMG activity. The first agonist burst, PA, is unaffected by vibration on either side. (Modified from Hannaford et al., 1985.)

position constant (Fig. 19.1, lower right). This yielded slower movements without the overshoot characteristic of the time-optimal movements produced by a control signal with three pulses. These changes are plotted in the upper right of Figure 19.1.

Tendon Vibration and Fast Head Movement Control

Vibration applied to the muscle tendon is known to strongly stimulate muscle spindles. By applying vibration to the tendon, one can thus alter the amount of spindle afference, and observe the effects on the control of fast movements. This paradigm probes the interaction between central commands (open-loop control) and reflex loops (closed-loop control) and encourages models of this interaction.

Continuously, i.e., predictably, applied vibration (Hannaford et al., 1985) (Fig. 19.2, right side) resulted in specific effects that increased or decreased EMG pulse areas, depending on which side was vibrated. The interesting exception was PA, which was not affected by continuous vibration. With continuous vibration the subject may be adapting his central commands to compensate for reflex effects of vibration. The effects of continuous vibration on dynamics were small except for a decrease in peak velocity with agonist continuous vibration. The vibration apparently activates the stretch reflex: the B-pulse increases with vibration of the antagonist (lower) and the C-pulse with vibration of the agonist (upper). The area of the A-pulse is not changed. This tells us that Stark's (1968) hypothesis that the stretch reflex loop is opened during a fast movement was largely correct. The question is, when does the proprioceptive loop close again, and when can the stretch reflex again modify the higher level, open-loop, preprogrammed descending controller signals? The answer seems to be: when we get to the B-pulse or the C-pulse, the stretch reflex can have an influence and can moderate something between 20 and 40% of the EMG pulse. This may be confirmed by modeling studies of the stretch reflex (Ramos and Stark, 1986).

With unpredictable vibration, applied at the time of the movement target transition, there are two principal effects (Fig. 19.3). One is an increase in PA amplitude accompanied by increases in peak velocity and displacement. The second is a reduction in reaction time. Both of these effects, which are independent of the side (agonist or antagonist) that is vibrated, appear to be related to alerting or arousing the subject rather than to alteration of spindle input (Hannaford, 1985; Hannaford et al., 1986a). Superimposed on the alerting effect is a modification of EMG pulse magnitudes; the pulses of activation appearing in the vibrated muscle increased in magnitude, and those appearing in the contralateral muscle decreased.

Another modeling technique is to invert the model in order to compute neurological control signals from trajectories of head movement (Fig. 19.4). Using the head velocity and assuming that agonist and antagonist muscles are not active concurrently, the signals to agonist and antagonist muscles can be estimated with an iterative computational method that successively reduces differences between the modeled and actual trajectory. Calculation for 20°, 40°, and 60° head rotations yields the predicted EMG patterns shown in Figure 19.4, lower right. Similar to the observed data, these patterns have three pulses. Furthermore, the relation be-

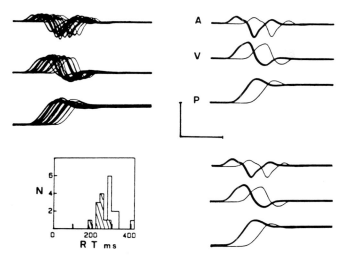

Figure 19.3.   Effects of unpredictable agonist tendon vibration on reaction time (RT) and movement dynamics. Overplot of movements (not synchronized; upper left panel) with (thick lines) and without (thin lines) vibration. Histogram (lower left) of reaction times for normal (open bars) and vibrated (hatched bars) movements shows reduction in reaction time with unpredictable vibration. The average of the two populations of movements (upper right) are synchronized at zero crossing of acceleration and plotted with a time shift of 79 msec, which is the average reduction in reaction time. Two typical responses (lower right) selected from the ensemble show that the averages are indeed representative of individual movements (Hannaford et al., 1986a).

tween height and width of these pulses and the movement trajectory is similar to the relationship observed experimentally (Fig. 19.4, lower left). This similarity indicates that the model accurately reproduces the important properties of the head movement system at both the EMG and movement trajectory levels. Since model elements correspond to actual physical entities, it should be possible to use the model to explore the causes of head movement abnormalities in various clinical disorders. The next section illustrates such an application of the model to torticollis.

CLINICAL ASPECTS: ASYMMETRIC COACTIVATION IN TORTICOLLIS

In torticollis spasmodicus (TS) there is often a significant asymmetrical activation and/or coactivation of muscles that rotate the head. The pathogenesis of TS is discussed in Chapter 20. This section will consider how head movement models can provide insight into the alterations in neck muscle activity that occur in this disorder.

Zangemeister and Stark (1982e, 1983) reported the patterns of neck muscle EMG and eye movements seen during head turns in patients with sustained tonic torticollis. Example records from a patient with 20° TS to the right are shown in Fig. 19.5A. The left sternocleidomastoid (whose EMG is shown in the trace la-

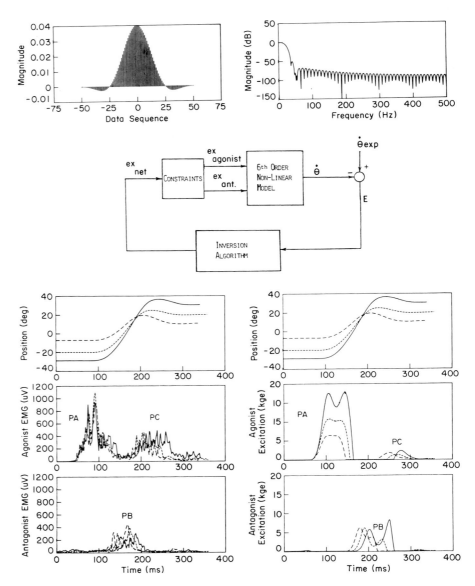

Figure 19.4. Inverse modeling process derives neurological control inputs from movement dynamics. The model (see Fig. 19.1) can be numerically inverted to compute neuromuscular control signals (lower right panel) from movement dynamics (lower left panel: EMGs plotted for comparison). The computation (block diagram, center) involves iteratively varying model input at each time sample to eliminate error (E) between experimentally measured velocity and model output. A constraint such as the reciprocal innervation constraint (suggested by the EMG evidence) is required to generate two control signals in this process. (Modified from Hannaford et al., 1986b.)

beled L ST) is one of the muscles that generates the tonic rightward head deviation. Correspondingly, it exhibits tonic activity in the rest position. It is further
activated during voluntary rotations to the left, exhibiting strong bursts of activity
during a rapid leftward rotation and sustained tonic activity when the leftward
head rotation is maintained. The right sternocleidomastoid (R ST) also exhibits
abnormal activity. It is silent in the rest position and is tonically activated throughout the period of leftward head rotation. There is no sign of the pause in agonist
activity that would normally occur in this muscle during the leftward movement.
The pattern is therefore one of sustained cocontraction of agonist and antagonist
muscles in which the phasic bursts of the normal three-pulse control pattern are
weak or absent.

The main sequence plot in Fig. 19.5B shows that the altered control pattern
in TS causes a marked increase of movement duration and decrease of peak acceleration and velocity. Rotations to the side contralateral to the TS position appear to be slower. Attempts have been made to reproduce these properties in
normal subjects by adding asymmetrical springlike compliance (K) to the head
(Zangemeister and Stark, 1982e, Hannaford et al., 1983). As demonstrated (Fig.
19.5C), the control signals (CSs) were increased and had a sustained tonic pattern
(single agonist pulse) for movements against the spring. As in TS, head movements to the side of the applied spring showed decreased bi/triphasic CSs, the
antagonist often starting earlier than the agonist. There was also a high amount
of cocontraction. We may infer from this evidence that asymmetrically changing
cocontraction and an asymmetrically added elastic load can cause two effects similar to those observed in TS. First, the CS changes to single pulse (first-order)
type with pulse width becoming more important than pulse height (see duration
increase in Fig. 19.5B). Second, muscle cocontraction becomes prominent. In-
terestingly this cocontraction does not always hinder movement performance, since
both elevated activity level of the muscles and positive initial velocity can contribute to a faster and shorter movement than usual.

The experimentally added spring resembled an increase of K_p, the parallel
elasticity. Although it is possible to simulate some of the characteristics of TS
behavior in this way (Zangemeister and Stark, 1982e), it appeared to be more
reasonable to try to simulate TS behavior by asymmetrically varying the series
elastic model parameter $(K_{s l/r})$ in the neck muscles (Fig. 19.6) since K_s has a much
greater influence on head movement characteristics than K_p (Zangemeister et al.,
1981b,c). Figure 19.6 compares experimental results from TS patients with length–
tension (L–T) characteristics of the model following appropriate changes of
$K_{s l/r}$ or the addition of asymmetric cocontraction. Three L–T curves are shown
for each muscle group (agonist vs antagonist) corresponding to the different levels
of tonic motoneuronal (MN) activation. In the curve labeled NORMAL + COC
only a minimum amount of tonic activity, corresponding to 20% cocontraction,
is present. Simulated movements for this condition (inset labeled NOR at upper
left) exhibit rapid position changes with relatively low torques. In the L–T curves
labeled TS-I and TS-C an asymmetrical cocontraction has been added that shifts
TS-I to the left and TS-C to the right. The result is a discontinuous L–T characteristic, which can be seen most clearly in the curves labeled 2 in the inset at
the lower right. Also illustrated in the inset is the large reduction in amplitude of

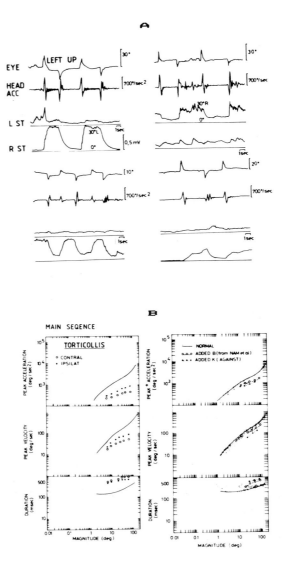

Figure 19.5. Clinical data from patients with torticollis spasmodicus. (A) High tonic EMG activity with head movements; (B) altered dynamics of fast head movements in TS patients.

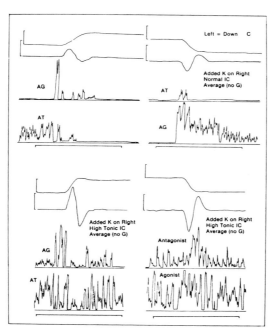

Figure 19.5. (C) Altered control signals in TS patients. Horizontal scale bar 1 sec; vertical bar 30°, 2200°/sec.

neck rotation produced by changing torque from T_0 to $-T_0$ that occurs in the cocontracted case (curves labeled 2) relative to the normal case with minimal cocontraction (curves labeled 1).

The asymmetrical shifting of curves TS-I and TS-C relative to the normal curve leads to two effects. First, small changes of head position might induce two very different reactions, that depend upon the direction of the movement. Trying to move *against* the TS′ direction results in high activation and force development of the then agonistic muscles due to the shift and therefore apparent stiffness increase of curve TS-I. Trying to move *with* the TS′ direction results in comparatively smaller force development, again due to the asymmetric L–T shift, here of curve TS-C.

The preceding analysis suggests that in pathological states such as torticollis spasmodicus, a primary cause (most likely centrally induced deviation of head position) may lead to secondary effects that are due to the asymmetric muscle activation in itself. More extensive studies may demonstrate a direction for rational treatment of TS through modifying asymmetric L–T characteristics. Given the biomechanical complexities of TS, it is likely that only proper synthesis of both clinical/experimental and modeling results will yield heuristic/diagnostic and, more important, therapeutically relevant insights into problems of tonic head deviation.

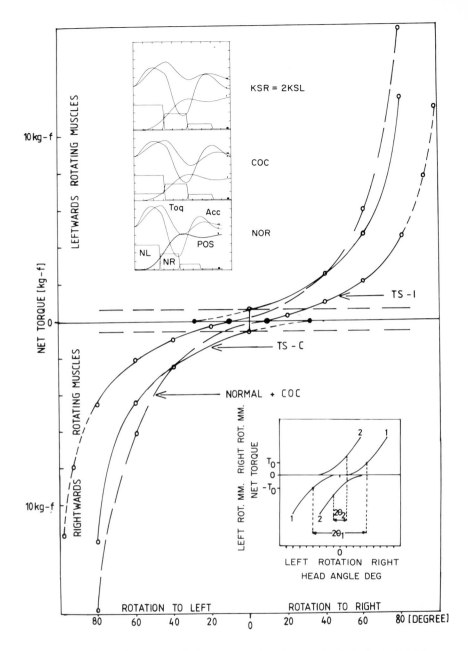

Figure 19.6.   Effect of asymmetrical cocontraction in sustained tonic torticollis spasmodicus compared to asymmetrical change of series elasticities. Net torque is plotted as
a function of head rotation amplitude and direction. Normal + COC (long dashed): Normal
subject with voluntary slight cocontraction of the neck muscles (about 20% of maximum).
TS-I: net torque for position ipsilateral to TS direction. TS-C: Net torque contralateral to
TS direction. Note: Slopes are very similar; short dashed lines are extrapolated from experimental data. Zero crossing of curve TS-C occurs around 20° to the right. Long dashed
lines parallel to the abscissa denote a continuous level of activation of both muscle groups.
Upper inset: Comparison of head model simulations for 25% cocontraction (COC), asym-

DISCUSSION

Medical therapy benefits strongly from a basic understanding of the underlying physical system. When we have this understanding, we have a model to which we can apply reason to deduce cause and effect. Two sources of this knowledge are experimental observation and quantitative modeling through computer simulation. In this chapter, both forms of evidence were used to gain insight into human pathology such as torticollis spasmodicus, in which head position is distorted tonically.

Experimental measurement focused primarily on fast voluntary, so called "time-optimal," head movements. These provide a useful experimental paradigm because the optimality constraint reduces variability of subject response. This encourages quantitative analysis of the dynamic trajectories of the movements (time functions of position, velocity, and acceleration) (Masek, 1963; Meiry, 1971; Morasso et al., 1977; Shirachi et al., 1978; Stark, 1968) and provides a repeatable baseline against which clinical data can be compared for diagnosis. For example, the relationship between movement magnitude and dynamic parameters (the main sequence diagram) (Zangemeister et al., 1981a; Zangemeister and Stark, 1982e; Hannaford et al., 1983, 1984) has been plotted for both normal and pathological cases (Figs. 19.1 and 19.5B). This comparison quantifies the dynamic effects of torticollis for movements with and against the deviation of static position.

Simulation has led to better insight into the neuromuscular sequence leading up to actual movement. By extending the homeomorphism of the sixth-order nonlinear model (Fig. 19.1, upper left) to constrain the control signal input to match recorded EMGs, simulations are possible that make explicit the effects of the control signal components (pulses) on movement dynamics (Hannaford et al., 1986). By using slightly more advanced numerical techniques, it is possible to calculate explicitly the control signal required to drive a given model to match actual movement dynamics (Hannaford et al., 1986b). This inverse modeling technique (see Fig. 19.4) allows us to estimate previously unmeasurable neurological control signals. The results of this technique of course depend on the model's structure and parameter values. The closest direct physiological measure of these signals, the EMG, provides a check on this method.

The head movement mechanisms studied, which are discussed in this chapter,

---

metrical series muscles elasticities (KSR = ANTAG; KSL = AGON), and normal model response (NOR). Note the greater forces, acceleration, and amplitude in asymmetrical Ks than in COC. Lower inset: Illustration of how a tonic cocontraction of antagonist muscle may lead to a significant increase in joint stiffness (modified from Humphrey and Reed, 1983). Length–tension curves for head horizontal rotation muscles (mostly sternomastoid and splenius). Increase in muscle activation does not change the slopes of the L–T curves, but instead shifts them toward shorter muscle lengths, or smaller head rotation amplitudes. The amplitude of an imposed torque disturbance is assumed to vary from $+T_0$ to $-T_0$. The rotations $2\theta_1$ and $2\theta_2$ are those resulting from this applied torque at low and high levels of antagonist muscle coactivation.

are involved in the control of gaze. Although this topic is beyond the scope of the present chapter, excellent work on voluntary shifts of gaze has been done (Bartz, 1965; Atkin and Bender, 1968; Zee, 1977; Barnes, 1979; Benson and Barnes, 1979; Kennard et al., 1982; Zangemeister and Stark, 1982b,c,d; Zangemeister and Mueller-Jensen, 1985; Stark et al., 1986). Quantitative models of gaze have also been put forward (Melvill-Jones, 1964; Jones and Milsum, 1965; Stark, 1968; Fleming et al., 1969; Gresty, 1974; Funk and Anderson, 1977; Gresty and Leech, 1977; Morasso et al., 1977; Fuller, 1980).

Reflexive maintenance of gaze, the vestibulooccular reflex (VOR), can also be observed quantitatively (Bartz, 1965; Atkin and Bender, 1968; Morasso et al., 1973; Barnes, 1979; Benson and Barnes, 1979; Fuller 1980a; Kennard et al., 1982; Zangemeister and Stark, 1982a,b,c,d,e) and analyzed or simulated numerically (Melvill-Jones, 1964; Jones and Milsum, 1965; Young, 1969; Young and Oman, 1969; Ormsby and Young, 1977; Raphan et al., 1977; Shirachi et al., 1978; Bock et al., 1979; Winters et al., 1984).

Similarly, the interaction of head movements with posture and locomotion has been studied (Nashner, 1977; Roberts, 1978; Stark et al., 1986). In both gaze-driven and postural head movements, adaptive processes are at work calibrating the interaction between head movements and other systems (Gilman and Bloedel, 1982; Mueller-Jensen et al., 1984). For this reason, head movements are an important paradigm for studying adaptation to changes such as added inertial, viscous, and elastic loads (Gauthier et al., 1981; Hannaford et al., 1983, 1984).

SUMMARY

This chapter describes a homeomorphic model of the neck in which each mathematical element corresponds to a physical structure. The model is used to investigate the properties of maximum speed, "time-optimal" head movements. The role of each of the muscle activity pulses in the typical triphasic EMG pattern that produces a head movement is analyzed and tendon vibration is used to see what role proprioceptive input plays in shaping these pulses. The model is also used to explore the causes of head movement abnormalities in torticollis spasmodicus.

20

Clinical Disorders of Head Movement

P. RONDOT

The normal behavior of cervical muscles is disturbed more or less selectively by diseases that alter the axis of the body or that cause abnormal movements of the limbs. For descriptive purposes, it is possible to distinguish three main functions of the cervical musculature: postural movements, orienting movements, and movements of expression. These types of movements appear to be disrupted or elicited inappropriately by a range of clinical disorders.

1. Postural movements. Maintaining the vertical position of the head seems to be a principal function of many neck muscles, but the strongest contribution is made by muscles at the back of the neck. The generalized dystonia that disturbs the axial posture of the body has severe effects on the position of the head. A localized dystonia, spasmodic torticollis (ST), is particularly disruptive to head posture.
2. Orienting movements. Like a hand that moves to explore the objects in its reach, the head also moves in order to place its visual and auditory receptors in the best position to receive maximum information. Choreas that disturb the movements of the limbs also interfere with the movements of the neck. They give the impression that the patient is leaning over in order to hear better or straightening up in order to see better.
3. Movements of expression. Neck muscles play a role in communication: shaking or nodding the head, tipping the head to one side in an expression of doubt, dropping the head in an attitude of sadness, pulling back the head in an attitude of scorn. These movements depend on sociocultural background and on geographical latitude; the apparent reserve of the anglo-saxon manner in opposition to the natural ebullience of the mediterranean people is well known. The tics that sometimes take over the cervical musculature caricature this form of expression.

Abnormal movements of the head can occur following lesions of the cerebral cortex or lesions of the basal ganglia. However, in the absence of any observable anatomical lesion, the head can also show abnormal movements of a particularly disabling nature, such as those caused by certain localized dystonias or by tics. These abnormal movements are probably due to a functional disturbance of the central mechanisms that modulate movements of the head.

CLINICAL ASPECTS OF ABNORMAL HEAD MOVEMENTS

Abnormal head movements vary in their clinical forms according to the site of the lesion.

Cortical Lesions

Cortical lesions produce the most stereotyped form of abnormal head movements and these are observed during localized epileptic fits. They are clonic or tonic movements of rotation, either to the same side or to the opposite side as that of the lesion. These localized fits are due to focal lesions located in the precentral gyrus. With the twisting of the head goes a turning of the eyes in the same direction. This association is characteristic of cortical lesions. It can be reproduced by stimulation of the primary frontal area (Penfield and Rasmussen, 1950) or the supplementary motor area (Penfield and Jasper, 1954). Hemorrhages, hematoma, or edematous softenings in the frontal area produce permanent deviations of the head and eyes in the same direction, toward the side of the lesion.

Lesions of the Basal Ganglia

Abnormal movements vary according to the region of the basal ganglia that is damaged. Two main types of abnormality can be distinguished from a clinical point of view: arrhythmical and rhythmical movements.

Arrhythmical Movements

Arrhythmical movements are characteristic symptoms of choreic and athetotic syndromes. *The choreic movement* is arrhythmic and involuntary. Quick, brusque, jerky, it does not follow a regular pattern, but varies in its amplitude and in its location. The cervical muscles are rarely the first involved. Usually the proximal limbs are the initial site of involuntary contractions. When chorea is very severe and the movements of the neck are very rapid, the movements of the eyes attempt to follow head movements but cannot find a point of focus. However, disorders in ocular movements can arise independently from neck movements and these further contribute to the choreic motor dysfunction. The character of the choreic movements is specific; as in the case of cortical movements, neck and eye movements are linked.

Lessened in a quiet environment and disappearing during sleep, choreic movements are increased by voluntary contractions. For example, choreic movements can be evoked by sticking out the tongue in some mild cases. They are enhanced when the patient concentrates on a mental task such as mental arithmetic. On EMG recordings, antagonistic muscles exhibit simultaneous arrhythmic contractions.

Huntington's chorea is due to striatal lesions, particularly caudate lesions. Choreic movements can be reproduced in monkeys by injecting γ-aminobutyric acid (GABA) antagonists into the putamen. A low level of GABA is the main biochemical characteristic of this disease.

Athetosis is rarely localized to the cervical musculature. When neck muscles are involved, athetosis is bilateral, and also affects the four limbs and the facial muscles, thus disturbing speech. In contrast to chorea, athetotic movements are slow, crawling-like behaviors that often cause a stretching of the neck. They are arrhythmical and are broken up by spasms that freeze the head and the limbs in abnormal postures for a few seconds. Augmented by effort, by sensory stimulation, and by emotions, they lessen with a calm environment and disappear during sleep.

The lesions that provoke this syndrome either occur at birth or appear during the first months or years. In contrast to the often localized disturbances in chorea, many cerebral structures may be injured. At the present time, we still cannot attribute this syndrome to any defect of neurotransmitter.

Rhythmical Movements of the Head

Rhythmical contractions of neck muscles occur in a number of situations. Most commonly, *tremor of the head* is idiopathic, and may or may not be hereditary; it is a postural tremor, most often of negation. The tremor may appear only late in life, when it is called senile tremor, although it sometimes occurs in young people. This tremor can either be localized to the neck or associated with a postural tremor of the limbs that precedes or follows the neck tremor. The eyes usually follow the tremor passively, causing a trembling vision. More rarely, a tremor of the eyes is synchronized with the tremor of the head but occurs in the opposite direction, thus stabilizing the visual image. Beta-blocker drugs are less effective on this tremor than on the tremors of the limbs.

The parkinsonian tremor only rarely involves the musculature of the neck (in contrast to the abnormal movements induced by levodopa, see below). "The head and the neck remain undamaged," according to Charcot (1886). When present, the tremor is one of approbation or negation. Its frequency is from 4 to 6 Hz and it responds favorably to the administration of levodopa (L-Dopa).

Another variety of rhythmical neck movement is produced by L-Dopa (L-Dopa-induced dyskinesia) as well as *neuroleptics* (tardive dyskinesia). Both types of dyskinesia are often localized in the neck, where they take the form of tonic contractions producing abnormal postures of the neck, similar to those of spasmodic torticollis. These tonic contractions are sometimes replaced by a low-frequency rhythmical activity of 0.5 to 2 Hz occurring sometimes in a synchronous manner in the synergistic rotational muscles (sternocleidomastoid on one side, splenius on the other) and sometimes in the extensor muscles (splenius on both sides) (Fig. 20.1).

The abnormal movements induced by L-Dopa are due to a supersensitivity to dopamine of the striatal dopaminergic receptors. Tardive dyskinesia results from blocking these same receptors, which then develop a supersensitivity related to their functional denervation. We have further suggested (Rondot and Bathien, 1986) that tardive dyskinesia could be caused by the reduced activity of the enzyme, glutamic acid decarboxylase, observed experimentally after long-term

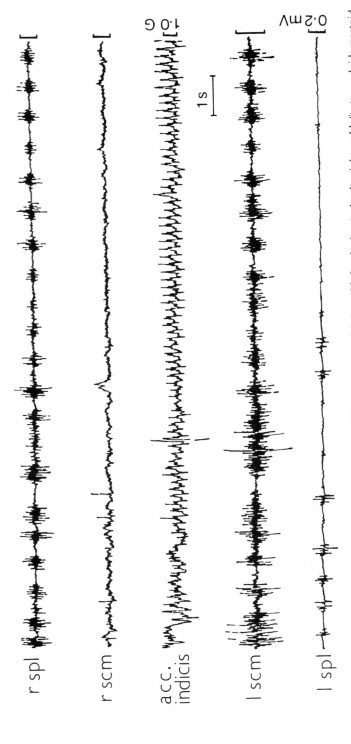

Figure 20.1.   L–Dopa dyskinesia. Parkinson's disease. EMG recordings of right and left splenius (r, l spl), right and left sternocleidomastoid (r, l scm), and acceleration of index tremor (acc. indicis). Rhythmical bursts were recorded from synergistic muscles (r spl, l scm) and from l spl.

administration of neuroleptics. This reduction tends to bring about a GABA-receptor supersensitivity resulting from disuse (Oberlander et al., 1977).

The Gilles de la Tourette's Syndrome and Spasmodic Torticollis (ST)

These deserve a special place because they are localized in the neck. No anatomical lesion has so far been identified to account for their development. Nevertheless, these diseases have a special importance since they are predominantly localized to the cervical region. They evolve in a chronic manner and they considerably modify the normal conditions of the sensory receptors of the head. This is particularly the case with ST, which will be discussed in greater detail.

Gilles de la Tourette's Syndrome

The spasms of Gilles de la Tourette's syndrome are very often localized in the cervical musculature. Nomura and Segawa (1982) estimate that approximately 24% of tics begin in the muscles of the dorsal neck. In most cases, they also spread to the face and sometimes are accompanied by vocal tests (throat clearing, vocalization, coprolalia). The movements caused by the tics resemble those of chorea because they are brusque and are localized in the proximal muscles of the limbs, in the neck, and in the face (Fig. 20.2). However, they differ because they are stereotyped, they resemble voluntary movements, and, when they are not too intense, they can be consciously interrupted for a brief period only to erupt again with increased intensity, as though suddenly liberated. Frequently, they develop along with psychobehavioral problems. No pathological lesions have been so far observed in this hyperkinetic syndrome. However, the fact that improvements follow administration of butyrophenone suggests that there is an abnormality in the dopaminergic system.

Spasmodic Torticollis (ST)

ST is a localized neck muscle dystonia that causes abnormal head postures. The abnormal postures can be classed into three basic groups according to the direction of deviation of the neck. The term "torticollis" refers to cases in which the head is rotated in a horizontal plane to the left or to the right, according to the direction in which the chin is turned. The term "antecollis" is used when the head is in flexion (bent forward), whereas "retrocollis" is used when the head is in extension (bent backward). If the vertical axis of the neck is inclined to one side, we use the term "laterocollis," left laterocollis if the left ear is inclined toward the left shoulder or right laterocollis in the opposite direction.

Often, as the result of the simultaneous occurrence of several abnormalities, the posture adopted by the patient is more complex. Most commonly, a "torticollis" on one side is combined with a "laterocollis" on the opposite side. In the great majority of cases, the direction of the dystonia remains the same for the same patient throughout the progression of the disorder and (where there is remission) in the relapse of the condition. However, in the case of more complex postures, one of the elements may progressively dominate. In the combination of torticollis and laterocollis, we have observed that the laterocollis becomes more dominant over time. In each of these deviations the eyes undergo a compensatory

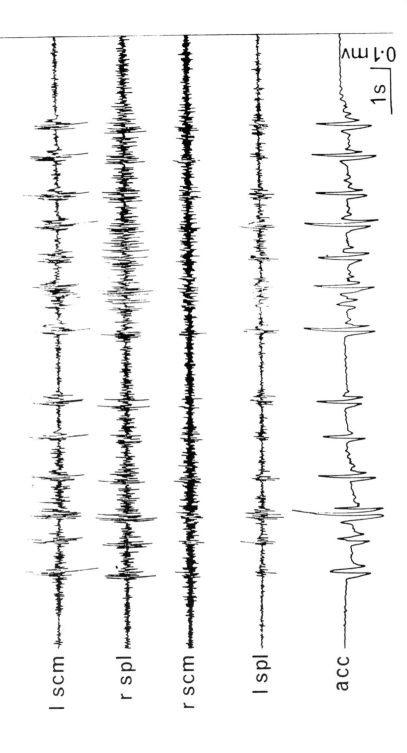

Figure 20.2. Tourette's syndrome. EMG recordings, bilaterally made from sternocleidomastoid (scm) and splenius (spl), show synchronous activation in the four muscles. The lower trace (acc) indicates the acceleration of horizontal head movement.

movement in the opposite direction so as to maintain the axis of vision in a sagittal plane.

The abnormal posture may be permanent throughout the day, as in the extreme forms of cervical dystonia in which the deviation of the neck is tonic and does not respond to reduction by a conscious effort. In other cases that are described more accurately by the term "spasmodic torticollis," we find that muscular spasms of the neck pull the head from its normal posture in either a jerky or a single movement. The spasm then abates after it has reached its maximum amplitude.

The tonic or spasmodic character of torticollis is not related to differences in the pathophysiology itself, but to differences in its degree of severity; when improvement occurs, tonic torticollis commonly becomes spasmodic. In fact Folz et al. (1959) have also noted that in animals, following an increase in intensity of stimulation, there occurs first clonic movements and then a tonic contraction of the neck muscles. In accordance with the severity of the disorder, a scale has been set up with five grades: intermittent movements without maintenance of an abnormal posture, intermittent movements interrupted by tonic deviations of short duration, development of an abnormal posture that can be corrected by voluntary movements, permanent deviation that cannot be corrected by voluntary movements, but can be restrained by a correcting countermovement (geste antagoniste), and permanent deviation that is completely unrestrainable.

Factors Capable of Modulating the Intensity of ST

Several factors can temporarily worsen ST: emotion, either pleasant or unpleasant, standing up and particularly walking, and cutaneous stimulation in the region of neck or the skull. Sometimes the reduction in torticollis that can be produced by lying down is counterbalanced by a worsening of spasms produced by contact of the occiput on the bed. However, in general, a reclining position favors muscular relaxation and the obvious symptoms of dystonia disappear during sleep. Nevertheless, sleep recordings show a number of abnormalities in patients with ST: the proportion of time spent in the waking state is high, over 20%, whereas the percentage of paradoxical sleep is clearly lowered (9–16%) (Rondot et al., 1981). The EMG of cervical muscles is abnormally active during sleep and the patterning of the muscular activity follows that of ST. Therefore, although sleep tends to lessen the dystonia, it cannot make it disappear completely.

Most patients have their own means of attenuating the spasms of torticollis. A correcting countermovement (geste antagoniste) usually consists of placing the hand on the cheek on the side to which the head is turned. However, the purpose of this maneuver is sometimes less simple to understand because the movement can be "paradoxical," and the hand becomes most effective when it is placed on the cheek on the side opposite to that of the torticollis. In retrocollis, the patient most often makes a movement that gives support to the occiput. Two factors may play a role in the subsequent improvement of the spasm: cutaneous stimulation and change of posture as a result of abduction of the shoulder, which can change the action of the trapezius muscle. Carrying a weight in the hand on the opposite side of the ST can provide relief (Tournay and Paillard, 1955), whereas the disorder can be worsened when the hand on the same side as the spasm is weighted down.

Abnormalities of Voluntary Contraction and Reflex Responses in ST

The data provided by clinical examination are supplemented by EMG recordings showing that neck muscles are activated simultaneously during voluntary movement directed to the side on which the torticollis occurs. When the patient attempts to move the head to the opposite side, the movement is often prevented by the tonic contraction of the antagonistic muscles responsible for the torticollis. The spasms provide not only a mechanical hindrance to the intended movement, but also a real reciprocal inhibition, for if the contraction of the antagonistic muscles is temporally suspended by anesthetic infiltration, the activity of the agonist muscles becomes increased (Fig. 20.3). This knowledge has led us to try alcoholization of the motor point of the most active muscles in ST, in order to enable rehabilitation.

The disorders in voluntary contraction should be compared to the changes observed in reflex responses (Fig. 20.4). In ST of medium intensity, passive stretch of the muscles responsible for the torticollis produces a recrudescence of activity, which rapidly gives way when the movement is continued. The exaggeration of the stretch reflex is thus rapidly controlled by an inhibition, possibly of tendon origin.

Another abnormality appears to us as though it may be more important in maintaining the abnormal posture; this is the shortening reaction. When a passive movement is carried out in the same direction as that of the torticollis, a considerable recrudescence of the activity of the muscles involved in the torticollis is observed (Rondot and Scherrer, 1966). In the case of ST toward the left, this abnormal activity is recorded in the right sternocleidomastoid muscle and in the left splenius muscle. The reaction to the passive shortening not only appears when the movement reproduces the pathological posture, but can also be observed at other times when the affected muscle is shortened. Thus in a right ST, abnormal activity is produced in the left sternocleidomastoid not only by rotating the head to the right but also by passively bending the neck. This activity occurs either in a tonic manner or in a clonic or rhythmical manner according to the type of torticollis. It does not depend on the rapidity of the passive movement, but on its amplitude. The same reaction is observed if the head is kept still, and the trunk is turned alternately from right to left. Thus, it does not depend on vestibular stimulation.

The shortening reaction is the exaggerated form of a reaction that is observed in the normal subject (Katz and Rondot, 1978). The reaction most frequently takes place in the muscles of the neck and tends to hold the head in a given position. Such reactions can be called "local posture reflexes," a name given by Foix and Thevenard (1929). The reactions are particularly pronounced in ST and appear to be responsible for provoking abnormal postures. They represent for us the principal pathophysiological factor underlying the origin of ST.

Evolution

The evolution of ST is chronic. Over the first 5 years relapses can occur: 23% reported by Jayne et al. (1984) and 12% by Friedmann and Fahn (1986). Spontaneous cures are possible but rare. The usual mode of progression follows the outline proposed by Meares (1971): an initial 5 years during which the ST usually

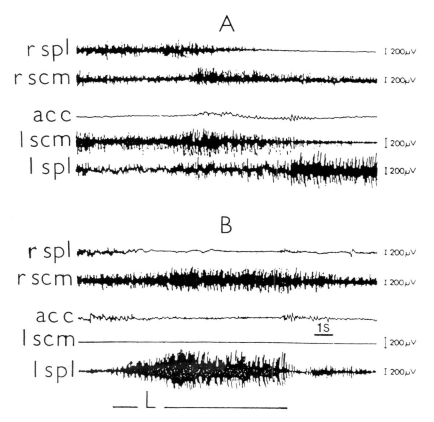

Figure 20.3.   Right spasmodic torticollis during active head rotation. (A) Inefficient attempts to rotate the head to the left are impeded by contraction of right splenius (spl) and left sternocleidomastoid (scm). (B) After anesthetic blockade of the r spl and l scm, free rotation becomes possible.

worsens but sometimes resolves, the following 5 years which show a stabilization, and then a period of greater or lesser duration in which a slight improvement occurs. No disorder in neurotransmitter function has been detected up to the present, which makes a therapeutic regimen difficult to design.

ST Associated with Other Extrapyramidal Diseases

ST is commonly associated with writer's cramp: it is present in 11% of the cases in our series. Writer's cramp often occurs at the same time as ST, but it can also precede the ST. In torsion dystonia one often observes a posture typical of torticollis, but it is rare for this generalized dystonia to begin with an ST (two cases in a series of 42 patients; Marsden and Harrison, 1974). Thus, it appears that we have two different disorders that vary both in their starting ages and in ways in which they evolve.

We frequently find that tremor is accompanied by an ST. In 40% of the cases

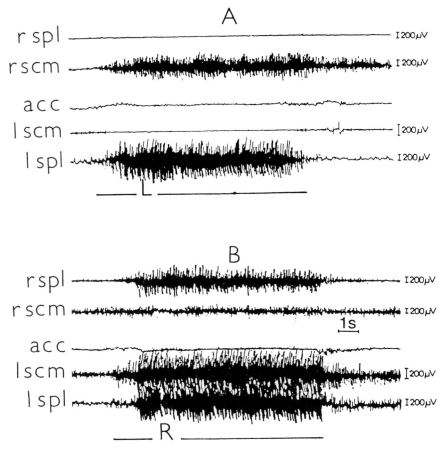

Figure 20.4.   Right spasmodic torticollis during passive head rotation. (A) Passive rotation of the head toward the left produces a shortening reaction in the right sternocleidomastoid (scm) and left splenius (spl) muscles. (B) Passive rotation toward the right produces a shortening reaction in the r spl and l scm muscles and a "stretch reflex" in the l spl.

in our series of patients with ST, we found a rhythmical activity of varying frequency; 0.5 to 1 Hz was recorded in the neck muscles. ST was associated less frequently with tremor of the upper limbs (in only 20% of our cases); it was more irregular than the essential tremor and did not spread in the same way as the latter. However, in an epidemiological study on essential tremor, Larsson and Sjogren (1960) did not find cases of dystonia in the past record of the essential tremor. This result argues for not making too close a connection between the two disorders.

Much more rarely ST is associated with other types of dysfunction: olivopontocerebellar atrophy, hereditary spastic paraplegia, Friedreich's disease, luysopallidal atrophy, and Parkinson's disease.

The Vestibular System and ST

Vestibular nuclei and muscles of the neck are closely connected (Wilson and Yoshida, 1969b). Lesions of the vestibular nuclei in the monkey are known to cause a transitory disorder of head posture (Tarlov, 1970). This observation has led several investigators to explore the vestibular function of patients suffering from ST. Their results do not agree. In 16 patients examined by Matthews et al. (1978), only 1 showed a directional asymmetry of labyrinthine function that favored the side to which the head was turned. No patient showed a significant directional preponderance of the nystagmus. More recently, new research by Bronstein and Rudge (1986) reached different conclusions in a group of 35 patients. Bronstein and Rudge found a directional preponderance in vestibular nystagmus opposite to the direction of the torticollis. This means that there is a tonic imbalance of muscle activity both in the neck and the extraocular system that tends to deviate the head and the eyes in the same direction. From these results, Bronstein and Rudge consider that the vestibular system has a primary involvement in ST. However, it is curious to note that the directional preponderance tends to decrease with time, whereas the ST persists or worsens. The evidence might suggest a secondary involvement of the vestibular system as a result of neck muscle contraction. This contraction itself might be able to produce an asymmetry of labyrinthine response that becomes compensated over the years, in the same way that asymmetries observed after labyrinthine lesions become compensated with time. The fact that an asymmetry of the vestibular response persists if the head is held still during the labyrinthine stimulation has been offered as an argument in favor of a primary involvement of the vestibular system. However, in such conditions, it is known that the muscles of patients afflicted with ST continue to contract and resist even more markedly when they encounter an obstacle that prevents the head from moving. It is thus possible that this directional preponderance may in fact be the consequence, if not of the head movement, at least of the contractions in neck muscles.

THE PATHOPHYSIOLOGY OF ABNORMAL HEAD MOVEMENTS

The location of the lesion determines the nature of abnormal head movements and so it is in terms of the location of the lesion that the abnormal head movements should be interpreted.

Contraversive movements caused by cortical lesions reproduce the voluntary movements of the head and eyes when the patient is made to look sideways. Stimulation of the precentral motor area elicits a similar movement and thus suggests that the disorder stems from discharge in the primary motor area. Most often the head is turned to the side opposite that of the lesion. However, sometimes the deviation occurs on the same side (Penfield and Jasper, 1954), thus suggesting that, in this primary motor area, there is a double representation of the neck muscles responsible for the contraversive movement. When the head is turned to the side of the lesion, as is noted during cerebral hemorrhages, the attitude is interpreted as being due to the release of rotation on the side of the healthy hemisphere in such a way that the actions of the muscles are no longer balanced by their contralateral antagonists whose motor centers are paralyzed by the lesions on the opposite side. The pathway that projects the appropriate motor commands to the brain stem probably passes through the ventral aspect of the pyramidal tract.

The most important lesions in Huntington's chorea are situated in the striatum and particularly in the caudate nucleus. The lesions are accompanied by a marked decrease of the neurotransmitter GABA, whereas the nigrostriate dopaminergic pathway remains intact. It is probable that the dysfunction of the GABAergic cells of the striatum removes their inhibitory influence on dopaminergic cells in the substantia nigra. Thus, the choreic movement would be due in part to the dopaminergic hyperactivity. Furthermore, administration of neuroleptics which block the dopaminergic receptors reduces the choreic movements, whereas administration of L-Dopa increases them. It is also possible that the dysfunction of striatal neurons interferes with the normal function of the globus pallidus and the subthalamic nucleus, which also receive a GABA input. A general somatotopic organization of movement-related cells was found in the globus pallidus as well as in the subthalamic nucleus (Delong et al., 1985). One may therefore suppose that choreic movements come about from changes in the control of limb and neck movements that are normally carried out by cells in the striatum.

Abnormal movements induced by L-Dopa are probably due to similar pathophysiological mechanisms: an excessive stimulation of the dopaminergic striatal receptors which disturbs the motor control normally carried out by the neurons of the striatum. In chorea, as in L-Dopa-induced dyskinesia, movements of the head would thus reveal a functional disturbance of motor processes normally transmitted by the cortico-striato-pallido-cortical circuit.

In the absence of anatomical lesions (Tarlov, 1970) or neurotransmitter abnormalities (Curzon, 1973; Lal et al., 1979) in ST, one must start with experimental studies in order to gain insight into its pathophysiology. Spasmodic torticollis was fortuitously produced in seven monkeys by Folz et al. (1959). The lesions common to all seven animals involved a portion of the decussation of the brachium conjunctivum, the medial longitudinal fasciculus, and a portion of the medial reticular formation. Poirier (1960) observed a tilting of the head toward the side opposite to that of unilateral lesions situated in the medial area of the tegmentum of the upper pons and midbrain. As a result of lesions in the pontine reticular formation, Cohen et al. (1968) have noted a tilting of the head in addition to a paralysis of horizontal gaze in an ipsilateral direction. Thus mesencephalic or pontine lesions are capable of producing torticollis.

More recently in an experimental study of hemiballismus, Crossman et al. (1984) have noted that injections of the GABA antagonist, bicuculline, in or near the zona incerta dorsal to the subthalamic nucleus produced a twisting of the head contralateral to the side that was injected with GABA antagonist. Through this zone pass the efferent pallidal pathways, and, in particular, the lenticular fasciculus that continues caudalward into the midbrain. One may suspect that ST is due to a functional deficiency of efferent mesencephalic pathways from the pallidum. A GABAergic involvement could lie at the root of its origin.

In conclusion, as for abnormal movements of the limbs, it is possible to differentiate abnormal movements of the neck according to the location of the lesion in cortical or subcortical structures. In the case of cortical lesions, lateral twisting movements of the head are most common; usually, they are associated with ocular movements in the same direction. When the basal ganglia or their efferent pathways are affected, no regular pattern can be observed and a lack of coordination between neck and eye movements can occur. ST can be considered as a functional disorder of the descending extrapyramidal pathways as far as suggested by the model found in monkeys by lesions in the zona incerta and in medial mesencephalic areas.

It would be useful for more detailed studies to be undertaken on neck movements, as up to now most observations of head-movement dysfunction have been included incidentally in the reports of experiments in other fields. One could then hope for greater efficacy in treating diseases that cause abnormal movements of the head and represent a severe handicap in spite of the attitude of a seventeenth-century poet who was afflicted with them.

> My neck is out of line
> And shrunken is my spine,
> But that suits me just fine,
> And I'm quite a handsome beau
> As torticollis go
> SCARRON

SUMMARY

A range of disorders can affect head movement. Some, such as athetosis or spasmodic torticollis, interfere primarily with the postural carriage of the head. Others, such as tics and choreic movements, interrupt or caricature the normal movements that occur during orienting behaviors or expression of mood. Commonly the nature of the abnormality can be related to specific lesions in the nervous system. Cortical lesions produce clonic or tonic head rotations, so that the head suddenly twists involuntarily and the eyes turn simultaneously in the same direction. Lesions of the basal ganglia can lead to a wider range of dysfunctions, including tremors, jerky choreic movements, or slow athetotic movements broken up by spasm. However, causative factors have yet to be identified for other disorders such as Gilles de la Tourette's syndrome and spasmodic torticollis.

Gilles de la Tourette's syndrome is characterized by localized, stereotyped contractions of neck muscles that occur rapidly and spontaneously. The muscular spasms characteristic of spasmodic torticollis are more prolonged and tend to pull or hold the head in an abnormal posture. In spasmodic torticollis, the affected muscles show abnormal reflex actions and have heightened EMG activity that persists even during sleep. A syndrome similar to spasmodic torticollis can be produced in experimental animals by localized lesions in the midbrain and pons, and by injection of antagonists to the transmitter GABA into the zona incerta. The evidence suggests that spasmodic torticollis may involve a dysfunction in motor pathways that relay through the midbrain from the basal ganglia.

References

Abbott, B.C., and D.R. Wilkie (1953). The relation between velocity of shortening and the tension–length curve of skeletal muscle. *J Physiol. (London)* **120**:214–223.

Abend, W. (1977). Functional organization of the superior vestibular nucleus of the squirrel monkey. *Brain Res.* **132**:65–84.

Abend, W. (1978). Response to constant angular acceleration of neurons in the monkey superior vestibular nucleus. *Exp. Brain Res.* **31**:459–473.

Abrahams, V.C., and S. Falchetto (1969). Hind leg ataxia of cervical origin and cervico-lumbar spinal interactions with a supratentorial pathway. *J Physiol. (London)* **203**:435–447.

Abrahams, V.C. (1971). Spino-spinal mechanisms in the chloralose anaesthetized cat. *J Physiol. (London)* **215**:755–768.

Abrahams, V.C. (1972). Neck muscle proprioceptors and a role of the cerebral cortex in postural reflexes in subprimates. *Rev. Can. Biol.* **31**:115–130.

Abrahams, V.C., and P.K. Rose (1975). Projections of extraocular, neck muscle, and retinal afferents to superior colliculus in the cat: Their connections to the cells of origin of the tectospinal tract. *J Neurophysiol.* **38**:10–18.

Abrahams, V.C., F.J.R. Richmond, and P.K. Rose (1975). Absence of monsynaptic reflex in dorsal neck muscles of the cat. *Brain Res.* **92**:130–131.

Abrahams, V.C., and F.J.R. Richmond (1977). Motor role of the spinal projections of the trigeminal system. In *Pain in the Trigeminal Region* (D.J. Anderson and B. Matthews, eds.), pp. 405–411. Elsevier/North Holland Biomedical Press, Amsterdam.

Abrahams, V.C., G. Anstee, F.J.R. Richmond, and P.K. Rose (1979). Neck muscle and trigeminal input to the upper cervical cord and lower medulla of the cat. *Can. J. Physiol. Pharmacol.* **57**:642–651.

Abrahams, V.C., and J. Keane (1984). Contralateral, midline, and commissural motoneurons of neck muscles: A retrograde HRP study in the cat. *J. Comp. Neurol.* **223**:448–456.

Abrahams, V.C., B. Lynn, and F.J.R. Richmond (1984a). Organization and sensory properties of small myelinated fibres in the dorsal cervical rami of the cat. *J. Physiol. (London)* **347**:177–187.

Abrahams, V.C., F.J.R. Richmond, and J. Keane (1984b). Projections from C2 and C3 nerves supplying muscles and skin of the cat neck: A study using transganglionic transport of horseradish peroxidase. *J. Comp. Neurol.* **230**:142–154.

Abrahams, V.C., and R.J. Clinton (1986). Unit response in the superior colliculus of the chloralose anaesthetised cat. Projections from vibration sensitive receptors. *J. Physiol. (London)* **371**:48P.

Abrahams, V.C., and J.E. Swett (1986). The pattern of spinal and medullary projections from a cutaneous nerve and a muscle nerve of the forelimb of the cat: A study using the transganglionic transport of HRP. *J. Comp. Neurol.* **246**:70–84.

Abzug, C., M. Maeda, B.W. Peterson, and V.J. Wilson (1974). Cervical branching of lumbar vestibulospinal axons. *J. Physiol. (London)* **243**:499–522.

Adamuk, E. (1870). Ueber die Innervation der Augenbewegungen. *Z. Medicin. Wissenschaft.* **5**:65–67.

Akaike, T. (1973). Comparison of neuronal composition of the vestibulospinal system between cat and rabbit. *Exp. Brain Res.* **18**:429–432.

Akaike, T., V.V. Fanardjian, M. Ito, M. Kumada, and H. Nakajima (1973a). Electrophysiological analysis of the vestibulospinal reflex pathway of rabbit. I. Classification of tract cells. *Exp. Brain Res.* **18**:446–463.

Akaike, T., V.V. Fanardjian, M. Ito, and H. Nakajima (1973b). Cerebellar control of the vestibulospinal tract cells in rabbit. *Exp. Brain Res.* **18**:446–463.

Akaike, T. (1983a). Electrophysiological analysis of cerebellar corticovestibular and fastiglovestibular projections to the lateral vestibular nucleus in the cat. *Brain Res.* **272**:223–235.

Akaike, T. (1983b). Neuronal organization of vestibulospinal system in the cat. *Brain Res.* **259**:217–227.

Albert, A. (1972). *Regression and the Moore–Penrose Pseudoinverse*. Academic Press, New York.

Alexander, R.M., and A. Vernon (1975). The dimensions of knee and ankle muscles and the forces they exert. *J. Human Movement Stud.* **1**:115–123.

Alstermark, B., M. Pinter, and S. Sasaki (1983a). Brainstem relay of disynaptic pyramidal EPSPS to neck motoneurons in the cat. *Brain Res.* **259**:147–150.

Alstermark, B., M. Pinter, and S. Sasaki (1983b). Convergence on reticulospinal neurons mediating contralateral pyramidal disynaptic EPSPS to neck motoneurons. *Brain Res.* **259**:151–154.

Alstermark, B., M. Pinter, and S. Sasaki (1983c). Monosynaptic trigeminospinal excitation of neck motoneurones. *Proc. Int. Union Physiol. Sci.* **15**:85.

Alstermark, B., A. Lundberg, and S. Sasaki (1984). Integration in descending motor pathways controlling the forelimb in the cat. 10. Inhibitory pathways to motoneurones via C3–C4 propriospinal neurones. *Exp. Brain Res.* **56**:279–292.

Altman, J., and M.B. Carpenter (1961). Fiber projections of the superior colliculus in the cat. *J. Comp. Neurol.* **116**:157–177.

Amano, N., J.W. Hu, and B.J. Sessle (1986). Responses of neurons in feline trigeminal subnucleus caudalis (medullary dorsal horn) to cutaneous intraoral and muscle afferent stimuli. *J. Neurophysiol.* **55**:227–243.

Ammann, B., J. Gottschall, and W. Zenker (1983). Afferent projections from the rat longus capitis muscle studied by transganglionic transport of HRP. *Anat. Embryol. (Berlin).* **166**:275–289.

Anastasopoulos, D., and T. Mergner (1982). Canal–neck interaction in vestibular nuclear neurons of the cat. *Exp. Brain Res.* **46**:269–280.

Anderson, J.H., and C. Pappas (1978). Neck motor responses to vertical rotations in the alert cat. *Soc. Neurosci. Abstr.* **4**:609.

Anderson, J.H., R.H.I. Blanks, and W. Precht (1978). Response characteristics of semicircular canal and otolith systems in cat. I. Dynamic responses of primary vestibular fibers. *Exp. Brain Res.* **32**:491–507.

Anderson, M.E., M. Yoshida, and V.J. Wilson (1971). Influence of superior colliculus on cat neck motoneurons. *J. Neurophysiol.* **34**:898–907.

Anderson, M.E. (1977). Segmental reflex inputs to motoneurons innervating dorsal neck musculature in the cat. *Exp. Brain Res.* **28**:175–187.

Andres, K.H., M. von During, and R.F. Schmidt (1985). Sensory innervations of the

Achilles tendon by group III and IV afferent fibers. *Anat. Embryol.* **172**:145–156.

Appenteng, K., M.J. O'Donovan, G. Somjen, J.A. Stephens, and A. Taylor (1978). The projection of jaw elevator muscle spindle afferents to fifth nerve motoneurons in the cat. *J. Physiol. (London)* **279**:409–423.

Armstrong, J.B., F.J.R. Richmond, and P.K. Rose (1982). Compartmentalization of motor units in the muscle biventer cervicis of the cat. *Soc. Neurosci. Abstr.* **8**:330.

Atkin, A., and M.B. Bender (1968). Ocular stabilization during oscillatory head movements. *Arch. Neurol. (Chicago).* **19**:559–566.

Bahill, T.A., M. Clark, and L. Stark (1975). The main sequence, a tool for studying human eye movements. *Math. Biosci.* **24**:191–204.

Baker, J., J. Goldberg, B. Peterson, and R. Schor (1982). Oculomotor reflexes after semicircular canal plugging in cats. *Brain Res.* **252**:151–155.

Baker, J., J. Goldberg, G. Hermann, and B.W. Peterson (1984a). Optimal response planes and canal convergence in secondary neurons in vestibular nuclei of alert cats. *Brain Res.* **294**:133–137.

Baker, J., J. Goldberg, G. Hermann, and B.W. Peterson (1984b). Spatial and temporal response properties of secondary neurons that receive convergent input in vestibular nuclei of alert cats. *Brain Res.* **294**:138–143.

Baker, J., J. Goldberg, C. Wickland, and B.W. Peterson (1984c). Spatial and temporal properties of vestibulo-neck reflex EMG. *Soc. Neurosci. Abstr.* **10**:162.

Baker, J., J. Goldberg, and B.W. Peterson (1985). Spatial and temporal response properties of the vestibulocollic reflex in decerebrate cats. *J. Neurophysiol.* **54**:733–756.

Bakker, D.A., and F.J.R. Richmond (1982). Muscle spindle complexes in muscles around upper cervical vertebrae in the cat. *J. Neurophysiol.* **48**:62–74.

Bakker, D.A., F.J.R. Richmond, and V.C. Abrahams (1984). Central projections from cat suboccipital muscles: A study using transganglionic transport of horseradish peroxidase. *J. Comp. Neuol.* **228**:409–421.

Bakker, D.A., F.J.R. Richmond, V.C. Abrahams, and J. Courville (1985). Patterns of primary afferent termination in the external cuneate nucleus from cervical axial muscles in the cat. *J. Comp. Neurol.* **241**:467–479.

Bakker, G.J., and F.J.R. Richmond (1981). Two types of muscle spindles in cat neck muscles: A histochemical study of intrafusal fiber composition. *J. Neurophysiol.* **45**:973–986.

Baldissera, F., H. Hultborn, and M. Illert (1981). Integration in spinal neuronal systems. In *Handbook of Physiology, Vol. II, Section 1: The Nervous System* (V.B. Brooks, ed.), pp. 509-545. American Physiological Society, Bethesda, MD.

Baloh, R.W., A.W. Sales, W.E. Kumley, and V. Honrubia (1975). Quantitative measurement of saccadic amplitude duration and velocity. *Neurology* **25**:1065–1070.

Banks, R.W., D. Barker, and M.J. Stacey (1982). Form and distribution of sensory terminals in cat hindlimb muscle spindles. *Phil. Trans. Roy. Soc. London Ser. B.* **299**:329–364.

Barany, R. (1906). Augenbewegungen durch Thoraxbewegungen ausgelost. *Z.B.I. Physiol.* **20**:298.

Barbas, H., and B. Dubrovsky (1981a). Excitatory and inhibitory interactions of extraocular and dorsal neck muscle afferents in cat frontal cortex. *Exp. Neurol.* **74**:51–66.

Barbas, H., and B. Dubrovsky (1981b). Central and peripheral effects of tonic vibratory stimuli to dorsal neck and extraocular muscles in the cat. *Exp. Neurol.* **74**:67–85.

Barker, D. (1974). The morphology of muscle receptors. In *Handbook of Sensory Phys-*

iology (C.C. Hunt, ed.), Vol. 3, pp. 1–190. Springer-Verlag, Heidelberg.

Barlow, D., and W. Freeman (1980). Cervico-ocular reflex in the normal adult. *Acta Otolaryngol.* **89**:487–496.

Barmack, N.H., M.A. Nastos, and V.E. Pettorossi (1981). The horizontal and vertical cervico-ocular reflexes of the rabbit. *Brain Res.* **224**:261–278.

Barnes, C.D., P. d'Ascanio, O. Pompeiano, and G. Stampacchia (1985). Chemical microstimulation of a cholinergic pontine reticular system enhances the gain of the vestibulospinal reflex. *4th. Capo Bio. Conf. Neurosci. Villasimius, Sardinia, Italy,* pp. 235.

Barnes, G.R. (1979). Vestibulo-ocular function during coordinated head and eye movements to acquire visual targets. *J. Physiol. (London)* **287**:127–147.

Barnes, G.R., and L.N. Forbat (1979). Cervical and vestibular afferent control of oculomotor response in man. *Acta Otolaryngol.* **88**:79–87.

Barone, R., C. Pavaux, P.C. Blin, and P. Cuq (1973). *Atlas d'Anatomie du Lapin,* pp. 45–50. Masson et Cie, Paris.

Bartz, J. (1965). Eye and head movements in peripheral vision: Nature of compensatory eye movements. *Science* **114**:1644–1645.

Basbaum, A.I., C.H. Clanton, and H.L. Fields (1978). Three bulbospinal pathways from the rostral medulla of the cat: An autoradiographic study of pain modulating systems. *J. Comp. Neurol.* **178**:209–224.

Basbaum, A.I., and H.D. Fields (1979). The origin of descending pathways in the dorsolateral funiculus of the spinal cord of the cat and rat: Further studies on the anatomy of pain modulation. *J. Comp. Neurol.* **187**:513–532.

Basmajian, J.V., and C.J. DeLuca (1985). *Muscles Alive: Their Functions Revealed by Electromyography,* 5th. ed. Williams & Wilkins, Baltimore, Maryland.

Batini, C., G. Moruzzi, and O. Pompeiano (1957). Cerebellar release phenomena. *Arch. Ital. Biol.* **95**:71–95.

Batini, C., and O. Pompeiano (1958). Effects of rostro-medial and rostro-lateral fastigial lesions on decerebrate rigidity. *Arch. Ital. Biol.* **96**:315–329.

Bazzet, H.C., and W.G. Penfield (1922). A study of the Sherrington decerebrate animal in the chronic as well as the acute condition. *Brain* **45**:185–266.

Becker, W., L. Deecke, and T. Mergner (1979). Neuronal responses to natural vestibular and neck stimulation in the anterior suprasylvian gyrus of the cat. *Brain Res.* **165**:139–143.

Bellman, R. (1965). *Dynamic Programming.* Princeton University Press, Princeton.

Bender, M.B., S. Shanzer, and I.H. Wagman (1964). On the physiologic decussation concerned with head turning. *Confin. Neurol. (Basel).* **24**:169–181.

Benson, A., and G. Barnes (1979). Vision during angular oscillation: The dynamic interaction of visual and vestibular mechanisms. *Aviat. Space Environ. Med.* **49**:340–342.

Berger, A.J., W.E. Cameron, D.B. Averill, R.C. Kramis, and M.D. Binder (1984). Spatial distributions of phrenic and medial gastrocnemius motoneurons in the cat spinal cord. *Exp. Neurol.* **86**:559–575.

Berman, A.L. (1968). *The brain stem of the cat. A cytoarchitectonic atlas with stereotaxic coordinates.* The University of Wisconsin Press, Madison.

Bernard, C. (1958). *Lecons sur la Physiologie et la Pathologie du Systeme Nerveux.* J.B. Bailliere, Paris.

Bernard, C. (1865). *An Introduction to the Study of Experimental Medicine.* Collier, New York.

Berthoz, A., and J.H. Anderson (1971). Frequency analysis of vestibular influence on extensor motoneurons. II. Relation between neck and forelimb extensors. *Brain Res.* **34**:376–380.

Berthoz, A. (1973). Biomechanical and neuromuscular responses to oscillating and transient forces in man and in the cat. In *Med. & Sport, Vol. 8,* pp. 249–260. Biomech. III, Karger, Basel.

Berthoz, A., and R. Llinás (1974). Afferent neck projections to the cat cerebellar cortex. *Exp. Brain Res.* **20**:385–401.

Berthoz, A., P.P. Vidal, and J. Corvisier (1982). Brain stem neurons mediating horizontal eye position signals to dorsal neck muscles of the alert cat. In *Physiological and Pathological Aspects of Eye Movements* (A. Roucoux, and M. Crommelinck, eds.), pp. 385–398. Junk, The Hague.

Berthoz, A., and A. Grantyn (1986). Neuronal mechanisms underlying eye-head coordination. In *Progress in Brain Research, Vol. 64* (H.-J. Freund, U. Büttner, B. Cohen, and J. Noth, eds.), pp. 325–343. Elsevier, Amsterdam.

Berthoz, A., A. Grantyn, and J. Droulez (1986). Some collicular efferent neurons code saccadic eye velocity. *Neurosci. Lett.,* **72**:289–294.

Bessou, P., and Y. Laporte (1961). Etude des recepteurs musculaires innerves par les fibres afferentes du group III (fibre myelinisees fines) chez le chat. *Arch. Ital. Biol.* **99**:293–321.

Bickley, W.G., and R.E. Gibson (1962). *Via Vector to Tensor.* John Wiley, New York.

Biemond, A. (1939). On a new form of experimental position-nystagmus in the rabbit and its clinical value. *Proc. Kon. Nederlandse Akad. Wetenschappen.* **42**:370–375.

Biemond, A. (1940). Further observations about the cervical form of positional-nystagmus and its anatomical base. *Proc. Kon. Nederlandse Akad. Wetenschappen.* **43**:901–906.

Biemond, A., and J. DeJong (1969). On cervical nystagmus and related disorders. *Brain* **92**:437–458.

Bilotto, G., J. Goldberg, B.W. Peterson, and V.J. Wilson (1982a). Dynamic properties of vestibular reflexes in the decerebrate cat. *Exp. Brain Res.* **47**:343–352.

Bilotto, G., R.H. Schor, Y. Uchino, and V.J. Wilson (1982b). Localization of proprioceptive reflexes in the splenius muscle of the cat. *Brain Res.* **238**:217–221.

Binder, M.D. (1981). Further evidence that the Golgi tendon organ monitors the activity of a discrete set of motor units within a muscle. *Exp. Brain Res.* **43**:186–192.

Birukow, G. (1937). Untersuchungen uber den optischen Drehnystagmus und uber die Sehscharfe beim Grasfrosch (*Rana temporaria*). *Z. Vergl. Physiol.* **25**:92–142.

Birukow, G. (1952). Studien uber statisch-optisch ausgeloste Kompensationsbewegungen und Koperhaltung bei Amphibien. *Z. Vergl. Physiol.* **34**:448–472.

Bizzi, E., and P. Schiller (1970). Single unit activity in the frontal eye fields of unanesthesized monkeys during eye and head movements. *Exp. Brain Res.* **10**:151–158.

Bizzi, E., R.E. Kalil, and V. Tagliasco (1971). Eye-head coordination in monkeys: Evidence for centrally patterned organization. *Science* **173**:452–454.

Bizzi, E., R.E. Kalil, and P. Morasso (1972a). Two modes of active eye-head coordination in monkeys. *Brain Res.* **40**:45–48.

Bizzi, E., R.E. Kalil, P. Morasso, and V. Tagliasco (1972b). Central programming and peripheral feedback during eye-head coordination in monkeys. *Bibl. Ophthal.* **82**:220–232.

Bizzi, E., A. Polit, and P. Morasso (1976). Mechanisms underlying achievement of final head position. *J. Neurophysiol.* **39**:435–444.

Bizzi, E., P. Dev, P. Morasso, and A. Polit (1978). Effect of load disturbances during centrally initiated movements. *J. Neurophysiol.* **41**:542–556.

Bizzi, E. (1981). Eye-head coordination. In *Handbook of Physiology Vol. II, Section I: the Nervous System* (V.B. Brooks, ed.), pp. 1321–1336. American Physiology Society, Bethesda, MD.

Blakemore, C., and M. Donaghy (1980). Coordination of head and eyes in the gaze changing behaviour of cats. *J. Physiol. (London)* **300**:317–335.

Blanks, R., I. Curthoys, and C. Markham (1972). Planar relationships of semicircular canals in the cat. *Am. J. Physiol.* **223**:55–62.

Blanks, R., I. Curthoys, and C. Markham (1975a). Planar relationships of the semicircular canals in man. *Acta Otolaryngol.* **80**:185–196.

Blanks, R., M. Estes, and C. Markham (1975b). The physiologic characteristics of vestibular first order canal neurons in the cat. II. Responses to constant angular acceleration. *J. Neurophysiol.* **38**:1250–1268.

Blanks, R.H.I., and W. Precht (1976). Functional characterization of primary vestibular afferents in the frog. *Exp. Brain Res.* **25**:369–390.

Blanks, R., I. Curthoys, M. Bennett, and C. Markham (1985). Planar relationships of the semicircular canals in rhesus and squirrel monkeys. *Brain Res.* **340**:315–324.

Bock, O., V. Koschitzky, and W.H. Zangemeister (1979). Vestibular adaptation to long term stimuli. *Biol. Cyber.* **33**:77–79.

Bohmer, A., V. Henn, and J. Suzuki (1985). Vestibulo-ocular reflexes after selective plugging of the semicircular canals in the monkey—response plane determinations. *Brain Res.* **326**:291–298.

Bolk, L. (1906). *Das Cerebellum der Saugetiere*. G. Fisher, Haarlem, Jena.

Botros, G. (1979). The tonic oculomotor function of the cervical joint and muscle receptors. *Adv. Otorhinolaryngol.* **25**:214–220.

Botterell, E.H., and J.F. Fulton (1938). Functional localization in the cerebellum of primates. II. Lesions of midline structures (vermis) and deep nuiclei. *J. Comp. Neurol.* **69**:47–62.

Botterman, B.R., M.D. Binder, and D.G. Stuart (1978). Functional anatomy of the association between motor units and muscle receptors. *Am. zool.* **18**:49–66.

Boyd, I.A. (1954). The histological structure of the receptors in the knee-joint of the cat correlated with their physiological response. *J. Physiol. (London)* **124**:476–488.

Boyd, I.A., and M.R. Davey (1968). *Composition of Peripheral Nerves*. Livingstone, Edinburgh.

Boyd, I.A. (1976). The mechanical properties of dynamic nuclear bag fibres, static nuclear bag fibres and nuclear chain fibres in isolated cat muscle spindles. *Brain Res.* **44**:33–47.

Boyd, I.A. (1981). The action of the three types of intrafusal fibre in isolated cat muscle spindles on the dynamic and length sensitivities of primary and secondary sensory endings. In *Muscle Receptors and Movement* (A. Taylor and A. Prochazka, eds.), pp. 17–32. Macmillan, London.

Boyd, I.A., and R.S. Smith (1984). The muscle spindle. In *Peripheral Neuropathy* (P.J. Dyck, P.K. Thomas, E.H. Lombert, R. Bunge, eds.), pp. 171–202. W.B. Saunders Company, London.

Boyd, I.A., and M.H. Gladden (1985). Morphology of mammalian muscle spindles. In *The Muscle Spindle* (I.A. Boyd and M.H. Gladden, eds.), pp. 3–22. Stockton Press, New York.

Boyle, R., and O. Pompeiano (1979a). Sensitivity of interpositus neurons to neck afferent stimulation. *Brain Res.* **168**:180–185.

Boyle, R., and O. Pompeiano (1979b). Frequency response characteristics of vestibulospinal neurons during sinusoidal neck rotation. *Brain Res.* **173**:344–349.

Boyle, R., and O. Pompeiano (1980a). Response characteristics of cerebellar interpositus and intermediate cortex neurons to sinusoidal stimulation of neck and labyrinth receptors. *Neuroscience* **5**:357–372.

Boyle, R., and D. Pompeiano (1980b). Reciprocal responses to sinusoidal tilt of neurons in Deiters' nucleus and their dynamic characteristics. *Arch. Ital. Biol.* **118**:1–32.

Boyle, R., and O. Pompeiano (1980c). Responses of vestibulospinal neurons to sinusoidal rotation of neck. *J. Neurophysiol.* **44**:633–649.

Boyle, R., and O. Pompeiano (1981a). Convergence and interaction of neck and macular vestibular inputs on vestibulospinal neurons. *J. Neurophysiol.* **45**:852–868.

Boyle, R., and O. Pompeiano (1981b). Response of vestibulospinal neurons to neck and macular inputs in the presence or absence of the paleocerebellum. *Ann. N.Y. Acad. Sci.* **374**:373–394.

Boyle, R., and O. Pompeiano (1981c). Relation between cell size and response characteristics of vestibulospinal neurons to labyrinth and neck inputs. *J. Neurosci.* **1**:1052–1066.

Boyle, R., and O. Pompeiano (1984). Discharge activity of spindle afferents from the gastrocnemius-soleus muscle during head rotation in the decerebrate cat. *Pflugers Arch.* **400**:140–150.

Bridgman, C.F. (1968). The structure of tendon organs in the cat. A proposed mechanism for responding to muscle tension. *Anat. Rec.* **162**:209–220.

Brink, E.E., N. Hirai, and V.J. Wilson (1980). Influence of neck afferents on vestibulospinal neurons. *Exp. Brain Res.* **38**:285–292.

Brink, E.E., K. Jinnai, N. Hirai, and V.J. Wilson (1981a). Cervical input to vestibulocollic neurons. *Brain Res.* **217**:13–21.

Brink, E.E., K. Jinnai, and V.J. Wilson (1981b). Pattern of segmental monosynaptic input to cat dorsal neck motoneurons. *J. Neurophysiol.* **46**:496–504.

Brink, E.E., E. Jankowska, and B. Skoog (1984a). Convergence onto interneurons subserving primary afferent depolarization of group I afferents. *J. Neurophysiol.* **51**:432–449.

Brink, E.E., I. Suzuki, S.J.B. Timerick, and V.J. Wilson (1984b). Directional sensitivity of neurons in the lumbar spinal cord to neck rotation. *Brain Res.* **323**:172–175.

Brink, E.E., I. Suzuki, S.J.B. Timerick, and V.J. Wilson (1985). Tonic neck reflex of the decerebrate cat: A role for propriospinal neurons. *J. Neurophysiol.* **54**:978–987.

Brink, E.E., and I. Suzuki (1987). Recurrent inhibitory connexions among neck motoneurones in the cat. *J. Physiol. (London),* **383**:301–326.

Brodal, A. (1957). The *Reticular Formation of the Brainstem.* Oliver and Boyd, Edinburgh.

Brodal, A., and B. Høvik (1964). Site and mode of termination of primary vestibulocerebellar fibres in the cat. An experimental study with silver impregnation methods. *Arch. Ital. Biol.* **102**:1–21.

Bronstein, A.M., and P. Rudge (1986). Vestibular involvement in spasmodic torticollis. *J. Neurol. Neurosurg. Psychiat.* **49**:290–295.

Brooks, V.B., and V.J. Wilson (1959). Recurrent inhibition in the cat's spinal cord. *J. Physiol. (London)* **146**:380–391.

Brown, A.G., P.K. Rose, and P.J. Snow (1976). The morphology of identified cutaneous afferent fibre collaterals in the spinal cord. *J. Physiol.* **263**:132–134P.

Burgess, P.R., and F.J. Clark (1969). Characteristics of knee joint receptors in the cat. *J. Physiol. (London)* **203**:317–335.

Burke, R.E., E. Jankowska, and G. ten Bruggencate (1970). A comparison of peripheral and rubrospinal synaptic input to slow and fast twitch motor units of triceps surae. *J. Physiol. (London)* **207**:709–732.

Burke, R.E., and P. Rudomin (1977). Spinal neurons and synapses. In *Handbook of Physiology, Vol. 1, Section 1: The Nervous System* (E.R. Kandel, ed.), pp. 877–944. American Physiological Society, Bethesda, MD.

Burke, R.E. (1981). Motor units: anatomy, physiology, and functional organization. In *Handbook of Physiology, Vol. II, Section 1: The Nervous System* (V.B. Brooks, ed.), pp. 345–422. American Physiological Society, Bethesda, MD.

Burke, R.E. (1985). Motor unit types: Functional specializations in motor control. In *The Motor System in Neurobiology* (E.V. Evarts, S.P. Wise, and D. Bousfield, eds.). Elsevier Biomedical Press, Amsterdam.

Büttner, U., J.A. Büttner-Ennever, and V. Henn (1977). Vertical eye movement related unit activity in the rostral mesencephalic reticular formation of the alert monkey. *Brain Res.* **130**:239–252.

Butz-Kuenzer, E. (1958). Optische und labyrinthare Auslosung der Lagereaktionen bei Amphibien. *Z. Tierpsychol.* **14**:429–447.

Campbell, S.K., T.D. Parker, and W. Welker (1974). Somatotopic organization of the externeal cuneate nucleus in albino rats. *Brain Res.* **77**:1–23.

Carpenter, M.B., J.W. Harbison, and P. Peter (1970). Accessory oculomotor nuclei in the monkey: projections and effects of discrete lesions. *J. Comp. Neurol.* **140**:131–154.

Carpenter, M.B., B.M. Stein, and P. Peter (1972). Primary vestibulocerebellar fibers in the monkey: Distribution of fibers arising from distinctive cell groups of the vestibular ganglia. *Am. J. Anat.* **135**:221–250.

Castiglioni, A.J., M.C. Gallaway, and J.D. Coulter (1978). Spinal projection from the midbrain in monkey. *J. Comp. Neurol.* **178**:329–346.

Cervero, F., and L.A. Connell (1983). Anatomical observations on the projections of somatic and visceral afferent fibres to the thoracic spinal cord of the cat. *J. Physiol. (London)* **343**:68–69P.

Cervero, F., and L.A. Connell (1984). Fine afferent fibers from viscera do not terminate in the substantia gelatinosa of the thoracic spinal cord. *Brain Res.* **294**:370–374.

Chambers, W.W. (1947). Electrical stimulation of the inferior of the cerebellum in the cat. *Am. J. Anat.* **80**:55–94.

Chambers, W.W., and J.M. Sprague (1955a). Functional localization in the cerebellum. I. Organization in longitudinal cortico-nuclear zones and their contribution to the control of posture, both extrapyramidal and pyramidal. *J. Comp. Neurol.* **103**:105–129.

Chambers, W.W., and J.M. Sprague (1955b). Functional localization in the cerebellum. II. Somatotopic organization in cortex and nuclei. *Arch. Neurol. Psychiat.* **74**:653–680.

Chan, Y.S., D. Manzoni, and O. Pompeiano (1982). Response characteristics of cerebellar dentate and lateral cortex neurons to sinusoidal stimulation of neck and labyrinth receptors. *Neuroscience* **7**:2993–3011.

Chan, Y.S., Y.M. Cheung, and J.C. Hwang (1985). Effect of tilt on the response of neuronal activity within the cat vestibular nuclei during slow and constant velocity rotation. *Brain Res.* **345**:271–278.

Charcot, J.M. (1886). *Lecons sur les Maladies du Systeme Nerveux*, Tome 1. Delahaye A. et Lecrosnier E., Paris.

Chevalier, G., and J.M. Deniau (1984). Spatio-temporal organization of a branched tecto-spinal/tecto-diencephalic neuronal system. *Neuroscience* **12**:427–439.

Chin, N.K., M. Cope, and M. Pang (1962). Number and distribution of spindle capsules in seven hindlimb muscles of the cat. In *Symposium on Muscle Receptors* (D. Barker, ed.). pp. 242. University Press, Hong Kong.

Chouet, B.A., and L.R. Young (1974). Tracking with head position using an electrooptical monitor. *IEEE Trans. Syst. Man. Cybern.* SMC **4**:192–204.

Clark, S.L. (1939). Responses following electrical stimulation of the cerebellar cortex in the normal cat. *J. Neurophysiol.* **2**:19–35.

Coburn, N. (1955). *Vector and Tensor Analysis.* Dover, New York.

Cochran, S.L., N. Dieringer, and W. Precht (1984). Basic optokineticocular reflex pathways in the frog. *J. Neurosci.* **4**:43–57.

Cohen, B., A. Komatsuzaki, and M.B. Bender (1968). Electro-oculographic syndrome in monkeys after pontine reticular formation lesions. *Arch. Neurol.* **18**:78–92.

Cohen, B., T. Uemura, and S. Takemori (1973). Effects of labyrinthectomy on optokinetic nystagmus (OKN) and optokinetic afternystagmus (OKAN). *Equilibrium Res.* **3**:88–93.

– Cohen, L.A. (1961). Role of eye and neck proprioceptive mechanisms in body orientation and motor coordination. *J. Neurophysiol.* **24**:1–11.

Cohen, B., J. Büttner-Ennever, D. Waitzman, and M.B. Bender (1981). Anatomical connections of a portion of the dorsolateral mesencephalic reticular formation of the monkey associated with horizontal saccadic eye movements. *Soc. Neurosci. Abstr.* **7**:132.

Cohen, B., V. Matsuo, T. Raphan, D. Waitzman, and J. Fradin (1982). Horizontal saccades induced by stimulation of the mesencephalic reticular formation. In *Physiological and Pathological Aspects of Eye Movements* (A. Roucoux, and M. Crommelinck, eds.), pp. 325–335. Junk, The Hague.

Collewijn, H. (1977). Eye- and head movements in freely moving rabbits. *J. Physiol. (London)* **266**:477–498.

Cook, G., and L. Stark (1968). The human eye movement mechanism. Experiments, modelling and model testing. *Arch. Ophthal.* **79**:428–436.

Cooke, J.D., B. Larson, D. Oscarsson, and B. Sjolund (1971). Origin and termination of cuneocerebellar tract. *Exp. Brain Res.* **13**:339–358.

Cooper, S., and P.M. Daniel (1956). Human muscle spindles. *J. Physiol. (London)* **133**:1–3P.

Cooper, S., and P.M. Daniel (1963). Muscle spindles in man, their morphology in the lumbricals and the deep muscles of the neck. *Brain* **86**:563–586.

Cooper, S. (1966). Muscle spindles and motor units. In *Control and Innervation of Skeletal Muscles* (B.L. Andrew, ed.), pp. 9–15. D.C. Thompson and Co. Ltd., Dundee.

Cope, S., and G.M.S. Ryan (1959). Cervical and otolith vertigo. *J. Laryngol. Otol.* **73**:113–120.

Corbin, K.B., and J.C. Hinsey (1935). Intramedullary course of the dorsal root fibres of each of the first four cervical nerves. *J. Comp. Neurol.* **63**:119–126.

Corbin, K.B., W.T. Lhamon, and D.W. Petit (1937). Peripheral and central connections of the upper cervical dorsal root ganglia in the rhesus monkey. *J. Comp. Neurol.* **66**:405–414.

Coulter, J.D., T. Mergner, and O. Pompeiano (1977). Integration of afferent inputs from neck muscles and macular labyrinthine receptors within the lateral reticular nucleus. *Arch. Ital. Biol.* **115**:332–354.

Coulter, J.D., R.M. Bowker, S.P. Wise, E.A. Murray, A.J. Castiglioni, and K.N. Westlund (1979). Cortical, tectal and medullary descending pathways to the cervical spinal cord. *Prog. Brain Res.* **50**:263–274.

Craig, A.D., and S. Mense (1983). The distribution of afferent fibers from the gastrocnemius-soleus muscle in the dorsal horn of the cat, as revealed by the transport of horseradish peroxidase. *Neurosci. Lett.* **41**:233–238.

Craigie, E.H. (1960). *Bensley's Practical Anatomy of the Rabbit.* University of Toronto Press, Toronto.

Crosby, E.C., R.C. Schneider, B.R. de Jonge, and P. Szonyi (1966). The alterations of tonus and movements through the interplay between the cerebral hemispheres and the cerebellum. *J. Comp. Neurol. (Suppl. 1)* **127**:1–91.

Crossman, A.R., M.A. Sambrook, and A. Jackson (1984). Experimental hemichorea/hemiballismus in the monkey. Studies of the intracerebral site of action in a drug-induced dyskinesia. *Brain* **107**:579–596.

Crouch, J.E. (1969). *Text-Atlas of Cat Anatomy.* Lea & Febiger, Philadelphia.

Cullheim, S., and J.O. Kellerth (1978). A morphological study of the axons and recurrent collaterals of cat motoneurones supplying different hind-limb muscles. *J. Physiol. (London)* **281**:285–299.

Curthoys, I.S., and C.H. Markham (1971). Convergence of labyrinthine influences on units in the vestibular nuclei of the cat. I. Natural stimulation. *Brain Res.* **35**:469–490.

Curthoys, I., E. Curthoys, R. Blanks, and C. Markham (1975). Orientation of semicircular canals in guinea pig. *Acta Otolaryngol.* **80**:197–205.

Curthoys, I.S., R.H.I. Blanks, and C.H. Markham (1977). Semicircular canal functional anatomy in cat, guinea pig and man. *Acta Otolaryngol.* **83**:258–265.

Curtis, D.R., K. Krnjevic, and R. Miledi (1958). Crossed inhibition of sacral motoneurones. *J. Neurophysiol.* **21**:319–326.

Curzon, G. (1973). Involuntary movements other than parkinsonism. Biochemical aspects. *Proc. R. Soc. Med.* **66**:873–875.

Darlot, C., P. Denise, and J. Droulez (1985). Modulation of horizontal eye position of the vestibulo-collic reflex induced by tilting in the frontal plane in the alert cat. *Exp. Brain Res.* **58**:510–519.

d'Ascanio, P., E. Bettini, and O. Pompeiano (1985a). Tonic inhibitory influences of locus coeruleus on the response gain of limb extensors to sinusoidal labyrinth and neck stimulations. *Arch. Ital. Biol.* **123**:69–100.

d'Ascanio, P., E. Bettini, and O. Pompeiano (1985b). Tonic facilitatory influences of dorsal pontine reticular structures on the response gain of limb extensors to sinusoidal labyrinth and neck stimulations. *Arch. Ital. Biol.* **123**:101–132.

DeJong, T.V.M., J.M.B.V. DeJong, B. Cohen, and L.B.W. Jongkees (1977). Ataxia and nystagmus induced by injection of local anesthetics in the neck. *Ann. Neurol.* **1**:240–246.

Delong, M.R., M.D. Crutcher, and A.P. Georgopoulous (1985). Primate globus pallidus and subthalamic nucleus: Functional organization. *J. Neurophysiol.* **53**:530–543.

Denoth, F., P.C. Magherini, O. Pompeiano, and M. Stanojevic (1979a). Responses of Purkinje cells of the cerebellar vermis to neck and macular vestibular inputs. *Pflugers Arch.* **381**:87–98.

Denoth, F., P.C. Magherini, O. Pompeiano, and M. Stanojevic (1979b). Neck and macular labyrinthine influences on the Purkinje cell of the cerebellar vermis in *Reflex Control of Posuture and Movement* (R. Granit and O. Pompeiano, ed.), pp. 515–527. Elsevier/North-Holland Biomedical Press, Amsterdam.

Denoth, F., P.C. Magherini, O. Pompeiano, and M. Stanojevic (1980). Responses of Purkinje cells of cerebellar vermis to sinusoidal rotation of neck. *J. Neurophysiol.* **43**:46–59.

Dichgans, J., E. Bizzi, P. Morasso, and V. Tagliasco (1973). Mechanisms underlying recovery of eye-head coordination following bilateral labyrinthectomy in monkeys. *Exp. Brain Res.* **18**:548–562.

Dichgans, J., E. Bizzi, P. Morasso, and V. Tagliasco (1974). The role of vestibular and neck afferents during eye-head coordination in the monkey. *Brain Res.* **71**:225–232.

Dieringer, N., and W. Precht (1982a). Compensatory head and eye movements in the frog and their contribution to stabilization of gaze. *Exp. Brain Res.* **47**:394–406.

Dieringer, N., and W. Precht (1982b). Dynamics of compensatory vestibular reflexes in the grassfrog, *Rana temporaria*. In *Physiological and Pathological Aspects of Eye Movements*. (A. Roucoux and M. Crommelinck, eds.), pp. 417–423. Junk, The Hague.

Dieringer, N., W. Precht, and A.R. Blight (1982). Resetting fast phases of head and eye and their linkage in the frog. *Exp. Brain Res.* **47**:407–416.

Dieringer, N., S.L. Cochran, and W. Precht (1983). Differences in the central organization of gaze stabilizing reflexes between frog and turtle. *J. Comp. Physiol.* **153**:495–508.

Dieringer, N., and W. Precht (1985). Coordination of fast phases of head and eye to intact and vestibularly lesioned unrestrained frogs. *Neurosci. Lett. Suppl.* **2**:479.

Dieringer, N. (1986). Vergleichende Neurobiologie der Organisation von blickstabilisierenden Reflexsystemen bei Wirbeltieren. *Naturwissenschaften* **73**:299–304.

Dieringer, N., and W.J. Daunicht (1986). Image fading—a problem for frogs? *Naturwissenschaften* **73**:330–332.

Dieringer, N., and W. Precht (1986). Functional organization of eye velocity and eye position signals in abducens motoneurons of the frog. *J. Comp. Physiol.* **158**:179–194.

Dieringer, N. (1987). The role of compensatory eye and head movements for gaze stabilization in the unrestrained frog. *Brain Res.*, **404**:33–38.

Dow, R.S. (1938). Effect of lesions in the vestibular part of the cerebellum in primates. *Arch. Neurol. Psychiat.* **40**:500–520.

Dow, R.S. (1970). Historical review of cerebellar investigation. In *The Cerebellum in Health and Disease* (W.S. Fiels and W.D. Willis, eds.), pp. 5–38. Warren H. Green, St. Louis.

Dubrovsky, B.O., and H. Barbas (1977). Frontal projections of dorsal neck and extraocular muscles. *Exp. Neurol.* **55**:680–693.

Duchenne, G.B.A. (1867). *Physiologie des Mouvements*. (Translated by E.B. Kaplan, 1949). Lippincott, Philadelphia.

Dunlap, K., and O.H. Mowrer (1931). Head movements and eye functions of birds. *J. Comp. Psychol.* **11**:99–113.

Dutia, M.B., and M.J. Hunter (1985). The sagittal vestibulocollic reflex and its interaction with neck proprioceptive afferents in the decerebrate cat. *J. Physiol. (London)* **359**:17–29.

Dykes, R.W., D.D. Rasmusson, D. Sretavan, and N.B. Rehman (1982). Submodality segregation and receptive-field sequences in cuneate, gracile and external cuneate nuclei of the cat. *J. Neurophysiol.* **47**:389–416.

Easter, S.S., Jr., P.R. Johns, and D. Heckenlively (1974). Horizontal compensatory eye movements in goldfish (*Carassius auratus*). I. The normal animal. *J. Comp. Physiol.* **92**:23–35.

Eccles, J.C., P. Fatt, and S. Landgren (1956). Central pathway for direct inhibitory action of impulses in largest afferent nerve fibres to muscle. *J. Neurophysiol.* **19**:75–98.

Eccles, J.C., R.M. Eccles, and A. Lundberg (1957a). Synaptic actions on motoneurones in relation to the two components of the group I muscle afferent volley. *J. Physiol. (London)* **136**:527–546.

Eccles, J.C., R.M. Eccles, and A. Lundberg (1957b). The convergence of monosyaptic excitatory afferents on to many different species of alpha motoneurones. *J. Physiol. (London)* **137**:22–50.

Eccles, J.C., R.M. Eccles, and A. Lundberg (1957c). Synaptic actions on motoneurones caused by impulses in Golgi tendon organ afferents. *J. Physiol. (London)* **138**:227–252.

Eccles, J.C., and A. Lundberg (1958). Integrative pattern of Ia synaptic actions on motoneurons of hip and knee muscles. *J. Physiol. (London)* **144**:271–298.

Eccles, R.M., and A. Lundberg (1959). Synaptic actions in motoneurones by afferents which may evoke the flexion reflex. *Arch. Ital. Biol.* **97**:199–221.

Eccles, J.C., R.M. Eccles, A. Iggo, and M. Ito (1961a). Distribution of recurrent inhibition among motoneurones. *J. Physiol. (London)* **159**:479–499.

Eccles, J.C., R.M. Eccles, A. Iggo, and A. Lundberg (1961b). Electrophysiological investigation on Renshaw cells. *J. Physiol. (London)* **159**:461–478.

Eccles, J.C., R.A. Nicoll, W.F. Schwarz, H. Taborikova, and T.J. Willey (1975). Reticulospinal neurons with and without monosynaptic inputs from cerebellar nuclei. *J. Neurophysiol.* **38**:513–530.

Edney, D.P., and J.D. Porter (1986). Neck muscle afferent projections to the brainstem of the monkey: Implications for the neural control of gaze. *J. Comp. Neurol.* **250**:389–398.

Edwards, S.B. (1975). Autoradiographic studies of the projections of the midbrain reticular formation: descending projections of nucleus cuneiformis. *J. Comp. Neurol.* **161**:341–358.

Edwards, S.B. (1977). The commissural projection of the superior colliculus in the cat. *J. Comp. Neurol.* **173**:23–40.

Edwards, S.B., and C.K. Henkel (1978). Superior colliculus connections with the extraocular motor nuclei in the cat. *J. Comp. Neurol.* **179**:451–468.

Ekerot, C.-F., B. Larson, and O. Oscarsson (1979). Information carried by the spinocerebellar paths. *Prog. Brain Res.* **50**:79–90.

Eldred, E., A. Maier, and C.F. Bridgman (1974). Differences in intrafusal fiber content of spindles in several muscles of the cat. *Exp. Neurol.* **45**:8–18.

Elliott, R. (1963). *Anatomy of the Cat*, 3rd. ed. Holt, Rinehart & Winston, New York.

Erway, L.C., B. Ghelarducci, O. Pompeiano, and M. Stanojevic (1978). Responses of cerebellar fastigial neurons to afferent inputs from neck muscles and macular labyrinthine receptors. *Arch. Ital. Biol.* **116**:173–024.

Escolar, J. (1948). The afferent connections of the 1st., 2nd. and 3rd. cervical nerves in the cat. *J. Comp. Neurol.* **89**:79–91.

Estes, M.S., R.H.I. Blanks, and C.H. Markham (1975). Physiological characteristics of vestibular first-order canal neurons in the cat. I. Response plane determination and resting discharge characteristics. *J. Neurophysiol.* **38**:1232–1249.

Evans, H.E., and G.C. Christensen (1979). *Miller's Anatomy of the Dog*, 2nd ed., pp. 303–316. W.B. Saunders Co., Philadelphia.

Evarts, E.V., and J. Tanji (1974). Gating of motor cortex reflexes by prior instruction. *Brain Res.* **71**:479–494.

Ewald, J.R. (1892). *Physiologische Untersuchungen uber das Endorgan des Nervus octavus*. Bergmann, Wiesbaden.

Ewert, J.P. (1967). Elektrische Reizung des retinalen Projektionsfeldes im Mittelhirn der Erdkröte (*Bufo bufo* L.): *Pflugers Arch.* **295**:90–98.

Ewing, C.L., and D.J. Thomas (1972). Human head and neck response to impact acceleration. NAMRL Monograph 21, Naval Aerospace Medical Res. Lab, Pensacola, FL.

Ezure, K., and S. Sasaki (1978). Frequency-response analysis of vestibular-induced neck reflex in cat. I. Characteristics of neural transmission from horizontal semicircular canal to neck motoneurons. *J. Neurophysiol.* **41**:445–458.

Ezure, K., S. Sasaki, Y. Uchino, and V.J. Wilson (1978). Frequency response analysis of vestibular-induced neck reflex in cat. II. Functional significance of cervical afferents and polysynaptic descending pathways. *J. Neurophysiol.* **41**:459–471.

Ezure, K., and V.J. Wilson (1983). Dynamics of neck-to-forelimb reflexes in the decerebrate cat. *J. Neurophysiol.* **50**:688–695.

Ezure, K., K. Fukushima, R.H. Schor, and V.J. Wilson (1983). Compartmentalization of the cervicocollic reflex in cat splenius muscle. *Exp. Brain Res.* **51**:397–404.

Ezure, K., and V.J. Wilson (1984). Interaction of tonic neck and vestibular reflexes in the forelimb of the decerebrate cat. *Exp. Brain Res.* **54**:289–292.

Fanardjian, V.V., and V.A. Sarkissian (1980). Spatial organization of the cerebellar corticovestibular projection in the cat. *Neuroscience* **5**:551–558.

Faulkner, R.F., and J.E. Hyde (1958). Coordinated eye and body movements evoked by brainstem stimulation in decerebrated cats. *J. Neurophysiol.* **21**:171–182.

Feldon, S., P. Feldon, and L. Kruger (1970). Topography of the retinal projection upon the superior colliculus of the cat. *Vision Res.* **10**:135–193.

Fernandez, C., and J.M. Goldberg (1971). Physiology of peripheral neurons innervating semicircular canals of the squirrel monkey. II. Response to sinusoidal stimulation and dynamics of peripheral vestibular system. *J. Neurophysiol.* **34**:661–675.

Fernandez, C., and J. Goldberg (1976a). Physiology of peripheral neurons innervating otolith organs of the squirrel monkey. I. Response to static tilts and to long-duration centrifugal force. *J. Neurophysiol.* **39**:970–984.

Fernandez, C., and J. Goldberg (1976b). Physiology of peripheral neurons innervating otolith organs of the squirrel monkey. II. Directional selectivity and force-response relations. *J. Neurophysiol.* **39**:985–995.

Fernandez, C., and J. Goldberg (1976c). Physiology of peripheral neurons innervating otolith organs of the squirrel monkey. III. Response dynamics. *J. Neurophysiol.* **39**:996–1008.

Ferraro, A., and S.E. Barrera (1935). Posterior column fibres and their termination in macacus rhesus. *J. Comp. Neurol.* **62**:507–530.

Ferrier, D. (1886). *The Functions of the Brain*, 2nd ed., London.

Fetz, E.E., E. Jankowska, T. Johannisson, and J. Lipski (1979). Autogenetic inhibition of motoneurones by impulses in group Ia muscle spindle afferents. *J. Physiol. (London)* **293**:173–195.

Fink, R.P., and L. Heimer (1967). Two methods for selective silver impregnation of degenerating axons and their synaptic endings in the central nervous system. *Brain Res.* **4**:369–374.

Fite, K.V., A. Reiner, and S.P. Hunt (1979). Optokinetic nystagmus and the accessory optic system of pigeon and turtle. *Brain Behav. Evol.* **16**:192–202.

Flament, D., and J. Hore (1986). Movement and electromyographic disorders associated with cerebellar dysmetria. *J. Neurophysiol.* **55**:1221–1233.

Flanders, M. (1985). Visually guided head movements in the african chameleon. *Vison Res.* **25**:935–942.

Fleming, D., W. Vossius, G. Bowman, and E. Johnstop (1969). Adaptive properties of eye tracking system as revealed by moving head and open loop studies. *Ann. N.Y. Acad. Sci.* **156**:825–850.

Fleming, F., and P.K. Rose (1983). Distribution axon collaterals of identified medial vestibulospinal axons in the upper cervical spinal cord of the cat. *Soc. Neurosci. Abstr.* **9**:663.

Fleshman, J.W., A. Lev-Tov, and R.E. Burke (1984). Peripheral and central control of flexor digitorum longus and flexor hallucis longus motoneurons: The synaptic basis of functional diversity. *Exp. Brain Res.* **54**:133–149.

Foix, Ch., and D.A. Thevenard (1929). Le reflexe de posture. *Rev. Neurol.* **30**:449–468.

Foltz, E.L., L.M. Knopp, and A.A. Ward (1959). Experimental spasmodic torticollis. *J. Neurosurg.* **36**:55–72.

Frankfurter, A., J.T. Weber, G.J. Royce, N.L. Strominger, and J.K. Harting (1976). An autoradiographic analysis of the tecto-olivary projection in primates. *Brain Res.* **118**:245–257.

Fredrickson, J.M., D. Schwarz, and H.H. Kornhuber (1966). Convergence and interaction of vestibular and deep somatic afferents upon neurons in the vestibular nuclei of the cat. *Acta Otolaryngol.* **61**:168–188.

Friedman, A., and S. Fahn (1986). Spontaneous remissions in spasmodic torticollis. *Neurology* **36**:398–400.

Friedman, S.M. (1970). *Visual Anatomy. Vol. 1. Head and Neck.* Harper & Row, New York.

Fritz, N. (1981). Ia Synergismus an der vorderen Extremitat der Katze. Dissertation. Ludwig-Maximilians-Universitat, Munchen, FRG.

Fuchs, A.F., and J. Kimm (1975). Unit activity in vestibular nucleus of alert monkey during horizontal angular acceleration and eye movement. *J. Neurophysiol.* **38**:1140–1161.

Fuchs, A.F., C.R.S. Kaneko, and C.A. Scudder (1985). Brainstem control of saccade eye movements. *Annu. Rev. Neurosci.* **8**:307–337.

Fukuda, J., S.M. Highstein, and M.Ito (1972). Cerebellar inhibitory control of the vestibulo-ocular reflex investigated in rabbit 3rd. nucleus. *Exp. Brain Res.* **14**:511–526.

Fukuda, T. (1983). *Statokinetic Reflexes in Equilibrium and Movement.* University of Tokyo Press, Tokyo.

Fukushima, K., N. Hirai, and S. Rapoport (1979a). Direct excitation of neck flexor motoneurons by the interstitiospinal tract. Brain Res. **160**:358–362.

Fukushima, K., N. Hirai, and S. Rapoport (1979b). Vestibulo-spinal, reticulospinal and interstitiospinal pathways in the cat. *Prog. Brain Res.* **50**:121–136.

Fukushima, K., B.W. Peterson, and V.J. Wilson (1979c). Vestibulospinal, reticulospinal and interstitiospinal pathways in the cat. *Prog. Brain Res.* **50**:121–135.

Fukushima, K., S. Murakimi, J. Matsushima, and M. Kato (1980a). Vestibular responses and branching of interstitiospinal neurons. *Exp. Brain Res.* **40**:131–145.

Fukushima, K., S. Murakami, M. Ohno, and M. Kato (1980b). Properties of mesencephalic reticulospinal neurons in the cat. *Exp. Brain Res.* **41**:75–78.

Fukushima, K., M. Ohno, S. Murakami, and M. Kato (1981). Effects of stimulation of frontal cortex, superior colliculus, and neck muscle afferents on interstitiospinal neurons in the cat. *Exp. Brain Res.* **44**:143–153.

Fukushima, K., K. Takahashi, J. Kudo, and M. Kato (1985). Interstitial-vestibular interaction in the control of head posture. *Exp. Brain Res.* **57**:264–270.

Fukushima, K. (1986). The interstitial nucleus of Cajal and its role in the control of movements of head and eyes. Progress in Neurobiol. (in press).

Fuller, J.H. (1978). Vestibular and neck sensory input to units in the vestibular nucleus of alert cats. *Soc. Neurosci. Abstr.* **4**:611.

Fuller, J.H. (1980a). The dynamic neck–eye reflex in mammals. *Exp. Brain Res.* **41**:29–35.

Fuller, J.H. (1980b). Linkage of eye and head movements in the alert rabbit. *Brain Res.* **194**:219–222.

Fuller, J.H. (1981). Eye and head movements during vestibular stimulation in the alert rabbit. *Brain Res.* **205**:363–381.

Fuller, J.H., H. Maldonado, and J. Schlag (1983). Vestibular-oculomotor interaction in cat eye–head movements. *Brain Res.* **271**:241–250.

Funk, C.J., and M.E. Anderson (1977). Saccadic eye movements and eye–head coordination in children. *Percept. Motor Skills* **44**:599–610.

Gans, C., and R.G. Northcutt (1983). Neural crest and the origin of vertebrates: A new head. *Science* **220**:268–274.

Gauthier, G.M., B. Martin, and L. Stark (1981). Effect of inertial loads on head–eye movements. *Proc. OMS '81*, California Institute of Technology, Pasadena, CA.

Georgopoulos, A.P., R. Caminiti, J.F. Kalaska, and J.P. Massey (1983). Spatial coding of movements: A hypothesis concerning the coding of movement direction by motor cortical populations. *Neural Coding of Motor Performance, Exp. Brain Res. (Suppl.)* **7**:327–336.

Gesell, A. (1938). The tonic neck reflex in the human infant. *J. Pediat.* **13**:455–464.

Gesell, A., and L.B. Ames (1950). Tonick-neck-reflex and symmetro-tonic behavior. *J. Pediat.* **36**:165–176.

Ghez, C., and D. Vicario (1978). The control of rapid limb movement in the cat. I. Response latency. *Exp. Brain Res.* **33**:173–189.

Gielen, C.C.A.M., and E.J. van Zuylen (1986). Coordination of arm muscles during flexion and supination: Application of the tensor analysis approach. *Neuroscience* **17**:527–539.

Gilman, J., and F. Bloedel (1982). *Diseases of the Cerebellum.* F.A. Davis Company, Philadelphia.

Gioanni, H. (1986). Quantitative study of optokinetic and vestibular responses of the eyes and of the head in the pigeon. *Neurosci. Lett. (Suppl.)* **26**:551.

Godlowski, W. (1938). Experimentelle Untersuchungen ueber die durch Reizung des Zwischen- und Mittelhirns hervorgerufenen assoziierten Augenbewegungen. *Z. ges. Neurol. Psychiat.* **162**:160–182.

Goel, V.K., C.R. Clark, D. McGoman, and S. Goyal (1984). An in-vitro study of the kinematics of the normal, injured and stabilized cervical spine. *J. Biomech.* **17**:363–376.

Goldberg, J., and B.W. Peterson (1986). Reflex and mechanical contributions to head stabilization in alert cats. *J. Neurophysiol.* **56**:857–875.

Goldberg, M.E., and R.H. Wurtz (1972). Activity of superior colliculus in behaving monkey. II. Effect of attention on neuronal responses. *J. Neurophysiol.* **35**:560–574.

Goldsmith, W. (1972). Biomechanics of head injury. In *Biomechanics, Its Foundations and Objectives* (Y.C. Fung, N. Perrone, and M. Anliker, eds.), pp. 585–634. Prentice Hall, Englewood Cliffs, NJ.

Gordon, A.M., A.F. Huxley, and F.J. Julian (1966). The variation isometric tension with sarcomere length in vertebrate muscle fibers. *J. Physiol. (London)* **184**:170–192.

Gottlieb, G.L., and G.C. Agarwal (1980). Response to sudden torques about ankle in man. III. Suppression of stretch-evoked responses during phasic contraction. *J. Neurophysiol.* **44**:233–246.

Graf, W., P.P. Vidal, and C. Evinger (1986). Biomechanical properties of the head movement system. In *The Control of Head Movement Abstracts.* Satellite Symposium of XXX IUPS Congress, Whistler, B.C.

Grant, G., J. Arvidsson, B. Robertson, and J. Ygge (1979). Transganglionic transport of horseradish peroxidase in primary sensory neurons. *Neurosci. Lett.* **12**:23–28.

Grant, G., M. Illert, and R. Tanaka (1980). Integration in descending motor pathways controlling the forelimb in the cat. 6. Anatomical evidence consistent with the existence of C3–C4 propriospinal neurones projecting to forelimb motor nuclei. *Exp. Brain Res.* **38**:87–93.

Grant, G., and J. Ygge (1981). Somatotopic organization of the thoracic spinal nerve in the dorsal horn demonstrated with transganglionic degeneration. *J. Comp. Neurol.* **202**:357–364.

Grantyn, A., and R. Grantyn (1976). Synaptic actions of tectofugal pathways on abducens motoneurons in the cat. *Brain Res.* **105**:269–285.

Grantyn, A., R. Grantyn, and K.-P. Robiné (1977). Neuronal organization of the tecto-oculomotor pathways. In Control of Gaze by Brain Stem Neurons (R. Baker, and A. Berthoz, eds.), pp. 197–206. Elsevier/North Holland Biomedical Press, Amsterdam, New York.

Grantyn, R., R. Baker, and A. Grantyn (1980). Morphological and physiological identification of excitatory pontine reticular neurons projecting in the cat abducens nucleus and spinal cord. *Brain Res.* 198:221–228.

Grantyn, A., and R. Grantyn (1982). Axonal patterns and sites of termination of cat superior colliculus neurons projecting in the tecto-bulbo-spinal tract. *Exp. Brain Res.* **46**:243–256.

Grantyn, A., R. Grantyn, A. Berthoz, and J. Ribas (1982). Tectal control of vertical eye movements: A search for underlying neuronal circuits in the mesencephalon. In Physiological and Pathological Aspects of Eye Movements (A. Roucoux, and M. Crommelinck, eds.), pp. 337–344. Dr. W. Junk Publishers, The Hague.

Grantyn, A., and A. Berthoz (1983). Discharge patterns of tecto-bulbo-spinal neurons during visuo-motor reactions in the alert cat. *Soc. Neurosci. Abstr.* **9**:751.

Grantyn, A., and A. Berthoz (1985). Burst activity of identified tecto-reticulo-spinal neurons in the alert cat. *Exp. Brain Res.* **57**:417–421.

Grantyn, A., A. Berthoz, and V. Ong-Meang (1985). Pontine reticulospinal neurons are a component of a reticular circuits controlling eye-head synergies. *Soc. Neurosci. Abstr.* **11**:1039.

Grantyn, A., and A. Berthoz (1987). Reticulo-spinal neurons participating in the control of synergic eye and head movements during orienting in the cat. I. Behavioral properties. *Exp. Brain Res.*, **66**:339–354.

Grantyn, A., V. Ong-Meang Jacques, and A. Berthoz (1987). Reticulospinal neurons participating in the control of synergic eye and head movements during orienting in the cat. II. Morphological properties as revealed by intra-axonal injections of horseradish peroxidase. *Exp. Brain Res.* **66**:355–377.

Greene, E.C. (1968). *Anatomy of the Rat.* Hafner, New York.

Gresty, M.A. (1974). Coordination of head and eye movements to fixate continuous and intermittent targets. *Vision Res.* **14**:395–403.

Gresty, M.A. (1975). Eye, head and body movements of the guinea pig in response to optokinetic stimulation and sinusoidal oscillation in yaw. *Pflugers Arch.* **353**:201–214.

Gresty, M.A. (1976). A reexamination of "neck reflex" eye movements in the rabbit. *Acta Otolaryngol.* **81**:386–394.

Gresty, M., and R. Baker (1976). Neurons with visual receptive field, eye movement and neck displacement sensitivity within and around the nucleus prepositus hypoglossi in the alert cat. *Exp. Brain Res.* **24**:429–433.

Gresty, M., and J. Leech (1977). Coordination of the head and eyes in pursuit of predictable and random target motion. *Aviat. Space Environ. Med.* **48**:741–744.

Grillner, S., and S. Lund (1968). The origin of a descending pathway with monosynaptic action of flexor motoneurons. *Acta Physiol. Scand.* **74**:274–284.

Grillner, S., T. Hongo, and S. Lund (1970). The vestibulospinal tract. Effects on alpha-motoneurones in the lumbosacral spinal cord in the cat. *Exp. Brain Res.* **10**:94–120.

Grillner, S., T. Hongo, and S. Lund (1971). Convergent effects on alpha motoneurones from the vestibulospinal tract and a pathway descending in the medial longitudinal fasciculus. *Exp. Brain Res.* **12**:457–479.

Guitton, D., M. Crommelinck, and A. Roucoux (1980). Stimulation of the superior colliculus in the alert cat. I. Eye movements and neck EMG activity evoked when the head is restrained. *Exp. Brain Res.* **39**:63–73.

Guitton, D., H. Buchtel, and R. Douglas (1982). Disturbances of voluntary saccadic eye movement mechanisms following discrete unilateral frontal lobe removals. In *Basis of Ocular Motility Disorders* (G. Lennerstrand, D.S. Zee, and E. Keller, eds.), pp. 497–499. Pergamon Press, Oxford.

Guitton, D., R.M. Douglas, and M. Volle (1984a). Rapid eye–head orienting movements in cat: Dependence of motor strategy on gaze amplitude. *J. Physiol.* **52**:1020–1030.

Guitton, D., M. Douglas, and M. Volle (1984b). Eye–head coordination cats. *J. Neurophysiol.* **52**:1030–1050.

Guitton, D., R.E. Kearney, N. Wereley, and B.W. Peterson (1986). Visual, vestibular and voluntary contributions to human head stabilization. *Exp. Brain Res.* **64**:59–69.

Guitton, D., and M. Volle (1987). Gaze control in humans: Eye-head coordination during orienting movements to targets within and beyond the oculomotor range. *J. Neurophysiol.* **58**:427–459.

Gura, E.V., and Yu.P. Limanskii (1976). Antidromic and synaptic potentials of motoneurons of the cat accessory nucleus. *Neurophysiology* **8**:246–248.

Haase, J., S. Cleveland, and H.-G. Ross (1975). Problems of postsynaptic autogenous and recurrent inhibition the mammalian spinal cord. *Rev. Physiol. Biochem. Pharmacol.* **73**:74–129.

Hagbarth, K.-E. (1952). Exitatory and inhibitory skin areas for flexor and extensor motoneurones. *Acta Physiol. Scand. Suppl. 94* **26**:1–58.

Hamm, T.M., W. Koehler, D.G. Stuart, and S. Vanden Noven (1985). Partitioning of monosynaptic Ia excitatory post-synaptic potentials in the motor nucleus of the cat semimembranosus muscle. *J. Physiol. (London)* **369**:379–398.

Hammond, P.H. (1956). The influence of prior instruction to the subject on an apparently involuntary neuro-muscular response. *J. Physiol. (London)* **132**:17–18.

Hampson, J.L., C.R. Harrison, and C.N. Woolsey (1946). Somatotopic localization in the cerebellum. *Fed. Proc.* **5**:41.

Hannaford, B., R. Maduel, M.N. Nam, V. Lakshminarayanan, and L. Stark (1983). Effects of loads on time optimal head movements: EMG, oblique, and main sequence relationships. *19th. Ann. Conf. Manual Control*, MIT, Cambridge, pp. 483–499.

Hannaford, B., and L. Stark (1984). Control strategies for neurologically ballistic movements. *Proc. 37th ACEMB*, Los Angeles, CA.

Hannaford, B., M.H. Nam, V. Lakshminarayanan, and L. Stark (1984). Electromyographic evidence of neurological controller signals with viscous load. *J. Motor Behav.* **16**:255–274.

Hannaford, B. (1985). *Control of fast movement: Human head rotation.* Ph.D. thesis, Department of Electrical Engineering and Computer Science, University of California, Berkeley.

Hannaford, B., and L. Stark (1985). Roles of the elements of the tri-phasic control signal. *Exp. Neurol.* **90**:619–634.

Hannaford, B., G. Cheron, and L. Stark (1985). The effects of applied vibration the triphasic EMG pattern in neurologically ballistic head movements. *Exp. Neurol.* **88**:447–460.

Hannaford, B., W.S. Kim, S.H. Lee, and L. Stark (1986). Neurological control of head movements: Inverse modeling and electromyographic evidence. *Math. BioSci.* **78**:159–178.

Harris, L.R. (1980). The superior colliculus and movements of the head and eyes in cats. *J. Physiol. (London)* **300**:367–391.

Harrison, P.J., and D. Zytnicki (1984). Crossed actions of group I muscle afferents in the cat. *J. Physiol. (London)* **356**:263–273.

Harting, J.K. (1977). Descending pathways from the superior colliculus: An autoradiographic analysis in the rhesus monkey (Macaca mulatta). *J. Comp. Neurol.* **173**:583–612.

Harting, J.K., M.F. Huerta, A.J. Frankfurther, N.L. Strominger, and G.J. Royce (1980). Ascending pathways from the monkey superior colliculus: An autoradiographic analysis. *J. Comp. Neurol.* **192**:853–882.

Hartman, C.G., and L. Straus, Jr. (1961). *The Anatomy of the Rhesus Monkey (Macaca mulatta).* Hafner, New York.

Hasan, Z., and J.C. Houk (1975). Transition in sensitivty of spindle receptors that occurs when muscle is stretched more than a fraction of a millimeter. *J. Neurophysiol.* **38**:673–689.

Hassler, R. (1956a). Die zentralen Apparate der Wendebewegungen. I. Ipsiversive Wendungen durch Reizung einer direkten vestibulothalamischen Bahn im Hirnstamm der Katze. *Arch. Psychiat. Nervenkr.* **194**:456–480.

Hassler, R. (1956b). Die zentralen Apparate der Wendebewegungen. II. Die neuronalen Apparate der vestibulären Korrekturwendungen und der Adversivbewegungen. *Arch. Psychiat. Nervenkr.* **194**:481–516.

Hassler, R., and W.R. Hess (1954). Experimentelle und anatomische Befunde über die Drehbewegungen und ihre nervösen Apparate. *Arch. Psychiat. Nervenkr.* **192**:488–526.

Hassler, R., and G. Diekmann (1970). Stereotactic treatment of different kinds of spasmodic torticollis. *Confin. Neurol.* **32**:135–143.

Hatze, H. (1978). A general myocybernetic control model of skeletal muscle. *Biol. Cybern.* **28**:143–157.

Hebel, R., and M.W. Stromberg (1976). *Anatomy of the Laboratory Rat.* Williams & Wilkins, Baltimore.

Hellebrandt, F.A., S.J. Houtz, M.J. Partridge, and C.E. Walters (1956). Tonic neck reflexes in exercises of stress in man. *Am. J. Phys. Med.* **35**:144–159.

Hellebrandt, F.A., M. Schade, and M.L. Carns (1962). Methods of evoking the tonic neck reflexes in normal human subjects. *Am. J. Phys. Med.* **41**:90–139.

Henneman, E., and L.M. Mendell (1981). Functional organization of motoneuron pool and its inputs. In *Handbook of Physiology, Vol. II, Section 1. The Nervous System* (V.E. Brooks, ed.), pp. 423–507. American Physiological Society, Bethesda, MD.

Hess, D.T. (1982). The tecto-olivo-cerebellar pathway in the rat. *Brain Res.* **250**:143–148.

Hess, W.R., S. Burgi, and V. Bucher (1946). Motorische Funktion des Tektal- und Tegmentalgebietes. *Mschr. Psychiat. Neurol.* **112**:1–52.

Hiatt, J.L., and L.P. Gartner (1982). *Textbook of Head and Neck Anatomy.* Appleton-Century-Crofts, New York.

Hikosaka, O., and M. Maeda (1973). Cervical effects on abducens motoneurons and their interaction with vestibulo-ocular reflex. *Exp. Brain Res.* **18**:512–530.

Hill, A.V. (1938). The heat of shortening and the dynamic constants of muscle. *Proc. Roy. Soc. Ser. B* **126**:136–195.

Hinoki, M., S. Hine, S. Okada, Y. Ishida, S. Koike, and S. Shizuki (1975). Optic organ and cervical proprioceptors in maintenance of body equilbrium. *Acta Otolaryngol. (Suppl.) (Stockholm)* **330**:169–184.

Hinsey, J.C., S.W. Ranson, and H.H. Dixon (1930). Responses elicited by stimulation of the mesencephalic tegmentum in the cat. *Arch. Neurol. Psychiat.* **24**:966–977.

Hirai, N., T. Hongo, and S. Sasaki (1978). Cerebellar projection and input organizations of the spinocerebellar tract arising from the central cervical nucleus in the cat. *Brain Res.* **157**:341–345.

Harai, N. (1983). Vestibular afferent inputs to lobules I and II of the cerebellar anterior lobe vermis in the cat. *Brain Res.* **277**:145–149.

Hirai, N., and Y. Uchino (1984). Floccular influence on excitatory relay neurones of vestibular reflexes of anterior semicircular canal origin in the cat. *Neurosci. Res.* **1**:327–340.

Hirai, N., T. Hongo, and S. Sasaki (1984a). A physiological study of identification, axonal course and cerebellar projection of spinocerebellar tract cells in central cervical nucleus of the cat. *Exp. Brain Res.* **55**:272–285.

Hirai, N., T. Hongo, S. Sasaki, M. Yamashita, and K. Yoshida (1984b). Neck muscle afferent input to spino-cerebellar tract cells of the central cervical nucleus of cat. *Exp. Brain Res.* **55**:286–300.

Hirai, N. (1987). Input–output relations of lobules I and II of the cerebellar anterior lobe vermis in connection with neck and vestibulospinal reflexes in the cat. *Neurosci. Res.* **4**:167–184.

Holmes, G. (1917). The symptoms of acute cerebellar injuries due to gunshot injuries. *Brain* **40**:461–535.

Holmqvist, B. (1961). Crossed spinal reflex actions evoked by volleys in somatic afferents. *Acta Physiol. Scand., Suppl. 181* **52**:1–66.

Holomanova, A., G. Cierny, and J. Zlatos (1972). Localization of the motor cells of the spinal root of the accessory nerve in the cat. *Folia Morphol.* **20**:232–234.

Holstege, G., H.G.J.M. Kuypers, and R.C. Boer (1979). Anatomical evidence for direct brainstem projections to the somatic motoneuronal cell groups and autonomic preganglionic cell groups in the cat spinal cord. *Brain Res.* **171**:393–433.

Holstege, G., and H. Collewign (1982). The efferent connections of the nucleus of the optic tract and the superior colliculus in the rabbit. *J. Comp. Neurol.* **209**:139–175.

Holstege, G., and H.G.J.M. Kuypers (1982). The anatomy of brain stem pathways to the spinal cord of the cat. A labelled amino acid tracing study. *Prog. Brain Res.* **57**:145–175.

Horridge, G.A. (1966). Direct response of the crab *Carcinus* to the movement of the sun. *J. Exp. Biol.* **44**:275–283.

Hosey, R.R., and Y.K. Liu (1982). A homeomorphic finite element model of the human head and neck. In *Finite Elements in Biomechanics* (R.H. Gallagher, B.R. Simon, P.C. Johnson, and J.F. Gross, eds.), pp. 379–401. John Wiley, New York.

Houk, J., and E. Henneman (1967). Responses of Golgi tendon organs to active contractions of the soleus muscle of the cat. *J. Neurophysiol.* **30**:466–481.

Huerta, M.F., and J.K. Harting (1982). Tectal control of spinal cord activity: Neuroanatomical demonstration of pathways connecting the superior colliculus with the cervical spinal cord grey. In *Progress in Brain Research, Vol. 57* (H.G.J.M. Kuypers and G.F. Martin, eds.), pp. 293–328. Elsevier Biomedical Press, Amsterdam.

Huizinga, E., and P. Van der Meulen (1951). Vestibular rotatory and optokinetic reactions in the pigeon. *Ann. Otol.-Rhinol.-Laryngol.* **60**:927–947.

Hulliger, M. (1984). The mammalian muscle spindle and its central control. *Rev. Physiol. Biochem. Parmacol.* **101**:1–110.

Hultborn, H., E. Jankowska and S. Lindstrom (1971). Relative contribution from different nerves to recurrent depression of Ia ipsps in motoneurones. *J. Phsyiol. (London)* **215**:637–664.

Humphry, D.R., and D.J. Reed (1983). Separate cortical systems for control of joint movement and joint stiffness: Reciprocal activation and coactivation of antagonist muscles. In *Motor Control Mechanisms in Health and Disease* (J. Desmedt, ed.), pp. 347–372. Raven Press, New York.

Huston, J.C., and C.E. Passerello (1978). Multibody dynamics including translation between the bodies—with application to head–neck systems. Office of Naval Res. Techn. Rept. No. ONR-CU-ES-0915 78-7.

Igarashi, M., B.R. Alford, T. Watanabe, and P.M. Maxian (1969). Role of neck proprioceptors for the maintenance of dynamic bodily equilibrium in the squirrel monkey. *Laryngoscope* **79**:1713–1727.

Igarashi, M., H. Isago, T. O-Uchi, and T. Kubo (1983). Uvulonodular lesion and eye–head coordination in squirrel monkeys. *Adv. Otol.-Rhinol.-Laryngol.* **31**:18–27.

Illert, M., A. Lundberg, and R. Tanaka (1976). Integration in descending motor pathways controlling the forelimb in the cat. 2. Convergence on neurones mediating disynaptic cortico-motoneuronal excitation. *Exp. Brain Res.* **26**:521-540.

Illert, M., A. Lundberg, and R. Tanaka (1977). Integration in descending motor pathways controlling the forelimb in the cat. 3. Convergence on propriospinal neurons transmitting disynaptic excitation from the corticospinal and other descending tracts. *Exp. Brain Res.* **29**:323–346.

Imai, Y., and T. Kusama (1969). Distribution of the dorsal root fibres in the cat. An experimental study with the Nauta method. *Brain Res.* **13**:338–359.

Ingram, W.R., S.W. Ranson, F.I. Hannett, F.R. Zeiss, and E.H. Terwilliger (1932). Results of stimulation of the tegmentum with the Horsley-Clarke stereotaxic apparatus. *Arch. Neurol. Psychiat.* **28**:513–541.

Ingvar, S. (1918). Zur Phylo- und Ontogenese des Kleinhirns nebst einem Versuch zur einheitlicher Erklarung der zerebellaren Lokalisation und Function. *Folia Neurobiol.* **11**:205–495.

Ingvar, S. (1923). On cerebellar localization. *Brain* **46**:301–335.

Ingvar, S. (1928). Studies in neurology. I. The phylogenetic continuity of the central nervous system. *Bull. Johns Hopkins Hosp.* **43**:315–337.

Ip, M.C. (1961). *The Number and Variety of Proprioceptors in Certain Muscles of the Cat.* M.Sc. Thesis, University of Hong Kong.

Isu, N., and J. Yokota (1983). Morphophysiological study of the divergent projection of axon collaterals of medial vestibular neurons in the cat. *Exp. Brain Res.* **53**:151–162.

Ito, M., and M. Yoshida (1964). The cerebellar-evoked monosynaptic inhibition of Deiters' neurones. *Experientia (Basel)* **20**:515–516.

Ito, M., N. Kawai, M. Udo, and N. Mano (1969). Axon reflex activation of Deiters' neurones from the cerebellar cortex through collaterals of the cerebellar afferents. *Exp. Brain Res.* **8**:249–268.

Ito, M., M. Udo, and N. Mano (1970). Long inhibitory and excitatory pathways converging onto cat reticular and Deiter's neurons and their relevance to reticulofugal axons. *J. Neurophysiol.* **33**:210–226.

Ito, M. (1972). Cerebellar control of the vestibular neurons: Physiology and pharmacology. *Prog. Brain Res.* **37**:377–390.

Ito, M. (1984). *The Cerebellum and Neural Control.* Raven Press, New York.

Jack, J.J.B. (1978). Some methods for selective activation of muscle afferent fibers. In *Studies in Neurophysiology, Essays in Honor of Professor A.K. McIntyre* (R. Porter, ed.), pp. 155–176. Cambridge University Press, Cambridge.

Jackson, J.H. (1907). Case of tumour of the middle lobe of the cerebellum—cerebellar paralysis with rigidity (cerebellar attitude)—occasional tetanus-like seizures. *Brain* **29**:425–440.

Jackson, R. (1977). *The Cervical Syndrome*, 4th ed. Charles C Thomas, Springfield, IL.

Jankowska, E., Y. Padel, and P. Zarzecki (1978). Crossed disynaptic inhibition of sacral motoneurones. *J. Physiol. (London)* **285**:425–444.

Jankowska, E., and A. Odutola (1980). Crossed and uncrossed synaptic actions on motoneurones of back muscles in the cat. *Brain Res.* **194**:65–78.

Jankowska, E., D. McCrea, P. Rudomin, and E. Sykova (1981). Observations on neuronal pathways subserving primary afferent depolarization. *J. Neurophysiol.* **46**:505–516.

Jankowska, E., and D. McCrea (1983). Shared neuronal pathways of reflex actions from Ib tendon organ afferents and Ia muscle spindle afferents in the cat. *J. Physiol. (London)* **338**:99–111.

Jayne, D., A.J. Lees, and G.M. Stern (1984). Remission in spasmodic torticollis. *J. Neurol. Neurosurg. Psychiat.* **47**:1236–1237.

Jeffreys, E. (1980). *Disorders of the Cervical Spine*. Butterworths, London.

Jofe, M.H., White, A.A., and M.M. Panjabi (1983). Physiology and biomechanics. In *The Cervical Spine* (The Cervical Spinal Research Soc., eds.), pp. 23–33. J.B. Lippincott Co., Philadelphia.

Johnson, J.I., W.I. Welker, and B.H. Pubols (1968). Somatotopic organization of raccoon dorsal column nuclei. *J. Comp. Neurol.* **132**:1–44.

Jones, A., S. Phillips, R. Kenyon, K. Kors, and L. Stark (1982). Head movements: A measure of multifocal reading performance. *Optomet. Monthly* **73**:104–106.

Jones, B.E., and T.-Z. Yang (1985). The efferent projections from the reticular formation and the locus coeruleus studied by anterograde and retrograde axonal transport in the rat. *J. Comp. Neurol.* **242**:56–92.

Jones, G.M., and J.H. Milsum (1965). Spatial and dynamic aspects of visual fixation. *IEEE Trans. Bio-Med. Eng.* **12**:54–62.

Kapandji, I.A. (1974). *The Phsyiology of the Joints, Vol. 3. The Trunk and the Vertebral Column*, 2nd ed. Churchill Livingston, New York.

Kasai, T., and D.S. Zee (1978). Eye–head coordination in labyrinthine-defective human beings. *Brain Res.* **144**:123–141.

Kasper, J., and U. Thoden (1981). Effects of natural neck afferent stimulation vestibulospinal neurons in the decerebrate cat. *Exp. Brain Res.* **44**:401–408.

Katz, R., and P. Rondot (1978). Muscle reaction to passive shortening in normal man. *EEG Clin. Neurophysiol.* **45**:90–99.

Kawamura, K., A. Brodal, and G. Hoddevik (1974). The projection of the superior colliculus onto the reticular formation of the brain stem. An experimental anatomical study in the cat. *Exp. Brain Res.* **19**:1–19.

Kawamura, K., and T. Hashikawa (1978). Cell bodies of origin of reticular projections from the superior colliculus in the cat: An experimental study with the use of Horseradish Peroxidase as tracer. *J. Comp. Neurol.* **182**:1–16.

Keane, J.M. (1981). *Peripheral organization the trapezius muscle complex in the cat*. M.Sc. Thesis, Queen's University, Kingston.

Keane, J., and F.J.R. Richmond (1981). Distribution of motoneurons supplying different heads of the cat trapezius muscle. *Physiologist* **23**:23.

Kearney, R.E., and I.W. Hunter (1982). Dynamics of human ankle stiffness: Variation with displacement amplitude. *J. Biomech.* **15**:753–756.

Keirstead, S.A., P.K. Rose, and S.J. Vanner (1982). Frequency and distribution of axon collaterals from upper cervical spinal motoneurons. *Soc. Neurosci. Abstr.* **8**:724.

Keirstead, S.A., and P.K. Rose (1983). Dendritic distribution of splenius motoneurons in the cat: Comparison of motoneurons innervating different regions of the muscle. *J. Comp. Neurol.* **219**:273–284.

Keirstead, S.A., and P.K. Rose (1984). Projection of muscle spindle afferents to dorsal neck muscle motoneurons revealed by spike triggered averaging. *Soc. Neurosci. Abstr.* **10**:745.

Kelly, J.P. (1985). Vestibular system. In *Principles of Neural Science,* (E.R. Kandel and J.H. Schwartz, eds.), 2nd ed., pp. 594. Elsevier, North-Holland, New York.

Kenins, P., H. Kikillus, and E.D. Schomburg (1978). Short and long-latency reflex pathways from neck afferents to hindlimb motoneurones in the cat. *Brain Res.* **149**:235–238.

Kennard, C., W.H. Zangemeister, S. Mellers, W.F. Hoyt, and L. Stark (1982). Eye–head coordination in patients with Parkinson's disease. In *Functional Basis of Ocular Motility Disorders* (G. Lennerstrand, D.S. Zee, and E. Keller, eds.), Vol. 37, pp. 517–524. Pergamon Press, Oxford and New York.

Kerr, F.W.L., and R. Olafson (1961). Trigeminal and cervical volleys: Convergence on single units in the spinal grey at C1 and C2. *Arch. Neurol.* **5**:171–178.

Kerr, F.W.L. (1971). Structural relation of the trigeminal spinal tract to upper cervical roots and the solitary nucleus in the cat. *Exp. Neurol.* **4**:134–148.

Kerr, F.W.L. (1972). Central relationships of trigeminal and cervical primary afferents in the spinal cord and medulla. *Brain Res.* **43**:561–572.

Khalil, T.B., and R.P. Hubbard (1977). Parametric study of head response by finite element modeling. *J. Biomech.* **10**:119–132.

Kilpatrick, I.C., G.L. Collingridge, and M.S. Starr (1982). Evidence for the participation of gamma-aminobutirate containing neurones in striatal and nigral derived circling in the rat. *Neuroscience* **7**:207–222.

King, W.M., S.G. Lisberger, and A.F. Fuchs (1976). Responses of fibres in medial longitudinal fasciculus (MLF) of alert monkeys during horizontal and vertical conjugate eye movements evoked by vestibular or visual stimuli. *J. Neurophysiol.* **39**:1135–1149.

King, W.M., W. Precht, and N. Dieringer (1980). Synaptic organization of frontal eye field and vestibular afferents to interstitial nucleus of Cajal in the cat. *J. Neurophysiol.* **43**:912–928.

King, W.M., A.F. Fuchs, and M. Magnin (1981). Vertical eye movement related responses of neurons in midbrain near interstitial nucleus of Cajal. *J. Neurophysiol.* **46**:549–562.

Kirkwood, P.A., T.A. Sears, and R.H. Westgaard (1981). Recurrent inhibition of intercostal motoneurones in the cat. *J. Physiol. (London)* **319**:111–130.

Kirkwood, P.A., and T.A. Sears (1982). Excitatory post-synaptic potentials from single muscle spindle afferents in external intercostal motoneurones of the cat. *J. Physiol. (London)* **322**:287–314.

Kopp, J., and G. Manteuffel (1984). Quantitative analysis of salamander horizontal head nystagmus. *Brain Behav. Evol.* **25**:187–196.

Körner, G. (1960). Untersuchungen über Zahl, Anordnung und Länge der Muskelspindeln in einigen Schulter-, den Oberarmmuskeln und im Musculus sternalis des Menschen. *Anat. Anz.* **108**:99–103.

Kotchabhakdi, N., and F. Walberg (1978). Primary vestibular afferent projections to the cerebellum as demonstrated by retrograde axonal transport of horseradish peroxidase. *Brain Res.* **142**:142–146.

Kubin, L., P.C. Magherini, D. Manzoni, and O. Pompeiano (1980). Responses of lateral reticular neurons to sinusoidal stimulation of labyrinth receptors in decerebrate cat. *J. Neurophysiol.* **44**:922–936.

Kubin, L., P.C. Magherini, D. Manzoni, and O. Pompeiano (1981a). Responses of lateral reticular neurons to sinusoidal rotation of neck in the decerebrate cat. *Neuroscience* **6**:1277–1290.

Kubin, L., P.C. Magherini, and O. Pompeiano (1981b). Responses of lateral reticular neurons to convergent neck and macular vestibular inputs. *J. Neurophysiol.* **46**:48–64.

Kubo, T., D.W. Jensen, M. Igarashi, and J.L. Homick (1981). Eye–head coordination during optokinetic stimulation in squirrel monkeys. *Ann. Otol.* **90**:85–88.

Kulak, R.F., T.B. Belytschko, A.B. Schultz, and J.O. Galanter (1976). Nonlinear behavior of the human intervertebral disc under axial load. *J. Biomech.* **9**:377–386.

Kuroki, T. (1958). Arrest reaction elicited from the brain stem. *Folia Psychiat. Neurol. Jap.* **12**:317–340.

Kuypers, H.G.J.M., and V.A. Maisky (1975). Retrograde axonal transport of horseradish peroxidase from spinal cord to brain stem cell groups in the cat. *Neurosci. Lett.* **1**:9–14.

Kuypers, H.G.J.M., and A.M. Huisman (1982). The new anatomy of the descending brain pathways. In *Brain Stem Control of Spinal Mechanisms* (B. Sjölund and A. Björklund, eds.), pp. 29–54. Elsevier Biomedical Press, Amsterdam.

Lacour, M., L. Borel, J. Barthelemy, S. Harlay, and C. Xerri (1987). Dynamic properties of the vertical otolith-neck reflexes in the alert cat. *Exp. Brain Res.* **65**:559–568.

Lal, S. (1979). Pathophysiology and pharmacotherapy of spasmodic torticollis. *J. Can. Sci. Neurol.* **6**:427–435.

Lal, S., K. Hoyte, M.E. Kiely, T.L. Sourkes, D.W. Baxter, K. Missala, and F. Andermann (1979). Neuropharmacological investigation and treatment of spasmodic torticollis. In *Advances in Neurology* (L.J. Poirier, T.L. Sourkes, and P.J. Bedard, eds.), Vol. 24, pp. 335–351. Raven Press, New York.

Land, M.F. (1975). Similarities in the visual behavior of arthropods and men. In *Handbook of Psychobiology* (M.S. Gazzaniga and C. Blakemore, eds.), pp. 49–72. Academic Press, New York.

Landgren, S., and H. Silfvenius (1968). Projections of the eye and the neck region of the anterior suprasylvian cerebral cortex of the cat. *Acta. Physiol. Scand.* **74**:340–347.

Landkof, B., W. Goldsmith, and J.L. Sackman (1976). Impact on a head–neck structure. *J. Biomech.* **9**:141–152.

Lanman, J., E. Bizzi, and J.E. Allum (1978). The coordination of eye and head movement during smooth pursuit. *Brain Res.* **153**:39–53.

Lannou, J., L. Cazin, and K.-F. Hamann (1980). Response of central vestibular neurons to horizontal linear acceleration in the rat. *Pflügers Arch.* **385**:123–129.

Larsell, O. (1953). The cerebellum of the cat and the monkey. *J. Comp. Neurol.* **99**:135–200.

Larsson, T., and T. Sjögren (1960). Essential tremor. A clinical and genetic population study. *Acta Psychiat. Neurol. Scand. (Suppl. 144)* **36**:1–176.

Laurutis, V.P., and D.A. Robinson (1986). The vestibulo-ocular reflex during human saccadic eye movements. *J. Physiol. (London)* **373**:209–233.

Lawrence, D.G., and H.G.J.M. Kuypers (1968). The functional organization of the motor system in the monkey. II. The effects of lesions of the descending brain stem pathways. *Brain* **91**:15–36.

Lazar, G., and P. Kolta (1979). The optokinetic head nystagmogram of the frog. *Acta Physiol. Acad. Sci. Hung.* **53**:479–486.

Lehman, S., and L. Stark (1979). Simulation of linear and nonlinear eye movement models: Sensitivity analysis and enumeration studies of time optimal control. *J. Cyber. Inf. Sci.* **4**:21–43.

Lestienne, F., P.P. Vidal, and A. Berthoz (1984). Gaze changing behaviour in head restrained monkey. *Exp. Brain Res.* **53**:349–356.

Levi-Civita, T. (1926). The absolute differential calculus. *Calculus of Tensors* (E. Persico, ed.). Dover, New York.

Lindsay, K.W., T.D.M. Roberts, and J.R. Rosenberg (1976). Asymmetric tonic labyrinth reflexes and their interaction with neck reflexes in the decerebrate cat. *J. Physiol. (London)* **261**:583–601.

Lipski, J., R.E.W. Fyffe, and J. Jodkowski (1985). Recurrent inhibition of cat phrenic motoneurons. *J. Neurosci.* **5**:1545–1555.

Liu, C.N. (1956). Afferent nerves to Clarke's and the lateral cuneate nuclei in the cat. *Arch. Neurol. Psychiat.* **75**:67–77.

Llinás, R. (1964). Mechanisms of supraspinal actions upon spinal cord activities. Differences between reticular and cerebellar inhibitory actions upon alpha extensor motoneurons. *J. Neurophysiol.* **27**:1117–1126.

Llinás, R., and J.W. Wolfe (1977). Functional linkage between the electrical activity in the vermal cerebellar cortex and saccadic eye movements. *Exp. Brain Res.* **29**:1–14.

Lloyd, D.P.C. (1941). Activity in neurons of the bulbospinal correlation system. *J. Neurophysiol.* **4**:115–134.

Lloyd, D.P.C., and V.J. Wilson (1959). Functional organization in the terminal segments of the spinal cord with a consideration of central excitatory and inhibitory latencies in monosynaptic reflex systems. *J. Gen. Physiol.* **42**:1219–1231.

Lockhart, R.D., G.F. Hamilton, and F.W. Fyfe (1959). *Anatomy of the Human Body.* Faber and Faber Ltd., London.

Loe, P., D. Tomko, and G. Werner (1973). The neural signal of angular head position in primary afferent vestibular nerve axons. *J. Physiol. (London)* **230**:29–50.

Loeb, G.E., and F.J.R. Richmond (1986). Synchronization of motor units in and among diverse neck muscles during slow movements in intact cats. *Soc. Neurosci. Abstr.* **16**:687.

Loeb, G.E., W.J. Yee, C.A. Pratt, C.M. Chanaud, and F.J.R. Richmond (1987). Cross-correlation of EMG reveals widespread synchronization of motor units during some slow movements in intact cats. *J. Neurosci. Methods,* in press.

Longet, F.A. (1845). Sur les troubles qui surviennent dans l'équilibration, la station et la locomotion des animaux, aprés la séction des parties molles de la nuque. *Gaz. Med. Paris* **13**:565–567.

Lopez-Barneo, J., C. Darlot, A. Berthoz, and R. Baker (1982). Neuronal activity in prepositus nucleus correlated with eye movement in the alert cat. *J. Neurophysiol.* **47**:329–352.

Lowenstein, O., and A. Sand (1940). The individual and integrated activity of the semi-circular canals of the elasmobranch labyrinth. *J. Physiol. (London)* **99**:89–101.

Lowenstein, O., and T. Roberts (1950). The equilibrium function of the otolith organs of the thornback ray. *J. Physiol. (London)* **110**:392–415.

Lund, S., and O. Pompeiano (1968). Monosynaptic excitation of alpha motoneurones from supraspinal structures in the cat. *Acta Physiol. Scand.* **73**:1–21.

Lund, S. (1980). Postural effects of neck muscle vibration in man. *Experientia* **36**:1398.

Lundberg, A. (1975). Control of spinal mechanisms from the brain. In *The Nervous System. Vol. 1. The Basic Neurosciences* (D.B. Tower, ed.), pp. 253–265. Raven Press, New York.

Lundberg, A., K. Malmgren, and E. Schomburg (1977). Comments on the reflex actions evoked by electrical stimulation of group II muscle afferents. *Brain Res.* **122**:551–555.

Lüscher, H.R., P. Ruenzel, and E. Henneman (1980). Topographic distribution of terminals of Ia and group II fibers in the spinal cord, as revealed by postsynaptic population potentials. *J. Neurophysiol.* **43**:968–985.

Lysell, E. (1969). Motion in the cervical spine. *Acta Orthop. Scand. Suppl.* No. 123.

Mabuchi, M., and T. Kusama (1970). Mesodiencephalic projections to the inferior olive and the vestibular and perihypoglossal nuclei. *Brain Res.* **17**:133–136.

Maeda, M., R.A. Maunz, and V.J. Wilson (1975). Labyrinthine influence on cat forelimb motoneurons. *Exp. Brain Res.* **22**:69–86.

Magni, F., and W.D. Willis (1964). Cortical control of brain stem reticular neurons. *Arch. Ital. Biol.* **102**:418–433.

Magnus, R. (1914). Welche Teile des Zentralnervensystems mussen fur das Zustandekommen der tonischen Hals und Labyrinthreflexe auf die Korpermuskulatur vorhanden sein? *Pflügers Arch.* **159**:224–250.

Magnus, R. (1924). *Korperstellung*, pp. XIII–740. Springer-Verlag, Berlin.

Magnus, R. (1926). Some results of studies in the physiology of posture. *Lancet* **211**:531–536.

Magoun, H.W., and R. Rhines (1946). An inhibitory mechanism in the bulbar reticular formation. *J. Neurophysiol.* **9**:165–171.

Mancia, M., A. Grantyn, G. Broggi, and M. Margnelli (1971). Synaptic linkage between mesencephalic and bulbo-pontine reticular structures as revealed by intracellular recording. *Brain Res.* **33**:491–494.

Manzoni, D., O. Pompeiano, and G. Stampacchia (1979). Tonic cervical influences on posture and reflex movements. *Arch. Ital. Biol.* **117**:81–110.

Manzoni, D., O. Pompeiano, U.C. Srivastava, and G. Stampacchia (1983a). Responses of forelimb extensors to sinusoidal stimulation of macular labyrinth and neck receptors. *Arch. Ital. Biol.* **121**:205–214.

Manzoni, D., O. Pompeiano, G. Stampacchia, and U.C. Srivastava (1983b). Responses of medullary reticulospinal neurons to sinusoidal stimulation of labyrinth receptors in decerebrate cat. *J. Neurophysiol.* **50**:1059–1079.

Manzoni, D., O. Pompeiano, U.C. Srivastava, and G. Stampacchia (1984). Gain regulation of vestibular reflexes in fore- and hindlimb muscles evoked by roll tilt. *Boll. Soc. Ital. Biol. Sper. (Suppl. 3).* **60**:9–10.

Marchand, A., D. Manzoni, O. Pompeiano, and G. Stampacchia (1987). Effects of stimulation of vestibular and neck receptors on Deiter's neurons projecting to the lumbosacral cord. *Pflügers Arch.* **409**:13–23.

Marchand, R., C.F. Bridgman, E. Shumpert, and E. Eldred (1971). Association of tendon organs with spindles in muscles of the cat's leg. *Anat. Rec.* **169**:23–32.

Markham, C.H., and I.S. Curthoys (1972). Convergence of labyrinthine influences on units in the vestibular nuclei of the cat. II. Electrical stimulation. *Brain Res.* **43**:383–396.

Marmarelis, P.E., and V.Z. Marmarelis (1978). *Analysis of Physiological Systems.* Plenum, New York.

Marsden, C.D., and M.J.G. Harrison (1974). Idiopathic torsion dystonia (Dystonia Musculorum Deformans). *Brain.* **97**:793–810.

Martin, G.F., A.O. Humberston, L.C. Laxson, and W.M. Panneton (1979a). Evidence for direction bulbospinal projections to laminae IX, X, and intermediolateral cell column. Studies using axonal transport techniques in the North American opossum. *Brain Res.* **170**:165–171.

Martin, G.F., L.C. Laxson, W.M. Panneton, and I. Tschismadia (1979b). Spinal projections from the mesencephalic and pontine reticular formation in the North American opossum: A study using axonal transport techniques. *J. Comp. Neurol.* **187**:373–400.

Martin, G.F., T. Cabana, A.O. Humbertson, Jr., L.C. Laxson, and W.M. Panneton (1981). Spinal projections from the medullary reticular formation of the North American opossum: Evidence for connectional heterogeneity. *J. Comp. Neurol.* **196**:663–682.

Masek, G.A. (1963). The role of head movements in human visual target pursuit. *Res. Lab. Electron MIT Quart. Prog. Rep.* **70**:348–351.

Matsushita, M., and N. Okado (1981). Spinocerebellar projections to lobules I and II of the cerebellar anterior lobe in the cat; as studied by retrograde transport of horseradish peroxidase. *J. Comp. Neurol.* **197**:411–424.

Matthews, P.B.C., and R.B. Stein (1969). The senstivity of muscle spindle afferents to small sinusoidal changes in length. *J. Physiol. (London)* **200**:723–743.

Matthews, P.B.C. (1972). *Mammalian Muscle Receptors and Their Central Actions.* Edward Arnold Ltd., London.

Matthews, W.B., P. Beasley, W. Parry-Jones, and G. Garland (1978). Spasmodic torticollis: A combined clinical study. *J. Neurol. Neurosurg. Psychiat.* **41**:485–492.

McCouch, G.P., I.D. Deering, and T.H. Ling (1951). Location of receptors for tonic neck reflexes. *J. Neurophysiol.* **14**:191–195.

McCrea, R.A., K. Yoshida, A. Berthoz, and R. Baker (1980). Eye movement related activity and morphology of second order vestibular neurons terminating in the cat abducens nucleus. *Exp. Brain Res.* **40**:468–473.

McCrea, R.A., and R. Baker (1985). Anatomical connections of the nucleus prepositus of the cat. *J. Comp. Neurol.* **237**:377–407.

McIlwain, J.T. (1986). Effects of eye position on saccades evoked electrically from superior colliculus of alert cats. *J. Neurophysiol.* **55**:97–112.

McIntyre, A.K. (1974). Central actions of impulses in muscle afferent fibers. In *Handbook of Physiology, Vol. III, Section 2, Muscle Receptors* (C.C. Hunt, ed.), pp. 235–288. Springer-Verlag, Berlin.

McKenzie, J.A., and J.F. Williams (1971). The dynamic behavior of the head and cervical spine during "whiplash." *J. Biomech.* **4**:477–490.

Meares, R. (1971). Natural history of spasmodic torticollis and effect of surgery. *Lancet* **2**:149–150.

Meiry, J.L. (1971). Vestibular and proprioceptive stabilization of eye movements. In *The Control of Eye Movements* (P. Bach-y-Rita and C.C. Collins, eds.), pp. 483–496. Academic Press, New York.

Melvill-Jones, G. (1964). Predominance of anti-compensatory oculomotor response during rapid head rotation. *Aerospace Med.* **35**:965–968.

Mendell, L.M., and E. Henneman (1971). Terminals of single Ia fibers: Location, density, and distribution within a pool of 300 homonymous afferents. *J. Neurophysiol.* **34**:171–187.

Mense, S., and H. Meyer (1985). Different types of slowly conducting afferent unit in cat skeletal muscle and tendon. *J. Physiol. (London)* **363**:403–417.

Mense, S. (1986). Slowly conducting afferent fibers from deep tissues: Neurobiological properties and central nervous actions. In *Progress in Sensory Physiology* (D. Ottoson, ed.), pp. 139–219. Springer-Verlag, Berlin.

Mergner, T., D. Anastasopoulos, and W. Becker (1982). Neuronal responses to horizontal neck deflection in the group x region of the cat's medullary brainstem. *Exp. Brain Res.* **45**:196–206.

Mergner, T., G.L. Nordi, W. Becker, and L. Deecke (1983). The role of canal–neck interaction for the perception of horizontal trunk and head rotation. *Exp. Brain Res.* **49**:198–208.

Merrill, T., W. Goldsmith, and Y.C. Deng (1984). Three-dimensional response of a lumped parameter head–neck model due to impact and impulsive loading. *J. Biomech.* **17**:81–95.

Mertz, H.J., and L.M. Patrick (1971). Strength and response of the human neck. *Proc. 15th Stapp Car Crash Conf.*, Soc. for Automotive Engineers, Calif., pp. 207–255.

Mertz, H.J. (1985). Anthropomorphic models. In *The Biomechanics of Trauma* (A.M. Nahum and J. Melvin, eds.), pp. 31–60, Appleton-Century-Crofts, Norwalk Conn.

Mesulam, M.-M., and J.M. Brushart (1979). Transganglionic and anterograde transport of horseradish peroxidase across dorsal root ganglia: A tetramethyl benzidine method for tracing central sensory connections of muscles and peripheral nerves. *Neuroscience* **4**:1107–1117.

Meyer, D.L., W. Graf, and U. von Seydlitz-Kurzbach (1979). The role of integrators in maintaining actively abnormal postures. A study of postural mechanisms in geckos. *J. Comp. Physiol.* **131**:235–246.

Miles, F., and D. Braitman (1980). Long-term adaptive changes in primate vestibulo-ocular reflex. II. Electrophysiological observations on semicircular canal primary afferents. *J. Neurophysiol.* **43**:1426–1436.

Miles, F.A., and B.B. Eighmy (1980). Long term adaptive changes in primate vestibuloocular reflex. I. Behavioral observations. *J. Neurophysiol.* **43**:1406–1425.

Miller, A.D., P.S. Roossin, and R.H. Schor (1982). Roll tilt reflexes after vestibulospinal tract lesions. *Exp. Brain Res.* **48**:107–112.

Monnier, M. (1943). Syndromes déviationnels provoqués par l'excitation et la destruction du système réticulaire bulbo-protubérantiel chez le chat. *Monatsschr. Psychiat. Neurol.* **107**:84–102.

Morasso, P., E. Bizzi, and J. Dichgans (1973). Adjustment of saccade characteristics during head movements. *Exp. Brain Res.* **16**:492–500.

Morasso, P., G. Sandini, and Z.R. Tagliasco (1977). Control strategies in the eye–head coordination system. *IEEE Trans. System Man. Cybern.* SMC **7**:639–647.

Morgan, C., I. Nadelhaft, and W. C. De Groat (1981). The distribution of visceral primary afferents from the pelvic nerve to Lissauer's tract and spinal grey matter and its relationship to the sacral parasympathetic nucleus. *J. Comp. Neurol.* **201**:415–440.

Mori, S., and A. Mikami (1973). Excitation of Deiters' neurons by stimulation of the nerves of neck extensor muscles. *Brain Res.* **56**:331–334.

Moruzzi, G. (1950). Effects at different frequencies of cerebellar stimulation upon postural tonus and myotatic reflexes. *Electroenceph Clin. Neurophysiol.* **2**:463–469.

Moschovakis, A.K., and A.B. Karabelas (1985). Observations on the somatodendritic morphology and axonal trajectory of intracellularly HRP-labeled efferent neurons located in the deeper layers of the superior colliculus of the cat. *J. Comp. Neurol.* **239**:276–308.

Mountcastle, V.B., ed. (1980). *Medical Physiology,* Vol. 1, 14th ed., pp. 824. C.V. Mosby Co., Toronto.

Mowrer, V.H. (1935). Some neglected factors with influence on the duration of the post-rotational nystagmus. *Acta Oto-Laryngol.* **22**:1–9.

Mueller-Jensen, A., W.H. Zangemeister, J. Kuechler, and H.D. Herrmann (1984). Haemangioblastome des Zentralnervensystems: Eine klinische Studie. *Eur. Arch. Psychiat. Neurol.* **234**:149–156.

Munoz, D., and D. Guitton (1985a). Tectospinal neurons in the cat have discharges coding gaze position error. *Brain Res.* **341**:184–188.

Munoz, D.P., and D. Guitton (1985b). Tecto-reticulo-spinal neurons have phasic discharge related to high but not low velocity saccadic gaze shifts. *Soc. Neurosci. Abstr.* **11**:287.

Munoz, D., and D. Guitton (1986). Presaccadic burst discharges of tecto-reticulo-spinal neurons in the alert head free and fixed cat. *Brain Res.* **398**:164–168.

Munson, J.B., and G.W. Sypert (1979a). Properties of single central Ia afferent fibres projecting to motoneurones. *J. Physiol. (London)* **296**:315–327.

Munson, J.B., and G.W. Sypert (1979b). Properties of single fibre excitatory post-synaptic potentials in triceps surae motoneurones. *J. Physiol. (London)* **296**:329–342.

Munson, J.B., J.W. Fleshman, and G.W. Sypert (1980). Properties of single fiber spindle group II epsps in triceps surae motoneurons. *J. Neurophysiol.* **44**:713–725.

Murakami, S., and M. Kato (1983). Central projection of nuchal group I muscle afferent fibers of the cat. *Exp. Neurol.* **79**:472–487.

Murray, E.A., and J.D. Coulter (1982). Organization of tectospinal neurons in the cat and rat superior colliculus. *Brain Res.* **243**:201–214.

Mussen, A.T. (1927). Experimental investigations on the cerebellum. *Brain* **50**:313–348.

Mussen, A.T. (1930). The cerebellum. A new classification of the lobes based on their reactions to stimulation. *Arch. Neurol. Psychiat.* **23**:411–459.

Mussen, A.T. (1931). The cerebellum. Comparison of symptoms resulting from lesions of individual lobes with reactions of the same lobes to stimulation: A preliminary report. *Arch. Neurol. Psychiat.* **25**:702–722.

Myers, E.R., and V.C. Mow (1983). Biomechanics of cartilage and its response to biomechanical stimuli. In *Cartilage* (B.K. Hall, ed.), Vol. 1, pp. 313–340. Academic Press, New York.

Mysicka, A., and W. Zenker (1981). Central projections of muscle afferents from the sternomastoid muscle in the rat. *Brain Res.* **211**:257–265.

Nachemson, A.L., and J.H. Evans (1968). Some mechanical properties of the third human lumbar interlaminar ligament (Ligamentum Flavum). *J. Biomech.* **1**:211–220.

Nadelhaft, I., J. Roppolo, C. Morgan, and W.C. De Groat (1983). Parasympathetic preganglionic neurons and visceral primary afferents in monkey sacral spinal cord revealed following application of horseradish peroxidase to pelvic nerve. *J. Comp. Neurol.* **216**:36–52.

Nakajima, K., M. Maeda, S. Ishii, and M. Miyazaki (1981). Neuronal organization of the tonic neck reflex. *Equilibrium Res.* **40**:195–201.

Nakao, S., S. Sasaki, R.H. Schor, and H. Shimazu (1982). Functional organization of premotor neurons in the cat medial vestibular nucleus related to slow and fast phases of nystagmus. *Exp. Brain Res.* **45**:371–385.

Nam, M.H., V. Lakshminarayanan, and L. Stark (1984). Effect of external viscous load on head movement. *IEEE Trans. Biomed. Eng. BME* **31**:303–309.

Nashner, L. (1977). Fixed patterns of rapid postural responses among leg muscles during stance. *Exp. Brain Res.* **30**:13–24.

Nauta, W.J.H., and P.A. Gygax (1954). Silver impregnation of degenerating axons in the central nervous system. A modified technique. *Stain Technol.* **29**:91–93.

Nelson, S.G., and L.M. Mendell (1978). Projection of single knee flexor Ia fibers to homonymous and heteronymous motoneurones. *J. Neurophysiol.* **41**:778–787.

Niemer, W.T., and H.W. Magoun (1947). Reticulo-spinal tracts influencing motor activity. *J. Comp. Neurol.* **87**:367–379.

Niimi, K., M. Miki, and S. Kawamura (1970). Ascending projections of the superior colliculus in the cat. *Okajimas Folia Anat. Jap.* **47**:269–287.

Nomura, Y., and M. Segawa (1982). Tourette syndrome in oriental children: Clinical and pathophysiological considerations. In *Gilles de la Tourette Syndrome* (A.J. Friedhoff and T.N. Chase, eds.), pp. 277–280. Raven Press, New York.

Norkin, C.C., and P.K. Levangie (1983). *Joint Structure and Function; A Comprehensive Analysis*, pp. 115–154. F.A. Davis, Philadelphia.

Nulsen, F.E., S.P.W. Black, and C.G. Drake (1948). Inhibition and facilitation of motor activity by the anterior cerebellum. *Fed. Proc.* **7**:86–87.

Nyberg, G., and A. Blomqvist (1984). The central projection of muscle afferent fibres to the lower medulla and upper spinal cord: An anatomical study in the cat with the transganglionic transport method. *J. Comp. Neurol.* **230**:99–109.

Nyberg-Hansen, R. (1964a). The location and termination of tectospinal fibers in the cat. *Exp. Neurol.* **9**:212–227.

Nyberg-Hansen, R. (1964b). Origin and termination of fibers from the vestibular nuclei descending in the medial longitudinal fasciculus. An experimental study with silver impregnation methods in the cat. *J. Comp. Neurol.* **122**:355–367.

Nyberg-Hansen, R. (1965). Sites and mode of termination of reticulospinal fibers in the cat: An experimental study with silver impregnation methods. *J. Comp. Neurol.* **124**:71–100.

Nyberg-Hansen, R. (1966). Sites of termination of interstitiospinal fibers in the cat. An experimental study with silver impregnation methods. *Arch. Ital. Biol.* **104**:98–111.

Oberlander, C., C. Dumont, and J.R. Boissier (1977). Rotational behavior after unilateral intranigral injection of muscimol in rats. *Eur. J. Pharmacol.* **43**:389–390.

Ommaya, A., and T. Gennarelli (1976). A physiopathologic basis for noninvasive diagnosis and prognosis of head injury severity. In *Head Injuries* (R. McLaurin, ed.), pp. 49–76. Grune & Stratton, New York.

Optican, L.M., and D.A. Robinson (1980). Cerebellar-dependent adaptive control of primate saccadic system. *J. Neurophysiol.* **44**:1058–1076.

Ormsby, C., and L.R. Young (1977). Integration of semicircular canal and otolith information for multisensory orientation stimuli. *Math. Biosci.* **34**:1–21.

Orne, D., and Y.K. Liu (1971). A mathematical model of spinal response to impact. *J. Biomech.* **4**:49–72.

Oscarsson, O. (1979). Functional units of the cerebellum—sagittal zones and microzones. *Trends Neurosci.* **2**:143–145.

Outerbridge, J.S., and G. Melvill-Jones (1971). Reflex vestibular control of head movement in man. *Aerospace Med.* **42**:935–940.

Paintal, A.S. (1960). Functional analysis of group III afferent fibres of mammalian muscles. *J. Physiol. (London)* **152**:250–270.

Panjabi, M.M., A.A. White, and R.A. Brand (1974). A note on defining body parts configurations. *J. Biomech.* **7**:385–387.

Panjabi, M.M., A.A. White, and R.M. Johnson (1975). Cervical spine biomechanics as a function of transection of components. *J. Biomech.* **8**:327–336.

Panjabi, M.M., R.A. Brand, and A.A. White (1976). The three-dimensional flexibility and stiffness properties of the thoracic spine. *J. Biomech.* **9**:185–192.

Patrick, L.M., and C.C. Chou (1976). Response of the human neck in flexion, extension and lateral flexion. *Vehicle Research Report VRI 7.3*, Soc. Automotive Engineers, New York.

Paynter, H.M. (1961). *Analysis and Design of Engineering Systems*. MIT Press, Cambridge.

Pélisson, D. and C. Prablanc (1986). Vestibulo-ocular reflex (VOR) induced by passive head rotation and goal directed saccadic eye movements do not simply add in man. *Brain Res.* **380**:397–400.

Pélisson, D. and C. Prablanc (1987). Gaze control in man: Evidence for vestibulo-occular reflex inhibition during goal directed saccade eye movements. In *Eye Movements: From Physiology to Cognition* (J.K. O'Regan and A. Lévy-Schoen, eds.). Elsevier, North-Holland, Amsterdam.

Pellionisz, A., and R. Llinás (1979). Brain modeling by tensor network theory and computer simulation. The cerebellum: Distributed processor for predictive coordination. *Neuroscience* **4**:323–348.

Pellionisz, A., and R. Llinás (1980). Tensorial approach to the geometry of brain function. Cerebellar coordination via a metric tensor. *Neuroscience* **5**:1761–1770.

Pellionisz, A. (1983). Sensorimotor transformation of natural coordinates via neuronal networks: Conceptual and formal unification of cerebellar and tectal models. In *COINS Technical Report 83-19*. II. *Workshop on Visuomotor Coordination in Frog and Toad—Models and Experiments* (R. Lara and M. Arbib, eds.). University of Massachusetts, Amherst, MA.

Pellionisz, A. (1984). Coordination: A vector-matrix description of transformations of overcomplete CNS coordinates and a tensorial solution using the Moore–Penrose generalized inverse. *J. Theoret. Biol.* **110**:353–375.

Pellionisz, A., and R. Llinás (1985). Tensor network theory of the metaorganization of functional geometries in the CNS. *Neuroscience* **16**:245–273.

Pellionisz, A., and B.W. Peterson (1985). Tensor models of primary sensorimotor systems, such as the vestibulo-collic reflex (VCR) and of the metaorganization of hierarchically connected networks. *Soc. Neurosci. Abst.* **11**:83.

Penfield, W., and Th. Rasmussen (1950). *The Cerebral Cortex of Man*. Macmillan, New York.

Penfield, W., and H. Jasper (1954). *Epilepsy and the Functional Anatomy of the Human Brain*. Little Brown and Company, Boston.

Perachio, A.A. (1981). Responses of neurons in the vestibular nuclei of awake squirrel monkeys during linear acceleration. In *The Vestibular System: Function and Morphology* (T. Gualtierotti, ed.), pp. 443–451. Springer-Verlag, New York, Heidelberg, Berlin.

Perl, E.R. (1958). Crossed reflex effects evoked by activity in myelinated afferent fibers of muscle. *J. Neurophysiol.* **21**:101–112.

Pernkopf, E. (1980). *Atlas of Topographical and Applied Human Anatomy, Vol. 1. Head and Neck* (H. Ferner, ed.). Urban and Schwarzenberg, Munich.

Peterson, B.W., M.E. Anderson, M. Filion, and V.J. Wilson (1971). Responses of reticulospinal neurons to stimulation of the superior colliculus. *Brain Res.* **33**:495–498.

Peterson, B.W., and L.P. Felpel (1971). Excitation and inhibition of reticulospinal neurons by vestibular, cortical and cutaneous stimulation. *Brain Res.* **27**:373–376.

Peterson, B.W., M.E. Anderson, and M. Filion (1974). Response of pontomedullary reticular neurons to cortical tectal and cutaneous stimuli. *Exp. Brain Res.* **21**:19–44.

Peterson, B.W., and C. Abzug (1975). Properties of projections from vestibular nuclei to medial reticular formation in the cat. *J. Neurophysiol.* **38**:1421–1435.

Peterson, B.W., M. Filion, L.P. Felpel, and C. Abzug (1975a). Responses of medial reticular neurons to stimulation of the vestibular nerve. *Exp. Brain Res.* **22**:335–350.

Peterson, B.W., R.A. Maunz, N.G. Pitts, and R. Mackel (1975b). Patterns of projection and branching of reticulospinal neurons. *Exp. Brain Res.* **23**:333–351.

Peterson, B.W. (1977). Identification of reticulospinal projections that may participate in gaze control. In *Control of Gaze by Brain Stem Neurons* (R. Baker and A. Berthoz, eds.), pp. 143–152. Elsevier Biomedical Press, Amsterdam.

Peterson, B.W., N.G. Pitts, K.Fukushima, and R. Mackel (1978). Reticulospinal excitation and inhibition of neck motoneurons. *Exp. Brain Res.* **32**:471–489.

Peterson, B.W., N.G. Pitts, and K. Fukushima (1979). Reticulospinal connections with limb and axial motoneurons. *Exp. Brain Res.* **36**:1–20.

Peterson, B.W., K. Fukushima, N. Hirai, R.H. Schor, and V.J. Wilson (1980). Responses of vestibulospinal and reticulospinal neurons to sinusoidal vestibular stimulation. *J. Neurophysiol.* **43**:1236–1250.

Peterson, B.W., G. Bilotto, J.H. Fuller, J. Goldberg, and B. Leeman (1981a). Interaction of vestibular and neck reflexes in the control of gaze. In *Progress in Oculomotor Research* (A. Fuchs and W. Becker, eds.), pp. 335–342. Elsevier, North-Holland, Amsterdam.

Peterson, B.W., G. Bilotto, J. Goldberg, and V.J. Wilson (1981b). Dynamics of vestibuloocular, vestibulocollic and cervicocollic reflexes. *Ann. N.Y. Acad. Sci.* **374**:395–402.

Peterson, B.W., and K. Fukushima (1982). The reticulospinal system and its role in generating vestibular and visuomotor reflexes. In *Brain Stem Control of Spinal Mechanisms* (B. Sjölund and A. Björklund, eds.), pp. 225–251. Elsevier, Amsterdam.

Peterson, B.W. (1984). The reticulospinal system and its role in the control of movement. In *Brainstem Control of Spinal Cord Function* (C.D. Barnes, ed.), pp. 27–86. Academic Press, New York.

Peterson, B., J. Baker, C. Wickland, and A. Pellionisz (1985a). Relation between pulling directions of neck muscles and their activation by the vestibulocollic reflex: Tests of a tensorial model. *Soc. Neurosci. Abstr.* **11**:83.

Peterson, B.W., J. Goldberg, G. Bilotto, and J.H. Fuller (1985b). Cervicocollic reflex: Its dynamic properties and interaction with vestibular reflexes. *J. Neurophysiol.* **54**:90–109.

Petras, J.M. (1966). Afferent fibres to the spinal cord the terminal distribution of dorsal root and encephalospinal axons. *Med. Ser. J. Can.* **22**:668–694.

Petras, J.M. (1967). Cortical, tectal and tegmental fiber connections in the spinal cord of the cat. *Brain Res.* **6**:275–324.

Petrovicky, P. (1976). Projections from the tectum mesencephali to the brain stem structures in the rat. I. The superior colliculus. *Folia Morphol.* **24**:41–48.

Pilyavsky, A.I. (1974). An analysis of monosynaptic cortico-reticular connections. *Neirofisiologia (Kiev)* **6**:103–105.

Poirier, J.L. (1960). Experimental and histological study of midbrain dyskinesia. *J. Neurophysiol.* **23**:534–551.

Pola, J., and D.A. Robinson (1978). Oculomotor signals in medial longitudinal fasciculus of the monkey. *J. Neurophysiol.* **41**:245–259.

Polacek, P. (1966). Receptors of the joints. Their structure, variability and classification. *Acta Fac. Med. Univ. Brun.* **23**:9–107.

Pollock, L.J., and L. Davis (1927). The influence of the cerebellum upon the reflex activities of the decerebrate animal. *Brain* **50**:277–312.

Pompeiano, O., and A. Brodal (1957). The origin of vestibulospinal fibers in the cat: An experimental–anatomical study with comments on the descending medial longitudinal fasciculus. *Arch. Ital. Biol.* **95**:166–195.

Pompeiano, O., and C.D. Barnes (1971). Effect of sinusoidal muscle stretch on neurons in medial and descending vestibular nuclei. *J. Neurophysiol.* **34**:725–734.

Pompeiano, O. (1974). Cerebello-vestibular interrelations. In *Handbook of Sensory Physiology.* (H.H. Kornhuber, ed.), Vol. VI/1., pp. 417–476. Springer-Verlag, Berlin.

Pompeiano, O. (1975). Vestibulo-spinal relationships. In *The Vestibular System* (R.F. Naunton, ed.), pp. 147–180. Academic Press, New York.

Pompeiano, O. (1979). Neck and macular labyrinthine influences on the cervical spinoreticulocerebellar pathway. *Prog. Brain Res.* **50**:501–514.

Pompeiano, O. (1980). Cholinergic activation of reticular and vestibular mechanisms controlling posture and eye movements. In *The Reticular Formation Revisited* (J.A.

Hobson and M.A.B. Brazier, eds.), pp. 473–512. Raven Press, New York.

Pompeiano, O. (1981). Neck and macular labyrinth inputs on lateral reticular nucleus and their influences on posture. In *Brain Mechanisms and Perceptual Awareness* (O. Pompeiano and C. Ajmone-Marsan, eds.), pp. 233–260. Raven Press, New York.

Pompeiano, O., D. Manzoni, U.C. Srivastava, and G. Stampacchia (1983a). Cholinergic mechanism controlling the response gain of forelimb extensor muscles to sinusoidal stimulation of macular labyrinth and neck receptors. *Arch. Ital. Biol.* **121**:285–303.

Pompeiano, O., D. Manzoni, U.C. Srivastava, and G. Stampacchia (1983b). Relation between cell size and response characteristics of medullary reticulospinal neurons to labyrinth and neck inputs. *Pflügers Arch.* **398**:298–309.

Pompeiano, O. (1984a). A comparison of the response characteristics of vestibulospinal and medullary reticulospinal neurons to labyrinth and neck inputs. In *Research Topics in Physiology, Vol. 6. Brainstem Control of Spinal Cord Function* (C.D. Barnes, ed.), pp. 87–140. Academic Press, Orlando.

Pompeiano, O. (1984b). Recurrent inhibition. In *Handbook of the Spinal Cord, Vol. 2 and 3. Anatomy and Physiology* (R.A. Davidoff, ed.), pp. 461–557. Marcel Dekker, New York.

Pompeiano, O., D. Manzoni, U.C. Srivastava, and G. Stampacchia (1984). Convergence and interaction of neck and macular vestibular inputs on reticulospinal neurons. *Neuroscience* **12**:111–128.

Pompeiano, O. (1985). Cholinergic mechanisms involved in the gain regulation of postural reflexes. In *Sleep. Neurotransmitters and Neuromodulators* (A. Wauquier, J.-M. Gaillard, J.M. Monti, and M. Radulovacki, eds.), pp. 165–184. Raven Press, New York.

Pompeiano, O., P. d'Ascanio, E. Horn, and G. Stampacchia (1985a). Gain regulation of the vestibulospinal reflex by the noradrenergic locus coeruleus system. *Soc. Neurosci. Abstr.* **11**:695.

Pompeiano, O., P. Wand, and U.C. Srivastava (1985b). Responses of Renshaw cells coupled with hindlimb extensor motoneurons to sinusoidal stimulation of labyrinth receptors in the decerebrate cat. *Pflügers Arch.* **403**:245–257.

Pompeiano, O., P. Wand, and U.C. Srivastava (1985c). Influence of Renshaw cells on the response gain of hindlimb extensor muscles to sinusoidal labyrinth stimulation. *Pflügers Arch.* **404**:107–118.

Pompeiano, O., D. Manzoni, A.R. Marchand, and G. Stampacchia (1987). Effects of roll tilt of the animal and neck rotation on different size vestibulospinal neurons in decerebrate cats with the cerebellum intact. *Pflügers Arch.* **409**:24–38

Pontryagin, L.S., V.C. Boltyanskii, R.V. Camkrendze, and E.F. Mischenko (1962). *The Mathematical Theory of Optimal Processes*. John Wiley, New York.

Poppele, R.E., and R.J. Bowman (1970). Quantitative description of linear behavior of mammalian muscle spindles. *J. Neurophysiol.* **39**:59–72.

Poppele, R.E., and D.C. Quick (1985). Effect of intrafusal muscle mechanics on mammalian muscle spindle sensitivity. *J. Neurosci.* **5**:1881–1885.

Powell, W.R. (1975). Static mechanical properties of the trachea and bronchial tree. *J. Biomech.* **8**:111–118.

Precht, W., R. Llinás, and M. Clarke (1971). Physiological responses of frog vestibular fibers to horizontal angular acceleration. *Exp. Brain Res.* **13**:378–407.

Precht, W., R. Volkind, M. Maeda, and M.L. Giretti (1976). The effects of stimulating the cerebellar nodulus in the cat on the responses of vestibular neurons. *Neuroscience* **1**:301–312.

Proske, U. (1981). The Golgi tendon organ. Properties of the receptor and reflex action of impulses arising from tendon organs. In *Neurophysiology IV—International Review of Physiology* (R. Porter, ed.), Vol. 25, pp. 127–171. University Park Press, Baltimore.

Pulaski, P.D., D.S. Zee, and D.A. Robinson (1981). The behaviour of the vestibulo-ocular reflex at high velocities of head rotation. *Brain Res.* **222**:159–163.

Rack, P.M., and D.R. Westbury (1974). The short range stiffness of active mammalian muscle and its effect on mechanical properties. *J. Physiol. (London)* **240**:331–350.

Ramón y Cajal, S. (1909). *Histologie du Système Nerveux de L'homme et des Vértébrés,* Vol. 2, pp. 712–717. Moline, Paris.

Ranson, S.W., H.K. Davenport, and E.A. Doles (1932). Intramedullary course of the dorsal root fibres of the first three cervical nerves. *J. Comp. Neurol.* **54**:1–12.

Raphan, T., B. Cohen, and V. Matsuo (1977). A velocity storage mechanism responsible for optokinetic nystagmus (OKN), OKAN, and vestibular nystagmus. In *Neuroscience. Vol. 1. Control of Gaze by Brain Stem Neurons* (J. Baker and A. Berthoz, eds.), pp. 37–47. Elsevier, North Holland, Amsterdam.

Rapoport, S., A. Susswein, Y. Uchino, and V.J. Wilson (1977a). Properties of vestibular neurones projecting to neck segments of the cat spinal cord. *J. Physiol. (London)* **268**:493–510.

Rapoport, S., A. Susswein, Y. Uchino, and V.J. Wilson (1977b). Synaptic actions of individual vestibular neurons on cat neck motoneurons. *J. Physiol. (London)* **272**:367–382.

Rapoport, S. (1978). Location of sternocleidomastoid and trapezius motoneurons in the cat. *Brain Res.* **156**:339–344.

Rapoport, S. (1979). Reflex connections of motoneurons of muscles involved in head movements in the cat. *J. Physiol. (London)* **289**:311–327.

Rasmussen, A.T. (1936). Tractus tecto-spinalis in the cat. *J. Comp. Neurol.* **63**:501–526.

Reber, J., and W. Goldsmith (1979). Analysis of large head–neck motions. *J. Biomech.* **12**:211–222.

Reighard, J., and H.S. Jennings (1963). *Anatomy of the Cat,* 3rd. ed. Holt, Rhinehart & Winston, New York.

Rexed, B. (1954). A cytoarchitectonic atlas of the spinal cord in the cat. *J. Comp. Neurol.* **100**:297–380.

Richmond, F.J.R., and V.C. Abrahams (1975a). Morphology and enzyme histochemistry of dorsal muscles of the cat neck. *J. Neurophysiol.* **38**:1312–1321.

Richmond, F.J.R., and V.C. Abrahams (1975b). Morphology and distribution of muscle spindles in dorsal muscles of the cat neck. *J. Neurophysiol.* **38**:1322–1339.

Richmond, F.J.R., G.C.B. Anstee, E.A. Sherwin, and V.C. Abrahams (1976). Motor and sensory fibres of neck muscle nerves in the cat. *Can. J. Physiol. Pharmacol.* **54**:294–304.

Richmond, F.J.R., D.A. Scott, and V.C. Abrahams (1978). Distribution of motoneurones to the neck muscles, biventer cervicis, splenius and complexus in the cat. *J. Comp. Neurol.* **181**:451–464.

Richmond, F.J.R., and V.C. Abrahams (1979a). Physiological properties of muscle spindles in dorsal neck muscles of the cat. *J. Neurophysiol.* **42**:604–617.

Richmond, F.J.R., and V.C. Abrahams (1979b). What are the proprioceptors of the neck? In *Reflex Control of Posture and Movement, Progress in Brain Research* (C.R. Granit and O. Pompeiano, eds.), pp. 245–254. Elsevier, North Holland, Amsterdam.

Richmond, F.J.R., and D.A. Bakker (1982). Anatomical organization and sensory receptor content of soft tissues surrounding upper cervical vertebrae in the cat. *J. Neurophysiol.* **48**:49–61.

Richmond, F.J.R., G.E. Loeb, and D. Reesor (1985a). Electromyographic activity in neck muscles during head movement in the alert, unrestrained cat. *Soc. Neurosci. Abstr.* **11**:83.

Richmond, F.J.R., D.R.R. Macgillis, and D.A. Scott (1985b). Muscle fiber compartmentalization in cat splenius muscles. *J. Neurophysiol.* **53**:868–885.

Richmond, F.J.R., M.J. Stacey, G.J. Bakker, and D.A. Bakker (1985c). Gaps in spindle physiology: Why the tandem spindle? In *The Mammalian Muscle Spindle* (I.A. Boyd and M. Gladden, eds.), pp. 75–81. Macmillan, London.

Richmond, F.J.R., G.J. Bakker, D.A. Bakker, and M.J. Stacey (1986). The innervation of tandem muscle spindles in the cat neck. *J. Comp. Neurol.* **245**:483–497.

Rispal-Padel, L., F. Cicirata, and C. Pons (1982). Cerebellar nuclear topography of simple and synergistic movements in the alert baboon (*Papio papio*). *Exp. Brain Res.* **47**:365–380.

Ritchie, L. (1976). Effects of cerebellar lesions on saccadic eye movements. *J. Neurophysiol.* **39**:1246–1256.

Roberts, T.D.M. (1978). *Neurophysiology of Postural mechanisms*, 2nd ed. Butterworths, London.

Robinson, D.A. (1975). Oculomotor control signals. In *Basic Mechanisms of Ocular Motility and Their Clinical Implications*, pp. 337–374. Pergamon, Oxford.

Robinson, T.E. (1978). Electrical stimulation of the brain stem in freely moving rats: I. Effects on behavior. *Physiol. Behav.* **21**:223–231.

Robinson, D.A. (1981). Control of eye movements. In *Handbook of Physiology, II: The Nervous System. Motor Control* (V.B. Brooks, ed.), pp. 1275–1320. Williams & Wilkins, Baltimore.

Robinson, D.A., and D.S. Zee (1981). Theoretical considerations of the function and circuitry of various rapid eye movements. In *Progress in Oculomotor Research* (A.F. Fuchs and W. Becker, eds.), pp. 3–9. Elsevier, North-Holland, Amsterdam.

Robinson, D.L., and C.D. Jarvis (1974). Superior colliculus neurons studied during head and eye movements of the behaving monkey. *J. Neurophysiol.* **37**:533–540.

Robinson, D.L., and M.E. Goldberg (1978). Sensory and behavioral properties of neurons in posterior parietal cortex of the awake, trained monkey. *Fed. Proc.* **37**:2258–2261.

Rondot, P., and J. Scherrer (1966). Contraction réflexe provoquée par le raccourcissement passif du muscle dans l'athétose et les dystonies d'attitude. *Rev. Neurol.* **114**:329–337.

Rondot, P., C.P. Jedynak, and G. Ferrey (1981). *Le Torticolis Spasmodique*. Masson et Cie, Paris.

Rondot, P., and N. Bathien (1986). Movement disorders in patients with coexistant neuroleptic-induced tremor and tardive dyskinesia: EMG and pharmacological study. *Adv. Neurol.* **45**:361–366.

Rose, P.K. (1981). Distribution of dendrites from biventer cervicis and complexus motoneurons stained intracellularly with horseradish peroxidase in the adult cat. *J. Comp. Neurol.* **197**:395–409.

Rose, P.K. (1982). Branching structure of motoneuron stem dendrites: A study of neck muscle motoneurons intracellularly stained with horseradish peroxidase in the cat. *J. Neurosci.* **2**:1596–1607.

Rose, P.K., and F.J.R. Richmond (1981). White-matter dendrites in the upper cervical spinal cord of the adult cat: A light and electron microscopic study. *J. Comp. Neurol.* **199**:191–203.

Rose, P.K., S.A. Keirstead, and S.J. Vanner (1985). A quantitative analysis of the geometry of cat motoneurons innervating neck and shoulder muscles. *J. Comp. Neurol.* **239**:89–107.

Rose, P.K., and S.A. Keirstead (1986). Segmental projection from muscle spindles: A perspective from the upper cervical spinal cord. *Can. J. Physiol. Pharmacol.* **64**:505–507.

Rosén, I. (1969). Localization in caudal brainstem and cervical spinal cord of neurones activated from forelimb group I afferents in the cat. *Brain Res.* **16**:55–71.

Rosén, I., and B. Sjölund (1973a). Organization of group I activated cells in the main and external cuneate nuclei of the cat: Identification of muscle receptors. *Exp. Brain Res.* **16**:221–237.

Rosén, I., and B. Sjölund (1973b). Organization of group I activated cells in the main and external cuneate nuclei of the cat: Convergence patterns demonstrated by natural stimulation. *Exp. Brain Res.* **16**:238–246.

Rosenberg, R.C., and D.C. Karnoop (1983). *Introduction to Physical System Dynamics.* McGraw-Hill, New York.

Ross, D. (1936). Electrical studies on the frog's labyrinth. *J. Physiol. (London)* **86**:117–146.

Rothmann, M. (1913). Die Funktion des Mittellappens des Kleinhirns. *Monatsshcr. Psychiatr. Neurol.* **34**:389–415.

Roucoux, A., and M. Crommelinck (1976). Eye movements evoked by superior colliculus stimulation in the alert cat. *Brain Res.* **106**:349–363.

Roucoux, A., and M. Crommelinck (1980). Eye and head fixation movements: Their coordination and control. In *Tutorials in Motor Behavior* (G.E. Stelmach and J. Requin, eds.), pp. 305–313. Elsevier, North-Holland, Amsterdam.

Roucoux, A., M. Crommelinck, J.M. Guerit, and M. Meulders (1980a). Two modes of eye–head coordination and the role of the vestibulo-ocular reflex in these two strategies. In *Progress in Oculomotor Research* (A.F. Fuchs and W. Becker, eds.), pp. 309–315. Elsevier, North-Holland, Amsterdam.

Roucoux, A., M. Crommelinck, and D. Guitton (1980b). Stimulation of the superior colliculus in the alert cat. II. Eye and head movements evoked when the head is unrestrained. *Exp. Brain Res.* **39**:75–85.

Roucoux, A., P.P. Vidal, C. Veraart, M. Crommelinck, and A. Berthoz (1982). The relation of neck muscle activity to horizontal eye position the alert cat. 1: Head fixed. In *Physiological and Pathological Aspects of Eye Movements* (A. Roucoux and M. Crommelinck, eds.), pp. 371–378. W. Junk, The Hague.

Roucoux, A., M. Crommelinck, M.F. Decostre, J. Cremieux, and A. Al-Ansari (1985). Gaze shift related neck muscle activity in trained cats. *Neurosci. Abstr.* **11**:83.

Rubin, A.M., J.H. Young, A.C. Milne, D.W.F. Schwarz, and J.M. Fredrickson (1975). Vestibular-neck integration in the vestibular nuclei. *Brain Res.* **96**:99–102.

Rubin, A.M., S.R.C. Liedgren, A.C. Milne, J.A. Young, and J.M. Fredrickson (1977). Vestibular and somatosensory interaction in the cat vestibular nuclei. *Pflügers. Arch.* **371**:155–160.

Rubin, A.M., S.R. Liedgren, L.M. Odkvist, A.C. Milne, and J.M. Fredrickson (1978). Labyrinthine and somatosensory convergence upon vestibulospinal neurons. *Acta Otolaryngol (Stockholm)* **85**:251–259.

Ryall, R.W., M.F. Piercey, and C. Polosa (1971). Intersegmental and intrasegmental distribution of mutual inhibition of Renshaw cells. *J. Neurophysiol.* **34**:700–707.

Ryall, R.W. (1981). Patterns of recurrent excitation and mutual inhibition of cat Renshaw cells. *J. Physiol. (London)* **316**:439–452.

Sahibzada, N., P. Dean, and P. Redgrave (1986). Movements resembling orientation or avoidance elicited by electrical stimulation of the superior colliculus in rats. *J. Neurosci.* **6**:723–733.

Sakai, K., J.P. Sastre, D. Salvert, M. Touret, M. Tohyama, and M. Jouvet (1979). Tegmentoreticular projections with special reference to the muscular atonia during paradoxical sleep in the cat: An HRP study. *Brain Res.* **176**:233–254.

Sakai, K. (1980). Some anatomical and physiological properties of ponto-mesencephalic tegmental neurons with special reference to the PGO waves and postural atonia during paradoxical sleep in the cat. In *The Reticular Formation Revisited* (J.A. Hobson and M.A.B. Brazier, eds.), pp. 427–447. Raven Press, New York.

Sances, A., R.C. Weber, S.J. Larson, J.S. Cusick, J.B. Myklebust, and P.R. Walsh (1981). Bioengineering analysis of head and spine injuries. *CRC Crit. Rev. Bioengng.* **6**:79–122.

Sanes, J.N., and V.A. Jennings (1984). Centrally programmed patterns of muscle activity in voluntary motor behavior in humans. *Exp. Brain Res.* **54**:23–32.

Sasaki, S., B. Alstermark, A. Lundberg, and M. Pinter (1983). Descending control and functional role of long C3–C4 propriospinal neurons. *Reflex Organization of the Spinal Cord and Its Descending Control Abstracts.* Canberra, Australia.

Schaefer, K.P. (1970). Unit analysis and electrical stimulation of the optic tectum of rabbits and cats. *Brain Behav. Evol.* **3**:222–240.

Schapiro, H., and D.C. Goodman (1969). Motor functions and anatomical basis in the forebrain and tectum of the alligator. *Exp. Neurol.* **24**:187–195.

Scheibel, M.E., and A.B. Scheibel (1958). Structural substrates for integrative patterns in the brain stem reticular core. In *Reticular Formation of the Brain* (H.H. Jasper, L.D. Proctor, R.S. Knighton, W.C. Noshay, and R.T. Costello, eds.), pp. 31–55. Little, Brown, Boston.

Schmidt, R.F. (1971). Presynaptic inhibition in the vertebrate central nervous system. *Ergebnisse Physiol. Biol. Chem. Exp. Pharmakol.* **63**:20–101.

Schmidt, R.F. (1973). Control of access of afferent activity to somatosensory pathways. In *Handbook of Physiology, Vol. II, Somatosensory System* (A. Iggo, ed.), pp. 151–206. Springer-Verlag, Berlin.

Schor, R.H. (1974). Responses of cat vestibular neurons to sinusoidal roll tilt. *Exp. Brain Res.* **20**:347–362.

Schor, R.H. (1981). Otolith contribution to neck and forelimb vestibulospinal reflexes. In *Progress in Oculomotor Research* (A. Fuchs and W. Becker, eds.), pp. 351–356. Elsevier North-Holland, New York and Amsterdam.

Schor, R.H., and A.D. Miller (1981). Vestibular reflexes in neck and forelimb muscles evoked by roll tilt. *J. Neurophysiol.* **46**:167–178.

Schor, R.H., and A.D. Miller (1982). Relationship of cat vestibular neurons to otolithspinal reflexes. *Exp. Brain Res.* **47**:137–144.

Schor, R.H., A.D. Miller, and D.L. Tomko (1984). Responses to head tilt in cat central vestibular neurons. I. Direction of maximum sensitivity. *J. Neurophysiol.* **51**:136–146.

Schor, R.H., A.D. Miller, S.J.B. Timerick, and D.L. Tomko (1985). Responses to head tilt in cat central vestibular neurons. II. Frequency dependence of neural response vectors. *J. Neurophysiol.* **53**:1444–1452.

Schor, R.H., I. Suzuki, S.J.B. Timerick, and V.J. Wilson (1986). Responses of interneurons in the cat cervical cord to vestibular tilt stimulation. *J. Neurophysiol.* **56**:1147–1156.

Schulze, M.L. (1955). Die absolute und relative Zahl der Muskelspindeln in den kurzen Daumenmuskeln des Menschen. *Anat. Anz.* **102**:290–291.

Schwarz, D.W.F., A.M. Rubin, R.D. Tomlinson, A.C. Milne, and J.M. Fredrickson

(1975). Studies on the integrative activity of the vestibular nuclei complex. *Can. J. Otolaryngol.* **4**:378–382.

Schwarz, D.W.F., and A.C. Milne (1976). Somatosensory representation in the vestibulocerebellum. *Brain Res.* **102**:181–184.

Scott, J.G., and L.M. Mendell (1976). Individual epsps produced by single triceps surae Ia afferent fibers in homonymous and heteronymous motoneurons. *J. Neurophysiol.* **39**:679–692.

Sears, T.A. (1964). Some properties and reflex connexions of respiratory motoneurones of the cat's thoracic spinal cord. *J. Physiol. (London)* **175**:386–403.

Segal, B.N., and A. Katsarkas (1986). Quick phase eye movements of goal directed vestibuloculomotor reflex reduce gaze error. *Soc. Neurosci. Abstr.* **12**:1090.

Sherrington, C.S. (1897). Decerebrate rigidity, and reflex coordination of movements. *J. Physiol. (London)* **22**:319–332.

Sherrington, C.S. (1906). *The Integrative Action of the Nervous System.* Yale University Press, New Haven.

Sherrington, C.S. (1909). On plastic tonus and proprioceptive reflexes. *Quart. J. Exp. Physiol.* **2**:109–156.

Sherrington, C.S. (1910). Flexion-reflex of the limb, crossed extension-reflex and reflex stepping and standing. *J. Physiol. (London)* **40**:28–121.

Shimamura, M., and R.B. Livingston (1963). Longitudinal conduction systems serving spinal and brain stem coordination. *J. Neurophysiol.* **26**:258–272.

Shimamura, M., and R.B. Livingston (1963). Longitudinal conduction systems serving spinal and brain stem coordination. *J. Neurophysiol.* **26**:258–272.

Shimamura, M., and I. Kogure (1979). Reticulospinal tracts involved in the spino-bulbo-spinal reflex in cats. *Brain Res.* **172**:13–21.

Shimazu, H., and W. Precht (1966). Inhibition of central vestibular neurons from the contralateral labyrinth and its mediating pathway. *J. Neurophysiol.* **29**:467–492.

Shimazu, H. (1983). Neuronal organization of the premotor system controlling horizontal conjugate eye movements and vestibular nystagmus. In *Motor Control Mechanisms in Health and Disease* (J.E. Desmedt, ed.), pp. 565–588. Raven Press, New York.

Shimizu, N., M. Naito, and M. Yoshida (1981). Eye–head coordination in patients with Parkinsonism and cerebellar ataxia. *J. Neurol. Neurosurg. Psychiat.* **44**:509–515.

Shinoda, Y., and K. Yoshida (1974). Dynamic characteristics of responses to horizontal head angular acceleration in the vestibulo-ocular pathway in the cat. *J. Neurophysiol.* **37**:653–673.

Shinoda, Y., T. Ohgaki, and T. Futami (1986). The morphology of single lateral vestibulospinal tract axons in the cervical spinal cord of the cat. *J. Comp. Neurol.* **249**:226–241.

Shirachi, D.K., D.L. Monk, and J.H. Black (1978). Head rotational spectral characteristics during two-dimensional smooth pursuit tasks. *IEEE Trans. Sys. Man. Cybern.* SMC **8**:715–724.

Shriver, J.E., B.M. Stein, and M.B. Carpenter (1968). Central projections of spinal dorsal roots in the monkey. I. Cervical and upper thoracic dorsal roots. *Am. J. Anat.* **123**:27–73.

Siegel, J.M., and K.S. Tomaszewski (1983). Behavioral organization of reticular formation: Studies in the unrestrained cat. I. Cells related to axial, limb, eye and other movements. *J. Neurophysiol.* **50**:696–716.

Simpson, J.I., and A. Pellionisz (1984). The vestibulo-ocular reflex in rabbit, as interpreted using the Moore–Penrose generalized inverse transformation of intrinsic coordinates. *Soc. Neurosci. Abst.* **10**:909.

Sirkin, D.W., T. Schallert, and P. Teitelbaum (1980). Involvement of the pontine reticular formation in head movements and labyrinthine righting in the rat. *Exp. Neurol.* **69**:435–357.

Skoglund, S. (1956). Anatomical and physiological studies of knee joint innervation in the cat. *Acta Physiol. Scand. (Suppl. 36)* **124**:1–101.

Skultety, F.M. (1962). Circus movements in cats following midbrain stimulation through chronically implanted electrodes. *J. Neurophysiol.* **25**:152–164.

Slijper, E.J. (1946). Comparative biologic-anatomical investigations on the vertebral column and spinal musculature of mammals. *Verhand. konink. Nederland. Akad. Wetenschappen, Natuurkunde, Tweede Sect. deel XLII,* **5**:1–128.

Soechting, J.F., and P.R. Paslay (1973). A model for the human spine during impact including musculature influence. *J. Biomech.* **6**:195–203.

Sprague, J.M., and W.W. Chambers (1953). Regulation of posture in intact and decerebrate cat. I. Cerebellum, reticular formation, vestibular nuclei. *J. Neurophysiol.* **16**:451–463.

Sprague, J.M., and W.W. Chambers (1954). Control of posture by reticular formation and cerebellum in the intact, anesthetized and unanesthetized and in the decerebrated cat. *Amer. J. Physiol.* **176**:52–64.

Srivastava, U.C., D. Manzoni, O. Pompeiano, and G. Stampacchia (1982). State-dependent properties of medullary reticular neurons involved during the labyrinth and neck reflexes. *Neurosci. Lett. (Suppl. 10).* **S461.**

Srivastava, U.C., D. Manzoni, O. Pompeiano, and G. Stampacchia (1984). Responses of medullary reticulospinal neurons to sinusoidal rotation of neck in the decerebrate cat. *Neuroscience* **11**:473–486.

Stacey, M.J. (1969). Free nerve endings in skeletal muscle of the cat. *J. Anat.* **105**:231–254.

Stampacchia, G., D. Manzoni, A.R. Marchand, and O. Pompeiano (1987). Convergence of neck and macular vestibular input on vestibulospinal neurons projecting to the lumbosacral segments of the spinal cord. *Arch. Ital. Biol.,* **125**:201–224.

Stanojević, M. (1981). Responses of cerebellar fastigial neurons to neck and macular vestibular inputs. *Pflügers Arch.* **391**:267–272.

Stark, L. (1968). *Neurological Control Systems.* Plenum Press, New York.

Stark, L., W.H. Zangemeister, B. Hannaford, and K. Kunze (1986). Use of models of brainstem reflexes for clinical research. In *Clinical Problems of Brainstem Disorders.* Thieme Stuttgart and New York.

Straschill, M., and P. Rieger (1973). Eye movements evoked by focal stimulation of the cat's superior colliculus. *Brain Res.* **59**:211–227.

Straschill, M., and F. Schick (1977). Discharges of superior colliculus neurons during head and eye movements of the alert cat. *Exp. Brain Res.* **27**:131–141.

Stauffer, E.K., D.G.D. Watt, A. Taylor, R.M. Reinking, and D.G. Stuart (1976). Analysis of muscle receptor connections by spike-triggered averaging. 2. Spindle group II afferents. *J. Neurophysiol.* **39**:1393–1402.

Stryker, M.P., and P.H. Schiller (1975). Eye and head movements evoked by electrical stimulation of monkey superior colliculus. *Exp. Brain Res.* **23**:103–112.

Stuart, D.G., C.G. Mosher, R.L. Gerlach, and R.M. Reinking (1972). Mechanical arrangement and transducing properties of Golgi tendon organs. *Exp. Brain Res.* **14**:274–292.

Sugi, N., and M. Wakakuwa (1970). Visual target tracking with active head rotation. *IEEE Trans. Sys. Sci. Cybern.* **6**:103–109.

Suzuki, D.A., H. Noda, and M. Kase (1981). Visual and pursuit eye movement-related activity in posterior vermis of monkey cerebellum. *J. Neurophysiol.* **46**:1120–1139.

Suzuki, I., S.J.B. Timerick, and V.J. Wilson (1985). Body position with respect to the head or body position in space is coded by lumbar interneurons. *J. Neurophysiol.* **54**:123–133.

Suzuki, I., B.R. Park, and V.J. Wilson (1986). Directional sensitivity of, and neck afferent input to, cervical and lumbar interneurons modulated by neck rotation. *Brain Res.* **367**:356–359.

Suzuki, J.-I., and B. Cohen (1964). Head, eye, body and limb movements from semicircular canal nerves. *Exp. Neurol.* **10**:393–405.

Syka, J., and T. Radil-Weiss (1971). Electrical stimulation of the tectum in freely moving cats. *Brain Res.* **28**:567–572.

Szebenyi, E.S. (1969). *Atlas of Macaca mulatta.* Farleigh Dickinson University Press, Rutherford.

Tait, J., and W.J. McNally (1934). Some features of the action of the utricular maculae (and of the associated action of the semicircular canals) of the frog. *Phil. Trans R. Soc. London, Ser. B.* **224**:241–268.

Tarlov, E. (1970). On the problem of the pathology of spasmodic torticollis in man. *J. Neurol. Neurosurg. Psychiat.* **33**:457–463.

Tauber, E.S., and A. Atkin (1968). Optomotor responses to monocular stimulation: Relation to visual system organization. *Science* **160**:1365–1367.

Ter Braak, J.W.G. (1936). Untersuchungen über denoptokinetischen Nystagmus. *Arch. Neerl. Physiol.* **21**:309–376.

Terry, C.T., and V.L. Roberts (1968). A viscoelastic model of the human spine subjected to +Gz accelerations. *J. Biomech.* **1**:161–168.

Terzuolo, C.A. (1959). Cerebellar inhibitory and excitatory actions upon spinal extensor motoneurones. *Arch. Ital. Biol.* **97**:316–339.

Thoden, U., R. Golsong, and J. Wirbitzky (1975). Cervical influence on single units of vestibular and reticular nuclei in cats. *Pflügers Arch.* **355**:R101.

Thoden, U., and J. Wirbitzky (1976). Influence of passive neck movements on eye position and brain stem neurons. *Pflügers Arch.* **362**:R37.

Thompson, J. (1970). Parallel spindle systems in the small muscles of the rat tail. *J. Physiol. (London)* **211**:781–799.

Tkaczuk, H. (1968). Tensile properties of human lumbar longitudinal ligaments. *Acta Orthop. Scand. Suppl.* **115**.

Tohyama, M., K. Sakai, D. Salvert, M. Touret, and M. Jouvet (1979a). Spinal projections from the lower brain stem in the cat as demonstrated by the horseradish peroxidase technique. I. Origins of the reticulo-spinal tracts and their funicular trajectories. *Brain Res.* **173**:383–403.

Tohyama, M., K. Sakai, M. Touret, D. Salvert, and M. Jouvet (1979b). Spinal projections from the lower brain stem in the cat as demonstrated by the horseradish peroxidase technique. II. Projections from the dorsolateral pontine tegmentum and raphe nuclei. *Brain Res.* **176**:215–231.

Tomko, D.L., R.J. Peterka, and R.H. Schor (1981a). Responses to head tilt in cat eighth nerve afferents. *Exp. Brain Res.* **41**:216–221.

Tomko, D.L., R.J. Peterka, R.H. Schor, and D.P. O'Leary (1981b). Response dynamics of horizontal canal afferents in barbiturate anesthetized cats. *J. Neurophysiol.* **45**:376–396.

Tomlinson, R.D., and D.A. Robinson (1984). Signals in vestibular nucleus mediating vertical eye movements in the monkey. *J. Neurophysiol.* **51**:1121–1136.

Tomlinson, R.D., and P.S. Bahra (1986a). Combined eye–head gaze shifts in the primate. I. Metrics. *J. Neurophysiol.* **56**:1542–1557.

Tomlinson, R.D., and P.S. Bahra (1986b). Combined eye–head gaze shifts in the primate. II. Interactions between saccades and the vestibulo-ocular reflex. *J. Neurphysiol.* **56**:1558–1570.

Torvik, A. (1956). Afferent connections to the sensory trigeminal nuclei, the nucleus of the solitary tract and adjacent structures. (An experimental study in the rat.). *J. Comp. Neurol.* **106**:51–142.

Torvik, A., and A. Brodal (1957). The origin of reticulospinal fibers in the cat: An experimental study. *Anat. Rec.* **128**:113–137.

Tournay, A., and J. Paillard (1955). Torticolis spasmodique et EMG. *Rev. Neurol.* **93**:347–355.

Uchino, Y., and N. Hirai (1984). Axon collaterals of anterior semi-circular canal-activated vestibular neurons and their coactivation of extraocular and neck motoneurons in the cat. *Neurosci. Res.* **1**:309–325.

Udo, M., and N. Mano (1970). Discrimination of different spinal monosynaptic pathways converging onto reticular neurons. *J. Neurophysiol.* **33**:227–238.

Ulfhake, B., and J.-O. Kellerth (1983). A quantitative morphological study of HRP-labelled cat motoneurons supplying different hindlimb muscles. *Brain Res.* **264**:1–20.

v. Holst, E., and H. Mittelstaedt (1950). Das Reafferenzprinzip. *Naturwissenschaften* **37**:464–476.

Vallois, H.V. (1922). Les transformations de la musculature de l'episome chez les vértébrés. *Arch. Morphol. Gen. Exp.* **13**:1–538.

Vanner, S.J., and P.K. Rose (1984). Dendritic distribution of motoneurons innervating the three heads of the trapezius muscle in the cat. *J. Comp. Neurol.* **226**:96–110.

Vidal, P.P., A. Roucoux, and A. Berthoz (1982). Horizontal eye position-related activity in neck muscles of the alert cat. *Exp. Brain Res.* **46**:448–453.

Vidal, P.P., J. Corvisier, and A. Berthoz (1983). Eye and neck motor signals in peri-abducens reticular neurons of the alert cat. *Exp. Brain Res.* **53**:16–28.

Vidal, P.P., W. Graf, and A. Berthoz (1986). The orientation of the cervical vertebral column in unrestricted awake animals. I. Resting position. *Exp. Brain Res.* **61**:549–559.

Viviani, P., and A. Berthoz (1975). Dynamics of the head–neck system in response to small perturbations: Analysis and modeling in the frequency domain. *Biol. Cybern.* **19**:19–37.

Voss, H. (1937). Untersuchungen über Zahl, Anordnung und Länge der Muskelspindeln in den Lumbricalmuskeln des Menschen und einiger Tiere. *Z. Mikr. Anat. Forsch.* **42**:509–524.

Voss, H. (1956). Zahl und Anordnung der Muskelspindeln in den oberen Zungenbein-muskeln, im M. trapezius und M. latissimus dorsi. *Anat. Anz.* **103**:443–446.

Voss, H. (1958). Zahl und Anordnung der Muskelspindeln in den unteren Zungenbein-muskeln, dem M. Sternocleido-mastoideus und den Bauchund tiefen Nackenmu-skeln. *Anat. Anz.* **105**:265–275.

Waldron, H.A., and D.G. Gwyn (1969). Descending nerve tracts in the spinal cord of the rat. I. Fibers from the midbrain. *J. Comp. Neurol.* **137**:143–154.

Walker, A.E., and T.A. Weaver (1942). The topical organization and termination of the fibers of the posterior columns in *Macaca mulatta*. *J. Comp. Neurol.* **76**:145–158.

Walters, R.L., and J.M. Morris (1973). An in-vitro study of normal and scoliotic inter-spinous ligaments. *J. Biomech.* **6**:343–348.

Walton, J.N. (1977). *Brain's Diseases of the Nervous System*, 8th ed. Oxford University Press, Oxford.

Warwick, R., and P.L. Williams, eds. (1973). *Gray's Anatomy*, 35th ed. Longman Pub. Co., London.

Watt, D.G.D., E.K. Stauffer, A. Taylor, R.M. Reinking, and D.G. Stuart (1976). Analysis of muscle receptor connections by spike-triggered averaging. *J. Neurophysiol.* **39**:1375–1392.

Weeks, O.T., and A.W. English (1985). Compartmentalization of the cat lateral gastrocnemius motor nucleus. *J. Comp. Neurol.* **235**:255–267.

Weeks, V.D., and J. Travell (1955). Postural vertigo due to trigger areas in the sternocleidomastoid muscle. *J. Pediat.* **47**:315–327.

Wenzel, D., and U. Thoden (1977). Modulation of hindlimb reflexes by tonic neck positions in cats. *Pflügers Arch.* **370**:277–282.

Wenzel, D., U. Thoden, and A. Frank (1978). Forelimb reflexes modulated by tonic neck positions in cats. *Pflügers Arch.* **374**:107–113.

Werner, G., H. Sacks, and J. Fierst (1969). Design and Evaluation of Experiments with Labyrinthine Statoreceptors. Technical Report, No. 2 to U.S. Air Force Office of Scientific Research. Arlington, VA.

Westheimer, G., and S.M. Blair (1975). Synkinese der Augen- und Kopfbewegungen bei Hirnstammreizungen am wachen Macacus-Affen. *Exp. Brain Res.* **24**:89–95.

White, A.A., and M.M. Panjabi (1978). *Clinical Biomechanics of the Spine*. J.B. Lippincott, Philadelphia.

Whittington, D.A., F. Lestienne, and E. Bizzi (1984). Behavior of preoculomotor burst neurons during eye–head coordination. *Exp. Brain Res.* **55**:215–222.

Wiksten, B. (1979). The central cervical nucleus in the cat. III. The cerebellar connections studied with anterograde transport of ^{3}H-leucine. *Exp. Brain Res.* **36**:175–189.

Wiksten, B., and G. Grant (1983). The central cervical nucleus in the cat. IV. Afferent fiber connections: An experimental anatomical study. *Exp. Brain Res.* **51**:405–412.

Wilkie, D.R. (1950). Relation between force and velocity in human muscle. *J. Physiol. (London)* **110**:249–280.

Willis, W.D., and R.E. Coggeshall (1978). *Sensory Mechanisms of the Spinal Cord*. Plenum, New York.

Wilson, V.J., and M. Yoshida (1969a). Comparison of effects of stimulation of Deiter's nucleus and medial longitudinal fasciculus on neck, forelimb, and hindlimb motoneurons. *J. Neurophysiol.* **32**:743–758.

Wilson, V.J., and M. Yoshida (1969b). Monosynaptic inhibition of neck motoneurons by the medial vestibular nucleus. *Exp. Brain Res.* **9**:365–380.

Wilson, V.J., M. Yoshida, and R.H. Schor (1970). Supraspinal monosynaptic excitation and inhibition of thoracic back motoneurons. *Exp. Brain Res.* **11**:282–295.

Wilson, V.J., and M. Maeda (1974). Connections between semicircular canals and neck motoneurons in the cat. *J. Neurophysiol.* **37**:346–357.

Wilson, V.J., M. Maeda, and J.I. Franck (1975a). Input from neck afferents to the cat flocculus. *Brain Res.* **89**:133–138.

Wilson, V.J., M. Maeda, and J.I. Franck (1975b). Inhibitory interaction between labyrinthine, visual and neck inputs to the cat flocculus. *Brain Res.* **96**:357–360.

Wilson, V.J., M. Maeda, J.I. Franck, and H. Shimazu (1976). Mossy fiber neck and second order labyrinthine projections to cat flocculus. *J. Neurophysiol.* **39**:301–310.

Wilson, V.J., R.R. Gacek, Y. Uchino, and A.M. Susswein (1978a). Properties of central vestibular neurons fired by stimulation of the saccular nerve. *Brain Res.* **143**:251–261.

Wilson, V.J., Y. Uchino, R.A. Maunz, A. Susswein, and K. Fukushima (1978b). Properties and connections of cat fastigial neurons. *Exp. Brain Res.* **32**:1–17.

Wilson, V.J., and G. Melvill-Jones (1979). *Mammalian Vestibular Physiology.* Plenum, New York.

Wilson, V.J., B.W. Peterson, K. Fukushima, N. Hirai, and Y. Uchino (1979). Analysis of vestibulocollic reflexes by sinusoidal polarization of vestibular afferent fibers. *J. Neurophysiol.* **42**:331–346.

Wilson, V.J., and B.W. Peterson (1981). Vestibulospinal and reticulospinal pathways. In *Handbook of Physiology, Vol. II, Section I, The Nervous System* (V.B. Brooks, ed.), pp. 667–702. American Physiological Society, Bethesda, MD.

Wilson, V.J., W. Precht, and N. Dieringer (1983). Responses of different compartments of cat's splenius muscle to optokinetic stimulation. *Exp. Brain Res.* **50**:153–156.

Wilson, V.J., K. Ezure, and S.J.B. Timerick (1984). Tonic neck reflex of the decerebrate cat: Response of spinal interneurons to natural stimulation of neck and vestibular receptors. *J. Neurophysiol.* **51**:567–577.

Wilson, V.J., R.H. Schor, I. Suzuki, and B.R. Park (1986). Spatial organization of neck and vestibular reflex acting on the forelimbs of the decerebrate cat. *J. Neurophysiol.* **55**:514–526.

Winters, J.M., and W. Goldsmith (1983). Response of an advanced head–neck model to transient loading. *J. Biomech. Eng.* **105**:63–70, 196–197.

Winters, J.M., M.H. Nam, and L. Stark (1984). Modeling dynamical interaction between fast and slow movements. Fast saccadic eye movement behavior in the presence of the slower VOR. *Math. Biosci.* **68**:159–185.

Winters, J.M., and L. Stark (1985). Analysis of fundamental human movement patterns through the use of in-depth antagonistic muscle models. *IEEE J. Biomed. Eng.* BME **32**:826–839.

Winters, J.M., and L. Stark (1987). Muscle models: What is gained and what is lost by varying model complexity. *Biol. Cybern.* **55**:403–420.

Worth, D. (1980). *Kinematics of the cranio-vertebral joints.* Ph.D. Dissertation, Victoria Institute of Colleges.

Wyke, B. (1967). The neurology of joints. *Ann. R. Coll. Surg. Engl.* **41**:25–50.

Wyke, B. (1979). Neurology of cervical spinal joints. *Physiotherapy* **65**:72–76.

Yamada, H. (1970). In *Strength of Biological Materials* (F.G. Evans, ed.). Williams & Wilkins, Baltimore.

Yee, J., and K.B. Corbin (1939). The intramedullary course of the upper five cervical dorsal root fibres in the rabbit. *J. Comp. Neurol.* **70**:297–304.

Yeow, M.B.L., and E.H. Peterson (1986a). Organization of motor pools supplying the cervical musculature in a cryptodyman turtle, pseudemys scripto elegans. I. Dorsal and ventral motor nuclei of the cervical spinal cord and muscles supplied by a single motor nucleus. *J. Comp. Neurol.* **243**:145–165.

Yeow, M.B.L., and E.H. Peterson (1986b). Organization of motor pools supplying the cervical musculature in a cryptodyman turtle, pseudemys scripto elegans. II. Medial motor nucleus and muscles supplied by two motor nuclei. *J. Comp. Neurol.* **243**:166–181.

Yin, T.C.T., and V.B. Mountcastle (1978). Mechanisms of neural integration in the parietal lobe for visual attention. *Fed. Proc.* **37**:2251–2257.

Young, L.R. (1969). The current state of vestibular system models. *Automatica* **5**:369–383.

Young, L.R., and C.M. Oman (1969). Models of vestibular adaptation to horizontal rotations. *Aerospace Med.* **40**:1076–1080.

Yu, J. (1972). The pathway mediating ipsilateral limb hyperflexion after cerebellar paravermal cortical ablation or cooling in cat. *Exp. Neurol.* **36**:549–562.

Zangemeister, W.H., A. Jones, and L. Stark (1981a). Dynamics of head movement trajectories: Main sequence relationship. *Exp. Neurol.* **71**:76–91.

Zangemeister, W.H., A. Jones, and L. Stark (1981b). Stimulation of head movement trajectories: Model and fit to main sequence. *Biol. Cybern.* **41**:19–32.

Zangemeister, W.H., S. Lehman, and L. Stark (1981c). Sensitivity analysis and optimization for a head movement model. *Biol. Cybern.* **41**:33–45.

Zangemeister, W.H., and L. Stark (1982a). Types of gaze movement: Variable interactions of eye and head movements. *Exp. Neurol.* **77**:563–577.

Zangemeister, W.H., and L. Stark (1982b). Gaze latency: Variable interactions of head and eye latency. *Exp. Neurol.* **75**:389–406.

Zangemeister, W.H., and L. Stark (1982c). Normal and abnormal gaze types with active head movements. In *Functional Basis of Ocular Motility Disorders* (G. Lennerstrand, D.S. Zee, and E. Keller, eds.), pp. 407–416. Pergamon Press, New York.

Zangemeister, W.H., and L. Stark (1982d). Gaze types: Interactions of eye and head movements in gaze. *Exp. Neurol.* **77**:563–577.

Zangemeister, W.H., and L. Stark (1982e). Understanding dynamics and control of normal and abnormal head movements by use of a parameterized head movement model. *Trans. IEEE Biomed. Soc. 82 CH1720* **3**:468–473.

Zangemeister, W.H., O. Meienberg, L. Stark, and W. Hoyt (1982a). Eye–head coordination in homonymous hemianopia. *Neurology* **225**:243–254.

Zangemeister, W.H., L. Stark, O. Meienberg, and T. Waite (1982b). Neural control of head rotation: Electromyographic evidence. *J. Neurological Sci.* **55**:1–14.

Zangemeister, W.H., and L. Stark (1983). Pathological types of eye and head gaze-coordination in neurological disorders. *Neuro-opthalmology* **3**:259–276.

Zangemeister, W.H., and A. Mueller-Jensen (1985). The coordination of gaze movements in Huntington's disease. *Neuro-ophthalmology* **5**:193–206.

Zangemeister, W.H., U. Phlebs, G. Huefner, and K. Kunze (1986). Active head rotations and correlated EEG potentials: Experimental and clinical aspects. *Acta Otolaryngol.* **101**:403–405.

Zee, D.S. (1977). Disorders of eye–head coordination. In *Eye Movements* (B. Brooks and F. Bajandas, eds.), pp. 9–39. Plenum, New York.

Zelena, J., and T. Soukup (1983). The in-series and in-parallel components in rat hindlimb tendon organs. *Neuroscience* **9**:899–910.

Zuk, A., D.G. Gwyn, and J.G. Rutherford (1982). Cytoarchitecture, neuronal morphology, and some efferent connections of the interstitial nucleus of Cajal (INC) in the cat. *J. Comp. Neurol.* **212**:278–292.

Index